Fri

Cardiac Anaesthesia

Oxford Specialist Handbooks published and forthcoming

General Oxford Specialist Handbooks

A Resuscitation Room Guide
Addiction Medicine
Hypertension
Perioperative Medicine, Second Edition
Post-Operative Complications, Second Edition

Oxford Specialist Handbooks in Anaesthesia

Cardiac Anaesthesia
General Thoracic Anaesthesia
Neuroanaethesia
Obstetric Anaesthesia
Paediatric Anaesthesia
Regional Anaesthesia, Stimulation and Ultrasound Techniques

Oxford Specialist Handbooks in Cardiology

Adult Congenital Heart Disease
Cardiac Catheterization and Coronary Intervention
Echocardiography
Fetal Cardiology
Heart Failure
Nuclear Cardiology
Pacemakers and ICDs

Oxford Specialist Handbooks in Critical Care

Advanced Respiratory Critical Care

Oxford Specialist Handbooks in End of Life Care

End of Life Care in Cardiology
End of Life Care in Dementia
End of Life Care in Nephrology
End of Life Care in Respiratory Disease
End of Life in the Intensive Care Unit

Oxford Specialist Handbooks in Neurology

Epilepsy
Parkinson's Disease and Other Movement Disorders
Stroke Medicine

Oxford Specialist Handbooks in Paediatrics

Paediatric Endocrinology and Diabetes
Paediatric Dermatology
Paediatric Gastroenterology, Hepatology, and Nutrition
Paediatric Haematology and Oncology
Paediatric Nephrology
Paediatric Neurology
Paediatric Radiology
Paediatric Respiratory Medicine

Oxford Specialist Handbooks in Psychiatry

Child and Adolescent Psychiatry
Old Age Psychiatry

Oxford Specialist Handbooks in Radiology

Interventional Radiology
Musculoskeletal Imaging

Oxford Specialist Handbooks in Surgery

Cardiothoracic Surgery
Hand Surgery
Hepato-pancreatobiliary Surgery
Oral Maxillofacial Surgery
Neurosurgery
Operative Surgery, Second Edition
Otolaryngology and Head and Neck Surgery
Plastic and Reconstructive Surgery
Surgical Oncology
Urological Surgery
Vascular Surgery

Oxford Specialist Handbooks in Anaesthesia
Cardiac Anaesthesia

Matthew Barnard

Consultant Anaesthetist,
The Heart Hospital,
London,
UK

Bruce Martin

Consultant Anaesthetist,
The Heart Hospital,
London,
UK

OXFORD
UNIVERSITY PRESS

OXFORD
UNIVERSITY PRESS

Great Clarendon Street, Oxford OX2 6DP

Oxford University Press is a department of the University of Oxford.
It furthers the University's objective of excellence in research, scholarship,
and education by publishing worldwide in

Oxford New York

Auckland Cape Town Dar es Salaam Hong Kong Karachi
Kuala Lumpur Madrid Melbourne Mexico City Nairobi
New Delhi Shanghai Taipei Toronto

With offices in

Argentina Austria Brazil Chile Czech Republic France Greece
Guatemala Hungary Italy Japan Poland Portugal Singapore
South Korea Switzerland Thailand Turkey Ukraine Vietnam

Oxford is a registered trade mark of Oxford University Press
in the UK and in certain other countries

Published in the United States
by Oxford University Press Inc., New York

British Library Cataloguing in Publication Data
Data available

Library of Congress Cataloging in Publication Data
Data available

Typeset by Glyph International., Bangalore, India
Printed in China
on acid-free paper through
Asia Pacific Offset Limited

ISBN 978–0–19–920910–1

10 9 8 7 6 5 4 3 2 1

Preface

We had two aims during the production of this book: to provide the information required for anaesthetic trainees looking after cardiac surgical patients and to provide a hands-on practical guide to what to do 'on the spot'. The latter means the tone of the book can be informal or even irreverent at times. This is intentional. The information content of the book aims to cover both the curriculum of post-graduate exams such as the FRCA and the knowledge one would wish to gain during a training attachment to a cardiac surgical unit.

The handbook has three sections. The first section covers the 'Cardiovascular system' and includes relevant aspects of basic sciences such as anatomy, physiology, and pharmacology. It also has a comprehensive account of the pathology, pathophysiology, and treatment of cardiovascular diseases. The second section covers aspects of organ systems that are relevant to all aspects of cardiac surgery. It incorporates both the importance of comorbidities in cardiac surgery and the effect of cardiac surgery on the major organ systems (renal, central nervous system etc.). It includes material that would otherwise overlap in many chapters. The third section contains the details of the conduct of assessment, anaesthesia, and post-operative care for cardiac surgery in general, as well as the major operations. The clinical chapters all follow a common structure. There is overlap of some key content in several chapters – this is deliberate so that each section can be conveniently studied independently.

Our aim is to provide a practical, useful, up-to-date account of current cardiac anaesthesia. As such this handbook should prove useful to anaesthetic trainees, cardiac surgical trainees and consultants, and allied professionals working in cardiac critical care and cardiac operating rooms. We have incorporated contributors from around the world, so that the UK perspective of the book is augmented by an international view.

Dr Matthew Barnard
Dr Bruce Martin

Contents

Detailed contents *ix*
Symbols and Abbreviations *xviii*
Contributors *xxvi*

Part 1 The cardiovascular system

Anatomy, pharmacology, physiology

1	The heart and its valves	**3**
2	Cardiac physiology	**13**
3	Cardiovascular drugs	**37**

Cardiovascular disease and treatment

4	Ischaemic heart disease, arrhythmias, and heart failure	**51**

Part 2 Organ system implications of cardiac surgery

5	Central nervous system	**73**
6	Haematology	**91**
7	The inflammatory response	**109**
8	Renal	**125**
9	Respiratory implications of cardiac surgery	**137**
10	Infection	**149**

Part 3 Clinical practice of cardiac anaesthesia

Cardiac interventions

11	Interventional cardiology and coronary artery disease	**165**

12 Interventions in congenital heart disease   179

13 Electrophysiological procedures   189

14 Cardiac surgery   195

    Anaesthesia for cardiac surgery and interventions

15 Preoperative assessment and investigations   207

16 Monitoring   223

17 Trans-oesophageal echocardiography   241

18 Cardiopulmonary bypass   261

19 Deep hypothermic circulatory arrest   273

20 Intra-aortic balloon counter-pulsation   28

21 Ventricular assist devices   29

22 Postoperative care   30

23 Anaesthesia for coronary artery disease   33

24 Off-pump surgery   34

25 Aortic valve surgery   35

26 Surgery of the thoracic aorta   37

27 Mitral valve surgery   39

28 Other valve disease   41

29 Paediatric congenital heart disease   42

30 Adult congenital heart disease   46

31 Hypertrophic cardiomyopathy   4

32 Anaesthesia for heart failure and transplantation   5

33 Urgent cardiac procedures   5

34 Anaesthesia for electrophysiology procedures   5

35 Cardiac disease in pregnancy   5

    Index 573

Detailed contents

Symbols and Abbreviations *xviii*
Contributors *xxvi*

Part 1 The cardiovascular system   **1**

Anatomy, pharmacology, physiology

1 The heart an its valves   **3**
The heart *4*
The cardiac valves *8*
Coronary arteries and veins *10*
Further reading *12*

2 Cardiac physiology   **13**
Introduction *14*
Electrophysiology *16*
Cardiac muscle *20*
The cardiac cycle *22*
Control of cardiac output *26*
Control of blood pressure *30*
Coronary circulation *32*
Further reading *35*

3 Cardiovascular drugs   **37**
Control of heart rate and rhythm *38*
Control contractility *40*
Control of preload and afterload *46*
Further reading *50*

Cardiovascular disease and treatment

**4 Ischaemic heart disease, arrhythmias,
and heart failure**   **51**
Ischaemic heart disease (IHD) *52*
Perioperative arrhythmias *60*

Heart failure (HF) *64*

Further reading *70*

Part 2 Organ system implications of cardiac surgery 71

5 Central nervous system 73

Introduction *74*

General considerations *76*

Incidence and etiology *78*

Prevention *82*

Management of established neurological complications *86*

Further reading *89*

6 Haematology 91

Heparin and protamine *92*

Preoperative antithrombotic drugs *94*

Bleeding and transfusion *96*

The postoperative bleeding patient *102*

Management of patients requiring postoperative anticoagulation *106*

Further reading *107*

7 The inflammatory response 109

The inflammatory response *110*

Activation of the inflammatory response *112*

Components of the inflammatory response *114*

Organ effects *118*

Modulation of the inflammatory response *120*

Further reading *123*

8 Renal 125

Acute renal failure *126*

Prevention *130*

A practical approach to perioperative renal protection *134*

Key points *135*

Further reading *136*

9 Respiratory implications of cardiac surgery   137
Introduction *138*
Preoperative assessment *140*
Intraoperative management of mechanical ventilation *141*
Postoperative respiratory function *142*
Further reading *147*

10 Infection   149
Infection risks *150*
Infection prophylaxis in cardiac surgery *152*
Infective endocarditis *154*
Sternal wound infections *160*
Further reading *162*

Part 3 **Clinical practice of cardiac anaesthesia**   163

Cardiac interventions

11 Interventional cardiology and coronary artery disease   165
What is coronary intervention? *166*
Pathophysiology of coronary artery disease *170*
The clinical spectrum of coronary heart disease *171*
Percutaneous coronary intervention *172*
PCI and non-cardiac surgery *176*
Anaesthetic support during a PCI *177*
Further reading *178*

12 Interventions in congenital heart disease   179
Background *180*
Interventions *181*
Further reading *187*

13 Electrophysiological procedures   189
Introduction *190*
Ablation *192*
Further reading *194*

14 Cardiac surgery   **195**

Risk assessment *196*

Conduct of surgery *198*

Emergency surgery *199*

Myocardial preservation *200*

Off-pump coronary artery bypass *203*

Minimally invasive cardiac surgery (MICS) *204*

Reoperative surgery *205*

New techniques in surgery *206*

Further reading *206*

Anaesthesia for cardiac surgery and interventions

15 Preoperative assessment and investigations   **207**

Preoperative evaluation *208*

Multifactorial risk indices *210*

Non-invasive testing and radionuclide studies *214*

Cardiac catheterization *219*

Further reading *222*

16 Monitoring   **223**

Perioperative electrocardiography *224*

Haemodynamic monitoring and invasive vascular access *228*

Cardiac output monitoring *236*

Temperature monitoring *238*

Neurologic monitoring *239*

Further reading *240*

17 Trans-oesophageal echocardiography   **241**

Ultrasound physics *242*

Imaging modes *244*

Uses and indications for trans-oesophageal echocardiography *248*

Monitoring applications *250*

Standard examination and views *252*

Complications of TOE *256*

Further reading *259*

18 Cardiopulmonary bypass   **261**

Cardiopulmonary bypass circuits *262*

Pre-bypass checklists *263*

Conduct of bypass *264*

Further reading *271*

19 Deep hypothermic circulatory arrest   **273**

Deep hypothermic circulatory arrest (DHCA) *274*

Cerebral metabolism and hypothermia *276*

Management of DHCA *278*

Outcome *284*

Further reading *285*

20 Intra-aortic balloon counter-pulsation   **287**

Principles *288*

Indications and contraindications *289*

Placement *290*

Management *292*

Further reading *296*

21 Ventricular assist devices   **297**

Principles *298*

Indications *299*

Types of VADs *300*

Anaesthetic management during VAD placement *302*

Complications *304*

Further reading *305*

22 Postoperative care   **307**

General principles *308*

Inotropes and cardiovascular medications *312*

Mechanical ventilation *316*

Abnormal gases *318*

The oliguric patient *320*

The hypotensive patient *322*

Atrial fibrillation *326*

Sedation and analgesia *328*

23 Anaesthesia for coronary artery disease 331
Pathology *332*
Pathophysiology of ischaemic disease *333*
Assessment *334*
Clinical presentation *336*
Preoperative investigations *337*
Haemodynamic goals *338*
Anaesthetic plan *340*
Adverse haemodynamics *342*
Therapeutic options *343*
Trans-oesophageal essentials *344*
Practice points *345*
Further reading *346*

24 Off-pump surgery 347
Background *348*
Managing the procedure *350*
Outcome *354*
Further reading *356*

25 Aortic valve surgery 357
Aortic stenosis *358*
Aortic regurgitation (AR) *362*
Surgical essentials and therapeutic options *366*
TOE essentials *370*
Practice points *374*
Further reading *375*

26 Surgery of the thoracic aorta 377
Introduction *378*
Thoracic aneurysms *380*
Ascending aortic aneurysms and aortic arch surgery *382*
Descending thoracic aneurysms *386*
Aortic dissection *390*
Practice points *395*
Further reading *396*

27 Mitral valve surgery 397

Introduction *398*

Mitral regurgitation *400*

Mitral stenosis (MS) *404*

Mixed mitral valve disease *408*

Practice points *409*

Further reading *410*

28 Other valve disease 411

Mixed valve lesions *412*

Tricuspid regurgitation *414*

Tricuspid stenosis *416*

Pulmonary stenosis and regurgitation *418*

Further reading *420*

29 Paediatric congenital heart disease 421

Foetal circulation *422*

Neonatal physiology *424*

Preoperative assessment and premedication *426*

Drugs used in paediatric cardiac anaesthesia *428*

Equipment and monitoring *429*

Management of cardiopulmonary bypass in children *430*

Coagulopathy after cardiac surgery in children *432*

Classification of congenital heart lesions *433*

'Simple' left to right shunts *434*

'Simple' right to left shunts *435*

Atrial septal defect *436*

Patent ductus arteriosus (PDA) *438*

Tetralogy of Fallot (TOF) *440*

Transposition of the great arteries (TGA) *442*

Truncus arteriosus *444*

Anomalous pulmonary venous connections *446*

Hypoplastic left heart syndrome *448*

Ventricular septal defect (VSD) and atrioventricular septal
defect (AVSD) *452*

Interrupted aortic arch *454*

Aortic stenosis (AS) *456*

Coarctation of the aorta *458*

Three common paediatric cardiac surgical procedures *460*

Cardiac catheterization and interventional cardiology *462*

Paediatric cardiac transplantation *464*

Further reading *467*

30 Adult congenital heart disease **469**

Introduction *470*

Assessment *471*

Terminology *472*

Classification *474*

Pathophysiology *476*

Specific lesions *478*

Sequelae *486*

Management *488*

Endocarditis *490*

Further reading *491*

31 Hypertrophic cardiomyopathy **493**

Pathology *494*

Therapeutic options *496*

Haemodynamic goals *497*

Anaesthetic plan and adverse haemodynamics *498*

TOE essentials *500*

Practice points *502*

Further reading *503*

32 Anaesthesia for heart failure and
transplantation **505**

Heart failure *506*

Anaesthesia for patients with severe heart failure *510*

Transplantation *514*

Anaesthetic management of heart transplantation *520*

Rejection and immunology *524*

The previously transplanted patient *526*

Further reading *527*

33 Urgent cardiac procedures   **529**

Cardiac tamponade *530*

Chest trauma *534*

Blunt trauma *536*

Aortic transection *538*

Pulmonary embolism *540*

Cardiac tumours *542*

Practice points *543*

Further reading *544*

34 Anaesthesia for electrophysiology procedures   **545**

Permanent and temporary pacemakers *546*

Anaesthesia for pacemaker and ICD insertion *550*

Indwelling pacemakers, ICDs, and anaesthesia *552*

Anaesthesia for DC cardioversion *554*

Anaesthesia for electrophysiology and catheter ablation procedures *556*

Further reading *561*

35 Cardiac disease in pregnancy   **563**

Background *564*

High-risk lesions *565*

The current spectrum of maternal heart disease *566*

Hierarchy of antenatal care (ANC) *568*

Practice points *570*

Further reading *571*

Index *573*

Symbols and abbreviations

~	approximately
↓	decreased
↑	increased
→	leading to
±	plus/minus
📖	refer to
AAI	atriapaced, atria sensed, inhibited
ABG	arterial blood gases
ACAB	atraumatic coronary artery bypass
ACC	American College of Cardiology
ACEI	angiotensin-converting enzyme inhibitors
ACS	acute coronary syndrome
ACT	activated clotting time
ADH	antidiuretic hormone
ADP	adenosine diphosphate
ADQI	Acute Dialysis Quality Initiative
AF	atrial fibrillation
AHA	American Heart Association
AICD	automated implantable cardioverter-defibrillator
ALI	acute lung injury
ANC	antenatal care
ANH	acute normovolaemic haemodilution
ANP	atrial natriuretic peptide
AP	action potential
AP	aortopulmonary
APA	atriopulmonary anastomosis
APR	acute phase reactant
aPTT	activated partial thromboplastin time
AR	aortic regurgitation
ARB	angiotensin receptor blocker
ARDS	acute respiratory distress syndrome
ARF	acute renal failure
AS	aortic stenosis
ASD	atrial septal defect

ASO	arterial switch operation
AT-III	antithrombin III
ATN	acute tubular necrosis
ATP	adenosine triphosphate
AV	atrioventricular
AVNRT	atrioventricular nodal re-entrant tachycardia
AVRT	atrioventricular re-entrant tachycardia
AVSD	atrioventricular septal defect
BCIS	British Cardiac Interventional Society
BiPAP	bilevel positive airway pressure
BIS	bi-spectral analysis monitor
BiVAD	biventricular assist device
BNP	B-type natriuretic peptide
BP	blood pressure
BSA	body surface area
BT	Blalock-Taussig
CABG	coronary artery bypass grafting
CAD	coronary artery disease
cAMP	cyclic adenosine monophosphate
CBF	coronary blood flow
CCS	Canadian Cardiovascular Society
CCSC	Canadian Cardiovascular Society Classification
CCTGA	congenitally corrected transportation of great arteries
CDC	Center for Disease Control
CEMACH	Confidential Enquiry into Maternal and Child Health
CFAM	cerebral function analysing monitor
CFE	complex fractionated electrogram
cGMP	cyclic guanosine monophosphate
CHD	congenital heart disease
CHF	congestive heart failure
CMR	cerebral metabolic rate
$CMRO_2$	cerebral metabolic rate of oxygen
cNOS	constitutive nitric oxide synthase
CNS	central nervous system
CO	cardiac output
CoA	coarctation of the aorta
COPD	chronic obstructive pulmonary disease
CPAP	continuous positive airway pressure
CPB	cardiopulmonary bypass
CPP	cerebral perfusion pressure

CPP	coronary perfusion pressure
CPR	cardiopulmonary resuscitation
CRF	chronic renal failure
CRP	C-reactive protein
CRT	cardiac resynchronization therapy
CSF	cerebrospinal fluid
CT	computed tomography
cTnc	troponin C
cTnl	troponin I
cTnT	troponin T
CVA	cerebrovascular accident
CVP	central venous pressure
CVR	coronary vascular resistance
CW	continuous wave
Cx	circumflex artery
CXR	chest X-ray
DA	ductus arteriosus
DC	direct current
DCM	dilated cardiomyopathy
DDD	dual paced, dual sensed, dual
DES	drug-eluting stents
DHCA	deep hypothermic circulatory arrest
DORV	double outlet right ventricle
DVT	deep vein thrombosis
EACA	ε-aminocaproic acid
ECG	electrocardiogram
ECMO	extracorporeal membrane oxygenation
ECT	ecarin clotting time
EDV	end diastolic volume
EEG	electroencephalogram
EF	ejection fraction
ELISA	enzyme-linked immunosorbent assay
EMG	electromyography
EPS	electrophysiology study
ERO	effective regurgitant orifice
ESC	European Society of Cardiology
ESR	erythrocyte sedimentation rate
ESRD	end-stage renal disease
ESV	end systolic volume
$ETCO_2$	end tidal carbondioxide

ETT	exercise tolerance test
EVAR	endovascular aneurysm repair
FAC	fractional area change
FBC	full blood count
FDA	Food and Drug Administration
FEV_1	forced expiratory volume in 1 second
FFP	fresh frozen plasma
FRC	functional residual capacity
GFR	glomerular filtration rate
GTN	glyceryl trinitrate (nitroglycerin)
Hb	haemoglobin
HCM	hypertrophic cardiomyopathy
HDU	high dependency unit
HF	heart failure
HIT	heparin-induced thrombocytopaenia
HITS	heparin-induced thrombocytopaenia syndrome
HLHS	hypoplastic left heart syndrome
HOCM	hypertrophic obstructive cardiomyopathy
HR	heart rate
HS	heart sound
IAA	interrupted aortic arch
IABP	intra-aortic balloon pump
ICC	interventional cardiac catheterization
ICD	implantable cardiac defibrillator
ICP	intracranial pressure
ICU	intensive care unit
IHD	ischaemic heart disease
IL	interleukin
IMA	internal mammary artery
iNO	inhaled nitric oxide
iNOS	inducible nitric oxide synthase
INR	international normalized ratio
IOCS	intraoperative cell salvage
IPPV	intermittent positive pressure ventilation
ITU	intensive therapy unit
IVC	inferior vena cava
JET	junctional ectopic tachycardia
JVP	jugular venous pressure
LA	left atrium
LAD	left anterior descending

RF	radio-frequency
RHD	rheumatic heart disease
RIND	reversible ischaemic neurological deficit
ROS	reactive oxygen species
RRT	renal replacement therapy
RV	right ventricle
RVAD	right ventricular assist device
RVEDP	right ventricular end-diastolic pressure
RVF	right ventricular failure
RVH	right ventricular hypertrophy
RVol	regurgitant volume
RVOT	right ventricular outflow tract
RVOTO	right ventricular outflow tract obstruction
RVSP	right ventricular systoliz pressure
RWMA	regional wall motion abnormality
SAM	systolic anterior motion
SAN	sinoatrial node
S_aO_2	arterial saturation
SBOS	Surgical Blood Ordering Schedule
SCD	sudden cardiac death
SCTS	Society of Cardiothoracic Surgeons of Great Britain and Ireland
SIMV	synchronized intermittent mandatory ventilation
SIRS	systemic inflammatory response syndrome
$S_{jv}O_2$	jugular venous oxygen saturation
SNP	sodium nitroprusside
$S_{PA}O_2$	pulmonary artery saturation
SPV	systolic pressure variation
$S_{PV}O_2$	pulmonary venous saturation
SSEP	somatosensory-evoked potential
S_vO_2	systemic venous saturation
STEMI	S-T elevation myocardial infarction
STS	Society of Thoracic Surgeons
SV	stroke volume
SVC	superior vena cava
SVR	systemic vascular resistance
TAPVC	total anomalous pulmonary venous connection
TAPVD	total anomalous pulmonary venous drainage
TAVI	transcutaneous aortic valve implantation
TCD	transcranial Doppler

TCI	target-controlled infusion
TCPC	total cavo-pulmonary connection
TDI	tissue Doppler imaging
TEA	thoracic epidural analgesia
TECAB	total endoscopic coronary artery bypass
TEG	thromboelastography/thromboelastogram
TGA	transposition of the great arteries
TIVA	total intravenous anaesthesia
TNF	tumour necrosis factor
TOE	trans-oesophageal echocardiography
TOF	tetralogy of Fallot
TPG	transpulmonary gradient
TR	tricuspid regurgitation
TTE	transthoracic echo
TV	tricuspid valve
UA	unstable angina
VAD	ventricular assist device
VAP	ventilator-associated pneumonia
VC	vena contracta
VF	ventricular fibrillation
VPB	ventricular premature beat
VSD	ventricular septal defect
VT	ventricular tachycardia
VTI	velocity time integral

Contributors

Professor R Anderson
Professor of Anatomy,
Institute of Child Health,
London,
UK

Dr S Allen
Consultant Anaesthetist,
Royal Hospitals,
Belfast,
UK

Dr J Arrowsmith
Consultant Anaesthetist,
Papworth Hospital,
Cambridge,
UK

Dr E Ashley
Consultant Anaesthetist,
The Heart Hospital,
London,
UK

Dr A Barbeito
Assistant Professor of
Anesthesiology,
Duke University,
North Carolina,
USA

Dr M Barnard
Consultant Anaesthetist,
The Heart Hospital,
London,
UK

Dr A Campbell
Consultant Anaesthetist,
The Heart Hospital,
London,
UK

Dr J Chikwe
Assistant Professor of Cardiac
Surgery,
Mount Sinai Hospital,
New York,
USA

Dr A Cohen
Consultant Anaesthetist,
Bristol Royal Infirmary,
Bristol,
UK

Dr S Cullen
Consultant Cardiologist,
The Heart Hospital,
London,
UK

Dr W Davies
Consultant Anaesthetist,
The Heart Hospital,
London,
UK

Dr C Dollery
Senior Lecturer in Cardiology,
The Heart Hospital,
London,
UK

Dr D Farran
Consultant Anaesthetist,
The Heart Hospital,
London,
UK

Dr A Gaunt
Consultant Anaesthetist,
Harefield Hospital,
London,
UK

Dr S George
Consultant Anaesthetist,
Harefield Hospital,
London,
UK

Dr J Gothard
Consultant Anaesthetist,
The Royal Brompton Hospital,
London,
UK

Dr K Grebenik
Consultant Anaesthetist,
John Radcliffe Hospital,
Oxford,
UK

Dr G Hopgood
Consultant Anaesthetist,
Tauranga Hospital,
New Zealand

Dr A Kelleher
Consultant Anaesthetist,
The Royal Brompton Hospital,
London,
UK

Dr L Kevin
Consultant Anaesthetist,
Galway Hospital,
Galway,
Ireland

Dr P Lambiase
Consultant Cardiologist,
The Heart Hospital,
London,
UK

Dr M Lees
Consultant Anaesthetist,
The Heart Hospital,
London,
UK

Dr M Lowe
Consultant Cardiologist,
The Heart Hospital,
London,
UK

Dr J Mackay
Consultant Anaesthetist,
Papworth Hospital,
Cambridge,
UK

Professor J Mark
Duke University,
North Carolina,
USA

Dr A McEwan
Consultant Anaesthetist,
Great Ormond Street Hospital,
London,
UK

Dr B Martin
Consultant Anaesthetist,
The Heart Hospital,
London,
UK

Dr M Patrick
Consultant Anaesthetist,
Wythenshaw Hospital,
Manchester,
UK

Dr A Rosenberg
Associate Professor of
Anesthesiology,
University of
Michigan,
USA

Dr A Smith
Consultant Anaesthetist,
The Heart Hospital,
London,
UK

Dr F Walker
Consultant Cardiologist,
The Heart Hospital,
London,
UK

Dr S Webb
Consultant Anaesthetist,
Papworth Hospital,
Cambridge,
UK

Dr M Westwood
Consultant Cardiologist,
The London Chest Hospital,
London,
UK

Dr P Wilson
Consultant Microbiologist,
University College London
Hospitals,
London,
UK

Dr B Woodcock
Clinical Assistant Professor of
Anesthesiology,
University of Michigan,
Michigan,
USA

Dr S Wright
Consultant Anaesthetist,
The Heart Hospital,
London,
UK

Mr J Yap
Consultant Cardiothoracic
Surgeon,
The Heart Hospital,
London,
UK

Part 1

The cardiovascular system

Anatomy, pharmacology, physiology

1	The heart and its valves	3
2	Cardiac physiology	13
3	Cardiovascular drugs	37

Cardiovascular disease and treatment

4	Ischaemic heart disease, arrhythmias, and heart failure	51

The heart and its valves

Professor R Anderson and
Dr J Chikwe

The heart 4
The cardiac valves 8
Coronary arteries and veins 10
Further reading 12

The heart

Introduction

The heart possesses atrial chambers, ventricles, and arterial trunks, one each for the right and left sides. The cardiac valves guard the inflows and the outflows to the ventricular mass.

The atrial chambers

Each atrium has a venous component, a body, an appendage, and a vestibule, and the two atria are separated by the septum. On the right side the venous component receives the superior and inferior caval veins, along with the coronary sinus, whilst the four pulmonary veins drain to the left atrium (LA). The right appendage is extensive and triangular, whilst the left one is narrow and tubular. The septum is limited to the oval fossa and its immediate surrounds, although infolded walls give the impression of a much greater septal area. The vestibules on both sides support the hinges of the atrioventricular valves.

Right atrium (Figure 1.1)

The right atrium (RA) receives venous drainage from four sources:

- The superior vena cava (SVC) superiorly, draining the azygous, jugular, and subclavian veins.
- The inferior vena cava (IVC) inferiorly, draining the lower body.
- The coronary sinus inferiorly, draining the heart.
- The anterior cardiac vein anteriorly, draining the front of the heart.

Running vertically downwards between the IVC and SVC is the crista terminalis, a muscular ridge marked externally by the sulcus terminalis. The sinus node lies at the superior end of the terminal groove, where the atrial appendage meets the SVC. The crista terminalis separates the smooth-walled posterior right atrium derived from the sinus venosus from the trabeculated appendage, derived from the foetal RA. The IVC and coronary sinus have rudimentary valves (the Eustachian and Thebesian valves respectively).

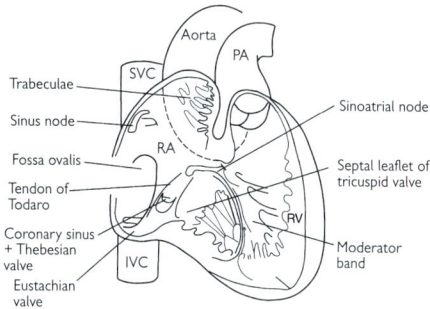

Figure 1.1 Interior of the right atrium and right ventricle showing the conduction system.

Left atrium

The left atrium is smaller than the right with thicker walls. It is long and narrow, compared to the wide-based RA. The four pulmonary veins open into the upper part of its posterior wall. On its septal surface there is a shallow depression and 'flap' valve, which corresponds to the fossa ovalis. The appendage is characterized by pectinate muscles.

Atrial septum

Although at first glance it looks as though the lateral RA wall between the IVC and SVC is the atrial septum, the true septum is virtually confined to the fossa ovalis. The superior rim of the fossa is commonly referred to as the septum secundum, but it is really an infolding between the right atrium and the pulmonary veins. Inferiorly the region around the coronary sinus is where the right atrial wall overlies the AV muscular septum. The anterior rim of the fossa ovalis overlies the aortic root.

The ventricles

Each ventricle has an inlet component, surrounding and supporting the atrioventricular valve, an apical trabecular component that acts as the pump to both circulations, and an outlet supporting the arterial valves.

Right ventricle (Figure 1.1)

The right ventricle (RV) consists of a large inlet (sinus) and a smaller outlet (conus) portion separated by the supraventricular crest. The inlet portion surrounds the tricuspid valve and its tension apparatus. The inflow tract is characterized by trabeculae carnae, from some of which papillary muscles project, attaching to the inferior border of the tricuspid valve leaflets via tendinae chordae. The moderator band is a muscular bundle crossing the ventricular cavity from the interventricular septum to the anterior wall, conveying the right branch of the AV bundle to the ventricular muscle. The outlet portion is smooth walled and consists of the infundibulum (a muscular structure that supports the pulmonary valve), the superior part of the septal band, and a very narrow portion superior to the trabecular septum. The thick, muscular supraventricular crest widely separates the pulmonary valve from the tricuspid valve.

Left ventricle

The left ventricle (LV) consists of a large trabeculated inlet (sinus) and a smaller smooth-walled outlet portion. In comparison to the well-separated pulmonary and tricuspid valves, the aortic and mitral valves are in fibrous continuity. Most of the inlet portion is finely trabeculated with anterolateral (anterior) and posteromedial (posterior) papillary muscles connecting to the mitral valve leaflets via tendinae chordae.

Ventricular septum

The ventricular septal surfaces are asymmetrical firstly because of the infundibular portion of the RV, secondly because of the differing long axis of RV (vertical) and LV (oblique), and thirdly because of the pressure differential between RV and LV. It is made up of a muscular septum, a membranous septum, and the atrioventricular septum. The atrioventricular septum lies between the right atrium and the left ventricle. The AV node lies in the atrial septum adjacent to the junction between the membranous and muscular portions of the atrioventricular septum, and the bundle of His passes toward the right trigone between these components.

The cardiac valves

The pulmonary valve is the most superior valve, while the tricuspid and mitral valves guard the diaphragmatic border of the cardiac short axis. Cradled between these three structures is the aortic valve, centrally located within the cardiac silhouette (Figure 1.2).

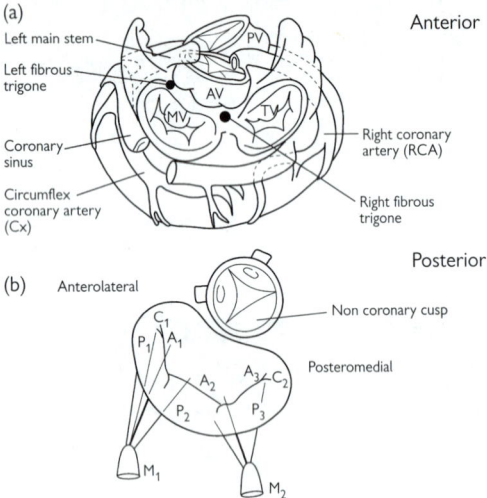

Figure 1.2 (a) Cardiac valves and their relationships viewed from above, with the atria removed. Note how the commissure of the left and the non-coronary sinuses of the aortic valve points at the midpoint of the anterior leaflet of the mitral valve. Note how the pulmonary valve commissure is adjacent to the commissure between the left and right coronary sinuses of the aortic valve. (b) The segmental classification used to describe mitral valve pathology in echocardiography and surgery.

Structure of the atrioventricular valves

Each atrioventricular valve possesses a hinge, leaflets, tendinous cords, and papillary muscles, which act in harmony to maintain the integrity of valvar function. The tricuspid valve has three leaflets positioned septally, anterosuperiorly, and inferiorly. The mitral valve has only anterior and posterior leaflets.

Tricuspid valve

This has an anterior, a septal, and a posterior leaflet. The orifice is triangular, larger than in the mitral valve, and the annulus is much less well defined. The leaflets and chordae are thinner than in the mitral valve. The chordae to the largest anterior leaflet arise from the anterior and medial papillary muscles. The posterior leaflet is the smallest and most inferior and is usually scalloped. The chordae to the septal leaflet arise from the posterior and septal papillary muscles. The conduction system is closely related to the septal leaflet.

Mitral valve

This bicuspid valve has a large anterior (aortic or septal) leaflet and a small posterior (mural or ventricular) leaflet. The leaflet area is much greater than the valve area, allowing a large area for coaptation, distinguished as a rough zone. The larger anterior leaflet inserts on only a third of the annulus, through which it is in fibrous continuity with the left half of the non-coronary cusp of the aortic valve. This fibrous sheet has distinct thickened lateral points known as the left and right trigones. The latter join with the membranous septum to form the central fibrous body of the heart. The smaller posterior leaflet inserts into two-thirds of the annulus and is scalloped. Each leaflet is segmented into three for the purposes of nomenclature. The chordae tendinae insert into both leaflets from the anterolateral and posteromedial papillary muscles. Three orders of chordae have been defined: first order insert onto the leaflet free margin; second order insert a few millimetres further back; and third order insert at the base of the posterior leaflet only. An alternative terminology is marginal cords, rough zone cords, and strut and basal cords.

The arterial valves

The arterial valves have ventricular support, sinuses, and leaflets, with all three needing to work together. There is no ring-like fibrous structure supporting the leaflets of the arterial valves, as there is for the atrioventricular valves. Instead, the hinges of the arterial valves extend in semilunar fashion from the ventricular support to the sinutubular junctions. The ventricular support is exclusively muscular in the right ventricle, but partly fibrous and partly muscular in the left. The leaflets themselves are simply pockets of fibrous tissue lined by endothelium. When closed, it is their shape and attachments that enable them to support the pressure of the diastolic column of arterial blood.

Aortic valve

The aortic valve is in fibrous continuity with the anterior leaflet of the mitral valve and the membranous septum. The free edge of each cusp is thickest and at the midpoint of each free edge is a fibrous nodulus of Aranti, bordered on either side by crescent-shaped lunulae that form the region of coaptation. The aortic sinuses (sinuses of Valsalva) are dilated, relatively thin-walled pockets of the aortic root, two of which give rise to the coronary arteries. Because of the shape of the cusps the annulus is crown-shaped. The cusps are called right, left, and non-coronary based on the origin of the coronary arteries.

Pulmonary valve

This is composed of right, left, and anterior (non-septal) leaflets. The structure of the pulmonary valve is similar to the aortic valve, with three differences. Firstly, the valve leaflets are flimsier than the aortic valve; secondly, coronary arteries do not originate from the sinuses; and thirdly, the valve is not in continuity with the anterior tricuspid valve leaflet.

The arterial trunks

The aortic valve is positioned posterior and to the right of the pulmonary valve, albeit that the trunks spiral as they course at right angles to each other to the margins of the pericardial cavity.

Coronary arteries and veins

The coronary arteries can be thought of as two main distributions (right and left), supplied by three vessels: right coronary artery (RCA), left anterior descending (LAD), and circumflex artery (Cx), which create four semicircles around the heart (Figure 1.3(a)).

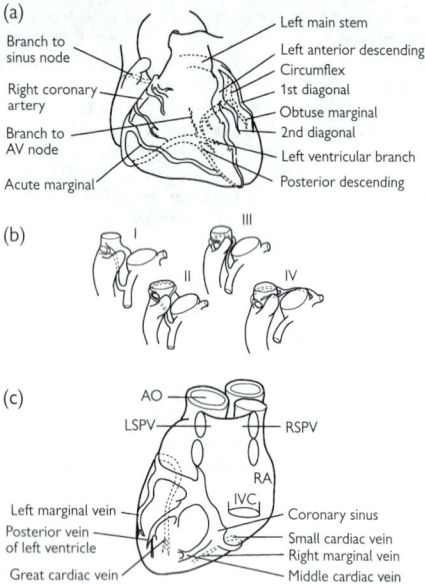

Figure 1.3 (a) Distribution of the coronary arteries. (b) Variations in the origin and course of the sinus node artery, which may arise from the right coronary artery (60%) and encircle the base of the superior vena cava in a clockwise (I), anticlockwise (II), or both (III) directions, or arise from the left coronary artery (40% of cases) (IV). (c) Distribution of the coronary veins.

Left main stem

The left main stem (LMS) arises from the ostium of the left sinus of Valsalva and travels between the pulmonary trunk anteriorly and the left atrial appendage to the left atrioventricular groove, dividing after 1–2 cm into LAD, Cx, and occasionally a third artery: the intermediate.

Left anterior descending

The LAD runs down the anterior interventricular groove to the apex of the heart, usually extending round the apex to the posterior interventricular groove and the territory of the posterior descending artery. A variable number of diagonals are given off over the anterior surface of the LV, small branches supply the anterior surface of the RV, and several branches are given off perpendicularly to supply the anterior two thirds of the interventricular septum. The first septal branch is the largest and can be used to identify the LAD on angiograms. Some of the right ventricular branches anastomose with infundibular branches of the proximal RCA.

Circumflex

The Cx originates at 90° from the LMS and runs medially to the LA appendage for 2–3 cm, continuing in the posterior left AV groove to the crux of the heart. In left dominant hearts (5–10%) the Cx turns 90° into the posterior interventricular groove to form the posterior descending artery (PDA). In 85–90% of hearts the PDA arises from the RCA (right dominant). About 5% of hearts are co-dominant. A variable number of obtuse marginals (OMs) arise from the Cx to supply the posterior LV. They are frequently intramuscular. The first branch of the Cx is the atrial circumflex, which courses round the LA near the AV groove.

Right coronary artery

The RCA arises from an ostium in the right sinus of Valsalva, and runs immediately into the deep right atrioventricular groove where it gives off branches to the anterior RV wall. The branch to the SA node is given off early. The acute marginal is a large branch that crosses the acute margin of the heart to travel to the apex. The origin of the PDA decides 'dominance'. In 90% of cases the RCA reaches the crux of the heart where it turns 90° to form the PDA. This runs towards the apex in the posterior interventricular groove. Septals that supply the posterior third of the interventricular septum arise at 90° from the PDA. The RCA supplies the right ventricle and a significant part of the left ventricle and septum. This has clinical implications if retrograde cardioplegia is used as Thebesian drainage into the right ventricle may compromise preservation of the left ventricle.

Venous drainage of the heart

This is shown in Figure 1.3(c). The coronary sinus runs in the posterior AV groove draining into the right atrium with the great cardiac vein. Thebesian veins empty directly into the heart chambers from the myocardium.

Variations in coronary anatomy

- Right dominant 90%, left dominant 5%, co-dominant 5%.
- Absent LMS with separate ostia for the Cx and the LAD (1%).
- Anomalous origin from pulmonary artery <0.01%.
- LAD represented by two separate parallel vessels (4%).
- SA node artery arising from the Cx (2–3%).
- SA node artery may travel round the SVC clockwise or anticlockwise, or bifurcate and travel in both directions (Figure 1.3(b)).
- AV node artery from RCA (55%), from Cx (45%).
- Two RCAs arising from sinus of Valsalva (10%).
- High diagonal (15%).

Further reading

1. Anderson R, Razavi R, Taylor A. Cardiac anatomy revisited. *Journal of Anatomy* 2004; 205: 159–177.
2. Lorenz C, von Berg J. A comprehensive shape model of the heart. *Medical Image Analysis* 2006; 10: 657–670.
3. Loukas M, Groat C, Khangura R, Gueorguieva Evans D, Anderson R. The normal and abnormal anatomy of the coronary arteries. *Clinical Anatomy* 2009; 22: 114–128.
4. Shane Tubbs R. Morphology of the heart. *Clinical Anatomy* 2009; 22: 1.

Cardiac physiology

Dr B Martin and Dr A Campbell

Introduction *14*
Electrophysiology *16*
Cardiac muscle *20*
The cardiac cycle *22*
Control of cardiac output *26*
Control of blood pressure *30*
Coronary circulation *32*
Further reading *35*

Introduction

The heart is a highly specialized organ with unique muscle combining the characteristics of both skeletal and smooth muscle, which allows it to contract up to 2.6 billion times during a lifetime. It has a specialized conducting system that allows a variable synchronized rhythm, carefully balances preload, afterload, and contractility and supplies the body's lifetime metabolic oxygen demand of 9.6 billion litres. When this system starts to fail tissue injury occurs. A thorough understanding of the basic principles that enable the heart to pump blood efficiently around the body and thus meet its demand for oxygen is essential for a cardiac anaesthetist.

Electrophysiology

Electrical conduction

There are two action potentials present in cardiac tissue: slow action potentials in specialized 'pacemaker' cells found in the conducting pathways and fast action potentials found throughout most of the remaining tissue making up the atria, ventricular, and Purkinje fibres.

   These two types of action potentials are different in:
- Their resting potentials.
- The rate of rise of depolarization.
- The propagation velocity.

Table 2.1 Action potentials in cardiac muscle

Feature	Slow action potentials	Fast action potentials
Resting potentials	−60 mV	−90 mV
Rate of rise of AP	Fast sodium channels absent	Fast sodium channels present
Propagation velocity	800 ms	200 ms

The resting membrane potential is dependent on:
- Permeability or leakiness to potassium ions.
- Impermeability or non-leakiness to sodium ions.
- Relative impermeability to calcium ions.

Potassium ions leak out of the cell and down a concentration gradient with fewer sodium ions moving in the opposite direction into the cell. This leads to a loss of positive intracellular charge and is further enhanced by a sodium/potassium ion ATPase pump, which keeps three potassium ions in the cell for every six sodium ions it pumps out. The result is a negative intracellular resting potential. This is an active process, requiring a large amount of the intracellular ATP.

Fast action potentials (Figure 2.1)

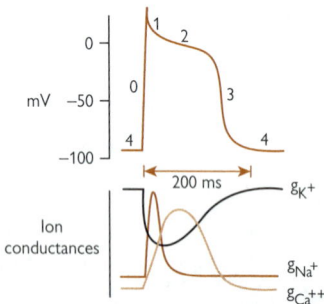

Figure 2.1 Fast action potentials.

- Phase 4: True resting potential is –90 mV; the slope at phase 4 moves towards a threshold of –70 mV where phase 0 is triggered. This positive change in charge is due to a reduction in potassium ion leakage out of the cell. The rate of change of this slope is under autonomic control with adrenergic ß1 receptors increasing the slope and therefore rate of depolarization. Cholinergic m2 fibres decrease the slope and slow the rate of depolarization.
- Phase 0: At –70 mV rapid depolarization occurs as double-gated fast sodium channels twist open accompanied by fast transient 'T' calcium channels causing a rapid influx of positive ions. At +30 mV the inner gates of the fast sodium channels rotate and close.
- Phase 1: Slower potassium channels open and allow leakage out of positive charge; there is brief partial repolarization.
- Phase 2: Dominated by slow calcium and slow sodium channels opening into the cell. Calcium release from the sarcoplasmic reticulum is the trigger for muscle contraction.
- Phase 3: Repolarization occurs with increased leakiness of potassium ions out of the cell and a decrease in positive calcium ions into the cell. The cell therefore becomes more negative, moving back towards its resting potential again.

Slow action potentials (Figure 2.2)

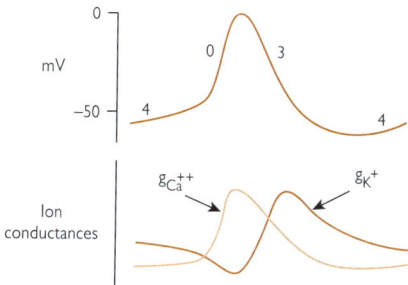

Figure 2.2 Slow action potentials.

- Phase 4: Resting potential is at –60 mV. Rhythmicity is dependent on the reduction in potassium leakage out of the cell and some positive sodium ion leakage inward. The rate of depolarization is again dependent on autonomic control.
- Phase 0: Depolarization occurs by the opening of slow sodium and slow calcium channels. Fast sodium channels are absent.
- There is no phase 1 or 2.
- Phase 3: repolarization occurs with regeneration of the negative resting potential by increased leakiness outwards of potassium and reduction of calcium leakage inwards.

Conduction pathway

- The sinoatrial (SA) node is made up of 'pacemaker' cells generating slow action potentials and is found in the roof of the right atrium lateral to the SVC ostia. It is connected to the atrioventricular (AV) node by anterior, middle, and posterior internodal pathways rather than discrete bundles. The anterior pathway is thought to be the main route.
- The AV node is found on the posterior inter-atrial septum close to the ostia of the coronary sinus. It has three discrete zones: atrial, nodal, and His. The first two zones delay conduction, accounting for the PR interval on the ECG and allowing time for ventricular filling.
- Once through the AV node the action potential passes along the right and left bundle branches either side of the ventricular septum, the left splitting further in anterior and posterior branches. Conduction then spreads out rapidly through the ventricles via an endocardial network of Purkinje fibres.

Cardiac muscle

- Cardiac muscle is unique in having characteristics of both skeletal and smooth muscle. The smallest unit or sarcomere is made up of myofibril filaments demarcated by Z lines seen on an electron micrograph. Hundreds of these myofibrils make up each muscle fibre, giving it a striated appearance. The myofibrils themselves are made of the protein chains actin and myosin (Figure 2.3).

- Actin is a long double helix made up of three protein molecules: primarily actin with every seventh molecule being a troponin complex held in place by tropomyosin. The cardiac troponin complex is also unique to cardiac muscle – it is the regulatory protein that initiates and inhibits the reaction between actin and myosin, allowing shortening and therefore contraction.

- Troponin C (cTnC) binds calcium and initiates contraction, troponin I (cTnI) inhibits this reaction, and troponin T (cTnT) binds the complex to tropomyosin. Detection of these subunits in the blood by immunoassay, following release into the circulation from tissue injury, allows accurate diagnoses of cardiac muscle damage.

- Myosin is a wider protein chain sitting centrally between the thinner actin chains. It is made up of four heavy and two light chains with hinged ATPase heads pointing outwards at 120° intervals, arranged in a spiral around the protein chain.

- If contraction starts with detachment of the myosin ATPase heads from actin, a wave of depolarization occurs during phase two of the fast action potential. Calcium is released from the sarcoplasmic reticulum and is bound by cTnC. This initiates contraction, causing the myosin ATPase heads to reattach to a new actin molecule, and force is then developed by the heads flexing, causing the sarcomere to shorten (Figure 2.3).

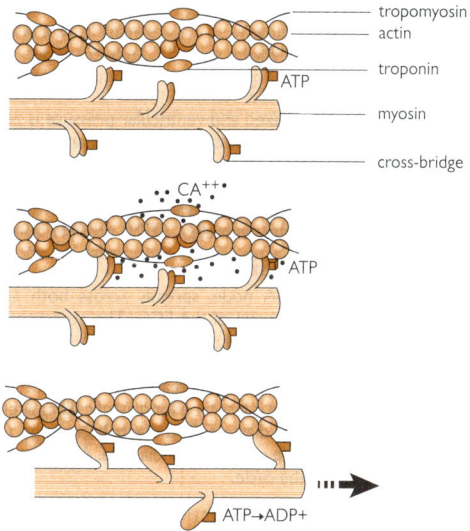

Figure 2.3 'Walk-along' mechanism for contraction of the muscle.

The pressure-volume loop (Figure 2.5)

The ventricular pressure-volume loop represents the events of the cardiac cycle. The cardiac cycle proceeds in an anticlockwise direction. End diastolic volume (EDV) and end systolic volume (ESV) are represented by points W and Y respectively. The area enveloped by the loop represents the stroke work (since work = pressure × volume).

The pressure-volume curve in diastole is initially quite flat, meaning that large increases in volume can be accommodated by only small increases in pressure. However, the ventricle becomes less distensible with greater filling, as shown by the sharp rise of the diastolic curve at large intraventricular volumes.

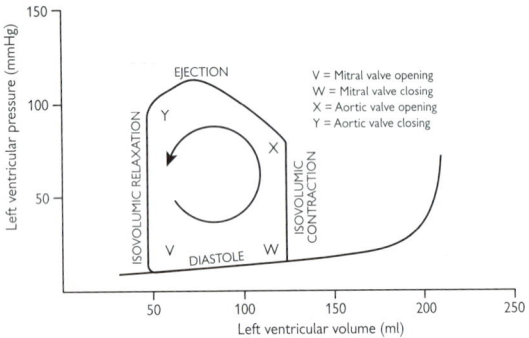

Figure 2.5 The pressure-volume loop.

Control of cardiac output

Cardiac output (CO) is the volume of blood pumped through the heart per minute, calculated by stroke volume × heart rate (CO = SV × HR). In a normal 70 kg person at rest this is about 5 l/min. Stroke volume is the difference between the ventricular end diastolic volume and the end systolic volume (the blood remaining after ejection). Any factor that alters either EDV or ESV will change SV.

Control of stroke volume

At a heart rate of 70 bpm the SV of a normal resting adult will be approximately 80 ml. The mean EDV at rest will normally range from ~110–130 ml. Ejection fraction = SV/EDV × 100% (normally around 70%).

There are three main factors that regulate EDV and ESV and therefore SV:
- Preload.
- Afterload.
- Contractility.

(1) Preload

Preload can be defined as the initial stretching of the cardiac myocytes just prior to systolic contraction and is determined by resting myocyte sarcomere length (not measured *in vivo*).

In an intact ventricle EDV is proportional to the preload. Measurement of EDV in patients is difficult in the perioperative situation. Echocardiography can be used to measure ventricular cavity radius and wall thickness, which together with the measured diastolic pressure allow calculation of the end diastolic wall stress, which correlates better with end diastolic fibre length than EDV. However, equating pressure with volume has limitations. The relationship between pressure and volume in diastole is curvilinear and changes when the ventricle moves along the P/V relationship. Also, acute changes in ventricular stiffness/compliance alter the relationship between pressure and volume. PCWP or CVP are used as less accurate surrogates for the filling pressure (LVEDP).

The heart has the intrinsic capacity to increase its force of contraction when preload is increased and therefore increases SV. This relationship between EDV and SV is known as **Starling's law of the heart** (Figure 2.6), which states that 'the energy of contraction of the muscle is proportional to the initial resting length of the muscle fibre' (note that it is not central venous pressure). Greater initial length of the muscle fibres increases the sensitivity of the myofibrils to calcium and may also increase Ca^{2+} release from the sarcoplasmic reticulum, thus resulting in increased force of contraction.

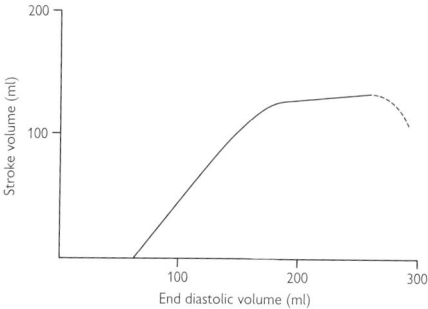

Figure 2.6 Starling curve. Sarcomeres cannot stretch indefinitely in response to pressure/volume.

Starling's Law ensures that the outputs of the LV and RV are matched as small differences in output occur all the time. It also ensures that SV is maintained against increases in afterload.

Factors increasing cardiac muscle fibre length (preload)
- Increased blood volume.
- Increased venous return including skeletal muscle pump, abdomino-thoracic pump – inspiration, gravity, lying down.
- Increased venous tone.
- Increased atrial activity.
- Decreased heart rate (more time for filling).
- Increased ventricular compliance.
- Valve stenosis, pulmonary hypertension (increased afterload).
- Systolic ventricular failure.

(2) Afterload

Afterload is the **systolic ventricular wall stress** and depends on arterial pressure, radius, and wall thickness. (**Law of Laplace**: ventricular wall stress ∝ ventricular pressure × ventricular radius/wall thickness.) It is the 'load' that the heart must eject blood against, i.e. the resistance to ventricular ejection.

Factors increasing afterload
- Anatomical obstruction (e.g. aortic stenosis).
- Increased SVR.
- Increased aortic pressure.
- Ventricular dilation.

An increase in afterload decreases the velocity of muscle fibre shortening. As there is a limited time for ejection, this reduces the rate of ventricular ejection and SV is reduced. Increased afterload results in increased myocardial work and O_2 consumption.

SV can be maintained when there is an increase in afterload. Increasing afterload initially reduces SV, but also increases LVEDP (i.e. increases preload). This occurs because the increase in ESV is added to the venous return into the ventricle, resulting in an increase in EDV. This increase in preload will stimulate the Starling mechanism and cardiac output returns to its original value over a few beats.

The right ventricle is much more sensitive to changes in afterload than the left ventricle because of its thinner wall.

The SV of a failing heart can be improved by decreasing the SVR, which decreases arterial pressure and decreases afterload, thus increasing SV.

(3) Contractility

Contractility is the ability of the heart to contract more forcefully without a change in myocyte sarcomere fibre length or stretch. Therefore, by definition Starling's Law does *not* cause an increase in contractility.

Factors affecting contractility include:

- Neurohormonal effects: sympathetic or parasympathetic systems or catecholamines – exercise, standing up, stress, haemorrhage. The sympathetic nervous system normally has the most important effect on contractility. The parasympathetic nervous system has a small effect on ventricular contractility.
- Chemical and pharmacological effects, e.g. blood K^+, Ca^{2+}, pH/intracellular acidosis, digoxin, β_1 agonists and antagonists, Ca^{2+} channel blockers.
- Pathological effects – ischaemia, bacteraemia.

In the normal circulation, a positive inotropic effect is commonly mediated through sympatho-adrenal discharge, which will improve cardiac performance in several ways; ventricular contraction is more rapid (increased Vmax and dP/dt) and is stronger. As a result the ventricles empty more completely (decreased ESV and increased SV), which will produce higher systolic pressure in the ventricle and aorta.

Changes in contractility change the ejection fraction, which is often used as a clinical index for contractility (Figure 2.7).

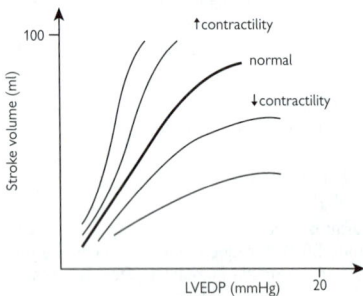

Figure 2.7 Effect of contractility on Starling Curve. Sympathetic stimulation moves the Starling curve upward and to the left.

Control of heart rate

- Changes in HR are more important than changes in SV in producing temporary adjustments in cardiac output.
- Heart rate is usually determined by the pacemaker of the sinoatrial node (SAN). This has an intrinsic rate of approximately 100 bpm and its rate is modulated by the autonomic nervous system. Normally at rest vagal parasympathetic nerves dominate and the resting heart rate is 60–80 bpm. A denervated (transplanted) heart beats at 100 bpm.
- Bowditch or 'interval-strength' effect – a direct intrinsic effect of rate on contractility – when HR increases there is a proportional increase in myocardial contractility.
- Increasing HR decreases diastolic filling time, but most ventricular filling occurs during the initial rapid filling phase so a modest increase in HR affects only diastasis (the late slower-filling phase) and so CO increases.
- Rapid HRs affect the rapid-filling phase and there is a decrease in CO.
- Severe bradycardia (<40 bpm) – the elevated SV is not enough to compensate for the decreased rate since most ventricular filling occurs in early diastole, and CO decreases.

Control of SVR

- Changes in small artery and arteriole resistances are the principal way in which organ blood flow and SVR are regulated.
- Because resistance depends on the fourth power of the radius, small changes in radius have a large effect on resistance (Poiseuille's law: resistance = $8VL/\pi r^4$; V = viscosity of fluid, L = vessel length, r = radius of vessel).
- Factors altering SVR: autonomic control (α-1 adrenergic constriction or β2 adrenergic vasodilatation), neurohormones e.g. angiotensin II, endothelial control (nitric oxide, endothelin).
- $SVR = 80 \times \dfrac{MAP - CVP}{CO}$

  Normal SVR = 900–1500 dynes/sec/cm^5
  (MAP and CVP in mmHg and CO in l/min.)

Control of blood pressure

MAP = (CO × SVR) + CVP

Systolic BP is modified mainly by changes in ejection velocity and SV. Diastolic BP is modified mainly by changes in SVR and the time available for blood to leave the arteries – the duration of diastole (which decreases as HR increases).

Immediate short-term control

Intrinsic characteristics of the heart:
- Starling's Law.
- Anrep effect – a sudden increase in afterload causes an increase in contractility after a drop in SV and a decrease in LVEDP.
- Bowditch effect – an increase in HR causes a small increase in contractility.

Autonomic control and baroreceptor reflexes

The nucleus solitarius in the medulla receives afferent fibres from the aortic arch and carotid sinus arterial baroreceptors via the vagus and glossopharyngeal nerves. Baroreceptors are mechanoreceptors sensitive to stretch of the vessel wall produced by increases in arterial blood pressure. At normal pressures baroreceptors inhibit sympathetic outflow and stimulate parasympathetic outflow from the medulla. With decreased blood pressure baroreceptor firing decreases and the sympathetic nervous system is activated producing increased contractility and vasoconstriction. Renal sympathetic nerve stimulation produces renin, angiotensin II, and aldosterone release, resulting in fluid retention and further vasoconstriction. The parasympathetic system is inhibited. MAP increases with tachycardia. The opposite occurs with acute increases in blood pressure.

- Arterial wall compliance is decreased in hypertension, atherosclerosis, and older age, thus reducing baroreceptor sensitivity.
- **Cardiopulmonary stretch receptors** – located mainly on the low pressure side of the circulation. They respond to changes in filling volumes. An increase in filling volume leads to inhibition of sympathetic outflow and decreased renin release.
- **Peripheral arterial chemoreceptors** (aortic and carotid bodies) – hypoxaemia and hypercapnia produce sympathetic stimulation.
- **Myogenic autoregulation** – see below.
- **Hormonal**:
  - Renin-angiotensin-aldosterone system.
  - Antidiuretic hormone (ADH) – very high ADH levels as in hypovolaemic shock cause arterial vasoconstriction.
  - Epinephrine and norepinephrine in sympathetic activation.

Intermediate/long-term control

This is mainly controlled by the kidneys, which alter total body water and sodium balance, thus altering blood volume.

Renin-angiotensin system

- Angiotensin causes:
  - Arterial vasoconstriction.
  - Release of aldosterone and ADH.
  - Thirst.
  - Cardiac and vascular hypertrophy/remodelling.
- **Aldosterone** – causes Na^+ and water retention by the kidneys.
- **ADH** is released from the posterior pituitary in response to decreased firing of cardiopulmonary baroreceptors, increased sympathetic activity and decreased arterial baroreceptor firing during hypotension, increased angiotensin II, and increased osmolarity detected by hypothalamic osmoreceptors. ADH increases permeability in renal collecting ducts with increased H_2O reabsorption and increased blood volume.
- **ANP** – released by the atria in response to atrial stretch and has a diuretic action as a result of a direct action and by inhibiting aldosterone. It decreases blood volume.

Coronary circulation

Coronary blood flow (CBF) is 250 ml/min. O_2 extraction at rest by the myocardium is high (65%) compared to other tissues (35%). The myocardium has a high capillary density (one capillary per myocyte) to satisfy the high energy requirement. As O_2 extraction is almost maximal, any increases in myocardial O_2 demand must be met mainly by increasing coronary flow. The heart has a high vasodilator capacity. Pathological mechanisms that impair CBF impair cardiac performance.

Factors influencing coronary blood flow (CBF)

- CBF = $\dfrac{CPP}{CVR}$

  CPP = coronary perfusion pressure
  CVR = coronary vascular resistance
- CPP = aortic diastolic pressure – LVEDP
- The heart has to produce its own perfusion pressure. The coronary circulation is unique in that it has an intermittent pattern of left coronary artery perfusion during systole due to mechanical compression of vessels by myocardial contraction. The subendocardium is most susceptible to ischaemia as its vessels are exposed to the highest compressive forces. Aortic root pressure = LVSP and reverse flow is seen during systole.
  In coronary artery stenosis there is increased systolic reverse flow and decreased diastolic forward flow. 85% of left coronary artery (LCA) flow occurs during diastole. LCA flow is limited by diastolic time (heart rate) and LVEDP.
- Right coronary artery flow occurs in systole and diastole as aortic root systolic pressure > RVSP.
- BP 130/80:
  - CPP – RV in systole is 130 – 25 = 105 mmHg.
  - CPP – RV in diastole = 80 – 0 = 80 mmHg.
  - So RCA flow rate is greatest in systole. But during the resting cardiac cycle diastole accounts for two thirds of its duration. 70% of RCA flow thus occurs during diastole.
- 80% of total coronary flow occurs in diastole.

Regulation of coronary vascular resistance

- The main source of CVR is arterioles <150 μm diameter.
- Vasomotor control of CVR occurs by several mechanisms as described below.

Metabolic control

- In the heart blood flow is closely linked to oxidative metabolism. Metabolic control is the main mechanism during increased myocardial work or ischaemia when vasodilator metabolites are produced and accumulate, thus increasing CBF.
- Metabolic control, however, is not thought to be significant in the maintenance of resting coronary artery tone.
- Adenosine produced from the metabolism of ATP appears to be the most important metabolite. Others include H^+, K^+, decreased PaO_2, and interstitial osmolarity. These metabolites particularly affect blood vessels in the 150–170 μm size range.

- A major part of this vasodilator action is mediated by opening of ATP-sensitive K^+ channels, which leads to relaxation of smooth muscle.
- Metabolic factors are also involved in the recruitment of capillaries.

Endothelial control

- Nitric oxide (NO) is the most important regulator of resting coronary artery tone and is also important during exercise, causing vasodilation.
- Nitric oxide plays an important role in flow-mediated control in the larger arterioles – increased blood flow leads to increased vascular shear stress and release of NO.
- Other vasodilators include prostacyclin and bradykinin.
- Platelet-derived substances such as serotonin are vasodilatory with normal endothelium, but vasoconstrict with damaged endothelium.
- When the endothelium is damaged vasoconstrictor substances can predominate, e.g. endothelin I and angiotensin II. Endothelial dysfunction occurs in hypertension, atherosclerosis, and diabetes.

Myogenic control (local)

- Myogenic control is an incompletely understood intrinsic property of vascular smooth muscle that leads to contraction and vasoconstriction when the lumens of blood vessels are stretched (intravascular pressure is increased), and relaxation when intravascular pressure is decreased.
- It is the dominant mechanism in autoregulation.
- The metabolic vasodilator response overrides the myogenic vasoconstrictor response, if present.

Autoregulation

- CBF is autoregulated between MAPs of 50–120 mmHg. CBF is relatively constant despite changes in arterial pressures in this range. Outside this range flow is directly dependent on perfusion pressure.
- Autoregulation is thought to be mediated by <150 μm diameter arterioles.
- Myogenic, metabolic, and endothelial factors are involved in control of vascular resistance during autoregulation, but myogenic factors dominate. Pathological mechanisms that decrease NO levels increase the lower limit of autoregulation and make the myocardium more vulnerable to hypoperfusion.

Neurogenic control

- Neurogenic control of coronary vascular resistance can be overcome by metabolic and myogenic controls.
- Sympathetic stimulation of the heart causes only temporary α-1 adrenergic vasoconstriction followed by vasodilation. Vasodilation occurs because sympathetic activation of the heart also causes β-1 mediated increases in HR and contractility, producing vasodilator metabolites. Metabolic vasodilation is restricted by α-receptor vasoconstriction. Parasympathetic stimulation causes mild coronary vasodilation.
- β-2 receptors are present in small numbers and thus play a minor role in coronary vascular control.

- **Myocardial O_2 delivery** = CBF × CaO_2
  CaO_2 = arterial O_2 content
  [CaO_2 = (1.39 × Hb × SaO_2) + (0.003 × PaO_2)]
- Fick equation: **myocardial O_2 consumption** = CBF × (CaO_2 − CvO_2).
  CvO_2 = venous O_2 content

Important factors affecting myocardial oxygen supply-demand balance

Supply
- Heart rate:
  - Diastolic time.
- Coronary perfusion pressure:
  - Aortic diastolic pressure.
  - Ventricular end diastolic pressure.
- Arterial oxygen content:
  - Arterial oxygen tension.
  - Haemoglobin concentration.
- Coronary vessel diameter.

Demand
- Basal requirements.
- Heart rate.
- Wall tension:
  - Preload (ventricular radius).
  - Afterload.
- Contractility.

Further reading

1. Carabello B. Evolution of the study of left ventricular function: Everything old is new again. *Circulation* 2002; 105: 2701.
2. Katz A. Ernest Henry Starling: His predecessors and the 'law of the heart'. *Circulation* 2002; 106: 2986.
3. Katz A. *Physiology of the Heart.* Fourth edition. Philadelphia, Lippincott-Raven 2006.
4. Klabunde RE. *Cardiovascular Physiology Concepts.* Philadelphia, Lippincott Williams & Wilkins 2004.
5. Opie L. *The Heart: Physiology, from cell to circulation.* Fourth edition. Philadelphia, Lippincott-Raven 2004.

Chapter 3

Cardiovascular drugs

Dr M Barnard and Dr M Lees

Control of heart rate and rhythm *38*
Control contractility *40*
Control of preload and afterload *46*
Further reading *50*

Control of heart rate and rhythm

Isoprenaline (isoproterenol)
- Synthetic catecholamine.
- Direct β-agonist (β1 > β2).
- Positive inotrope and positive chronotrope.
- Metabolized partly by liver and partly excreted unchanged. Short half-life (2 minutes), therefore titratable.
- Increased heart rate and contractility, vasodilation, bronchodilation:
  - Heart rate   increase
  - Contractility   increase
  - Cardiac output   increase
  - Blood pressure   variable, often falls due to reduced SVR
  - SVR   decrease
  - PVR   decrease
- Can induce ischaemia due to tachycardia, inotropy, and hypotension.
- Can provoke supraventricular arrhythmias.
- Indications:
  - Low cardiac output, resistant to atropine, pacing not available.
  - Low cardiac output with fixed stroke volume (transplant).
  - Pulmonary hypertension, RV failure with bradycardia.
  - Beta-blocker overdose.
  - Temporary therapy in AV block (not second degree where block may increase).
- Dose: 0.02–0.5 µg/kg/minute. As bolus 10 to 20 µg and repeat.
- Beware! Isoprenaline comes in two very different formulations. One is 100 µg in 10 ml; the other is 1 mg/ml. Do not confuse the two (the first is for single boluses, the second for infusions).

Atropine
- Competitive antagonist at muscarinic cholinergic receptors.
- Minimal metabolism, 80–90% renal elimination. Lasts 15–30 minutes.
- Increases heart rate.
- Can exacerbate bradycardia at low doses (<0.2 mg).
- Adverse effects:
  - CNS – sedation and confusion in children/elderly.
  - Urinary retention.
  - Increased intra-ocular pressure.

Amiodarone
- Vasodilating and negative inotropic effects (α- and β-antagonist).
- Potassium channel blocker and prolongs QT interval.
- May cause bradycardia or heart block.
- Long-term treatment risks pulmonary fibrosis, thyroid disorder, corneal deposits, and photosensitivity.
- May increase the effects of oral anticoagulants and digoxin.

- Dose: 300 mg over 1 hour, followed by infusion of approximately 1 g/day (1 mg/min for 6 hours followed by 0.5 mg/min). Ideally administered via central or large peripheral vein as drug solution is irritant.
- High lipid solubility and hence tissue accumulation. Therefore patients on chronic therapy do not need 'reloading' when doses are missed perioperatively.

Control contractility

Beta-agonists and dopaminergic agonists

Dobutamine
- Direct β1-agonist, limited β2 and α1 agonism.
- Positive inotropy, vasodilator, can increase heart rate.
- Plasma half-life 2 minutes. Partly redistributed, partly hepatic metabolism and conjugation.
  - Contractility   increase
  - Heart rate   increase
  - Cardiac output   increase
  - Blood pressure   variable, can increase
  - SVR   decrease
  - PVR   decrease
- Clinical usage:
  - 'Inodilator' properties increase cardiac output, while increase in myocardial oxygen requirement is offset by vasodilator properties. Myocardial oxygen consumption increases less than with other catecholamines.
  - Tachycardia less at low doses than with dopamine.
  - Tachycardia and arrhythmias can limit use, particularly at high doses.
  - Tachycardia more than Epinephrine (adrenaline) to achieve same effect on CO.
  - Afterload reduction can be useful in failing heart.
  - Vasodilation means hypotension may occur.
  - Vasodilation is non-selective – skeletal muscle can 'steal' from other vascular beds.
  - Tachyphylaxis after 72 hours.
  - Dose: 2.5–20 µg/kg/min.

Dopamine
- Direct agonist at α1, β1, β2, and dopamine-1.
- Indirect release of neuronal Norepinephrine (noradrenaline).
- Redistributed, metabolized, and taken up by nerve terminals.
- Renal and mesenteric blood flow increase at 1–3 µg/kg/min.
  - Contractility   increase
  - Blood pressure   increase
  - Heart rate   increase
  - Cardiac output   increase 3–10 µg/kg/min, decrease >10 µg/kg/min
  - SVR   decrease <10 µg/kg/min, increase >10 µg/kg/min
  - PVR   increase depending on α-agonism.
- Clinical use:
  - Increases salt and water excretion, but no longer used for renal 'protection' or renal benefit. May be nephrotoxic.
  - Renal, splanchnic, and pulmonary vasoconstriction at high doses.
  - Dose-dependent effects outlined above demonstrate considerable variability between individuals.
  - Maximal effect (efficacy) less than Epinephrine (adrenaline).
  - Increases myocardial oxygen consumption.

- Can be used at low doses for modest increase in cardiac output, particularly where SVR low and phosphodiesterase (PDE) inhibitors would cause hypotension.
- Switch to Epinephrine (adrenaline) or PDE if inadequate response at <10 µg/kg/min.
- Dose: 1–20 µg/kg/min. In practice <10 µg/kg/min.
- Traditionally combined with glyceryltrinitrate to produce 'inodilator' effect. This can be effective, but largely superseded by PDE.

Epinephrine (adrenaline)
- Direct α1, α2, β1, and β2-agonist.
- Rapid metabolism and neuronal uptake:
  - Heart rate   increase
  - Contractility   increase
  - SVR   decrease low dose, increase high dose
  - PVR   decrease low dose, increase high dose
  - Cardiac output   usually increase, can decrease at high doses
  - Blood pressure   increase
- Efficacy (maximal effect) greater than dopamine and dobutamine, with less tachycardia.
- Clinical usage:
  - Increases myocardial work and oxygen consumption. Can precipitate ischaemia.
  - Causes tachycardia and arrhythmias.
  - Acidosis and elevation of plasma glucose and lactate occur. Most frequently in patients with hypertrophied left ventricles.
  - Agent of choice in anaphylaxis.
  - Low dose infusion can be very effective in post-CPB bronchospasm.
  - Dose: 0.01–0.2 µg/kg/min. Cardiac arrest: 0.5–1.0 mg (high dose no longer recommended).
  - Combination of low dose with low dose enoximone/milrinone is very effective, with minimal adverse effects due to low doses of each agent.

Norepinephrine (noradrenaline)
- 📖 see also p. 46 – Vasopressors.

Isoprenaline (isoproterenol)
- 📖 see also p. 38 – Control of heart rate and rhythm.

Phosphodiesterase inhibitors
- Phosphodiesterase inhibitors (PDEIs) inhibit cyclic adenosine monophosphate (cAMP)-specific phosphodiesterase (PDE III) in cardiac and smooth muscle.
- Increased cAMP enhances inotropy, lusitropy (improved diastolic relaxation), chronotropy, dromotropy (AV conduction), and electrical automaticity.

- Enoximone and milrinone are two agents mainly used in the UK:
  - Heart rate   no change, slight increase
  - Cardiac output   increase
  - Blood pressure   often decrease
  - SVR   decrease
  - PVR   decrease
  - Myocardial work unchanged or slight increase
- Favourable profile on myocardial oxygen requirements useful in patients with coronary disease.
- No action on β-receptors, so tachyphylaxis does not occur and retains efficacy in chronic heart failure (β-receptor down-regulation).
- Fewer arrhythmias than with adrenergic agonists.
- Clinical use:
  - Vasodilation may cause significant hypotension. Counteracting with vasopressors is often necessary.
  - Very useful in severe low cardiac output syndrome, or difficult weaning from CPB.
  - Used as bridge to transplantation or temporary support of severe cardiomyopathy.
  - Will wean some patients from CPB who otherwise would have required intra-aortic balloon pump.
  - Very useful and effective synergism with β-agonists (e.g. epinephrine).
  - Milrinone: loading dose 25–50 µg/kg. Maintenance 0.375–0.75 µg/kg/min.
  - Enoximone: loading dose 0.5–1.0 mg/kg (typically 0.5 mg/kg). Maintenance 0–20 µg/kg/min. Typically start at 2.5 µg/kg/min.
  - Milrinone and enoximone have very different pharmacokinetics. Half-life of milrinone is 30–60 minutes; enoximone much longer. Therefore do not 'titrate' enoximone like adrenergic agents. Choose a dose and assess response. Change dose over period of hours not minutes.
  - Enoximone will precipitate with dextrose infusions. It is therefore usually given by a dedicated lumen on a central line.

cAMP-independent agents

Calcium

- Unbound calcium ion is physiologically active.
- Normally 50% unbound.
- Increases contractility and SVR. Blood pressure increases.
- Rapid action, duration 10 to 15 minutes.
- Ischaemic cells sequestrate intracellular calcium. Administration of extracellular calcium can exacerbate cellular damage in this situation.
- Useful in:
  - Hypocalcaemia (CPB-induced dilution).
  - Hyperkalaemia (excess cardioplegia).
  - Overdose of calcium channel blockers.
  - Hypermagnesaemia.

- In practice a bolus is often given on separation from CPB, to 'jump start' cardiac contraction. While this is largely historical, it may not be deleterious as long as ischaemia or reperfusion injury are not prominent.
- Clinical use:
  - 10% calcium chloride 10 ml contains 272 mg or 13.6 mEq calcium. 10% calcium gluconate 10 ml contains 93 mg or 4.6 mEq elemental calcium.
  - Usual dose is 3–10 ml bolus of 10% calcium chloride.

Levosimendan
- Increases sensitivity of the heart to calcium.
- Binds to troponin C in a calcium-dependent manner.
- Effects greatest when intracellular calcium concentrations highest (early systole).
- PDE III inhibitor:
  - Heart rate   increase
  - Cardiac output   increase
  - SVR   decrease
  - Blood pressure   variable, unchanged
- Independent of cAMP (so no interaction with β-agonists and PDEI, and possibly fewer arrhythmias).
- Has been used in setting of severe post-cardiotomy acute heart failure.
- Dose 8–24 μg/kg/min.

β-adrenergic antagonists
- Reduce heart rate, contractility, and myocardial oxygen requirements.
- Bradycardias and heart block possible. May precipitate bronchospasm.
- Useful in ischaemia:
  - Blunt reflex tachycardias.
  - Reduce increases in contractility.
  - Prolong duration of diastole, and hence LV coronary blood flow.
  - Antiarrhythmic.
  - Reduce arterial wall stress in dissection by decreasing ejection velocity.
  - Reduce outflow tract gradients in hypertrophic cardiomyopathy.
  - May not improve cardiovascular outcomes in a variety of disease scenarios.

Esmolol
- Selective β1-antagonist.
- Titratable – ultra-short acting due to metabolism by plasma esterases.
- Half-life 9 minutes.
- Dose: 0.25–0.5 mg/kg loading bolus, followed by infusion of 50–200 μg/kg/min.
- Titrate to effect.

Labetalol
- Combined α- and β-antagonist (ratio 1:7 for IV use).
- Half-life 3–8 hours.
- Useful for vasodilation without reflex tachycardia.

- Duration of action useful pre- and post-operatively but limits titratability.
- Dose: 5–20 mg bolus and repeat every 10 to 15 minutes until desired effect.

Calcium channel blockers

- Calcium channel blockers reduce intracellular calcium in myocardial cells, vascular smooth muscle, and cardiac conduction tissue.
- Selectivity for these three effects varies considerably between agents. Therefore the spectrum of the following effects will reflect this selectivity:
  - Vasodilation.
  - Myocardial depression.
  - Reduction in myocardial ischaemia (increased coronary flow and reduced heart rate, reduced contractility, reduced afterload).
  - Conduction system effects – AV node conduction depressed. Sinus rate reduced. Ventricular ectopy suppressed.
- Arterial vasodilation predominates, with minimal venous dilation.
- Coronary vasodilation is prominent.

Amlodipine
- Dihydropyridine.
- Predominantly vasodilator.
- Little negative inotropy.
- Dose: 5–10 mg daily.

Diltiazem
- Selective coronary vasodilator.
- Decreases heart rate.
- Used in rate control of SVT.
- Afterload reduction means better tolerated (compared with verapamil) in poor LV function.
- Use with caution in patients with heart block or on β-blockers.
- No long-term outcome benefit in chronic therapy.
- Dose: 20 mg over 2 minutes loading. Repeat with increments of 25 mg.
- Half-life 3–5 hours.

Nifedipine
- Dihydropyridine, profound vasodilator, including coronary arteries.
- Little myocardial depression.
- No conducting system effects.
- No available intravenous formulation. Sublingual formulation has been withdrawn in UK.
- Worse outcomes in treatment of chronic hypertension.

Verapamil
- Vasodilator and negative inotrope.
- Long half-life: 3–10 hours.
- Chronic therapy increases digoxin levels.
- May not be tolerated in presence of poor LV function.
- Dose: 5–15 mg bolus slowly. Repeat after 30 minutes if required.
- Hypotension may be treated with phenylephrine – although beware heart rate.

Control of preload and afterload

Vasopressors

Adrenergic agents: selective agonists

Phenylephrine
- Synthetic non-catecholamine.
- α1 agonist.
- Indicated in hypotension and low SVR states.
- Particularly useful when heart rate is high.
- Mainly arterial vasoconstriction:

HR	reflex decrease
Contractility	no direct effect
Cardiac output	decrease
Blood pressure	increase
SVR	increase
PVR	increase

- Myocardial oxygen requirements not increased if hypertension avoided.
- Cardiac output may increase if due to low coronary perfusion.
- Stroke volume may decrease due to increased SVR.
- Renal and splanchnic perfusion may be compromised.
- Rapid enzyme metabolism.
- Clinical use:
  - IV bolus 1–10 μg/kg. In practice dilute to either 1 mg/ml (high strength) or 1 mg in 10 ml (low strength). For low dose boluses give 50 μg at a time.
  - In severe hypotension or during CPB give high dose boluses up to 500–1000 μg at a time.
  - Infusion: 0.5–10 μg/kg/min.
  - Phenylephrine probably agent of choice for immediate correction of vasodilation in most patients with coronary disease or aortic stenosis.

Metaraminol
- Primary effect as an α1-agonist but with weak α2, β1, and β2 effects.
- In addition causes release of norepinephrine at the nerve terminal.
- Increases in blood pressure predominantly caused by α1 effects but increase in cardiac output and release of norepinephrine contribute at clinically relevant doses.
- Replaces norepinephrine in storage vesicles after prolonged use (5 hours). Efficacy is one tenth that of norepinephrine.

Adrenergic agents: mixed agonists

Dopamine: 📖 see also Beta-agonists and dopaminergic agonists p. 40.
Epinephrine: (adrenaline): 📖 see also Beta-agonists and dopaminergic agonists p. 40.

Norepinephrine (noradrenaline)

- Direct α1, α2, and β1 agonist. Limited β2 agonist.
- Redistributed, neuronal uptake and enzyme metabolism.
- Efficacy (maximal effect) greater than phenylephrine (α1 only).
  - HR   variable, reflex decrease
  - Contractility   increased
  - Cardiac output   variable
  - Blood pressure   increased
  - SVR   increased
  - PVR   increased
- Risk of reduced organ perfusion (e.g. renal, hepatic, splanchnic).
- Clinical use:
  - Low SVR conditions (sepsis, 'vasoplegia' following CPB).
  - Increase in SVR desired as well as positive inotropy.
  - Phenylephrine ineffective.
  - Dose: 0.01–0.3 µg/kg/min.

Vasopressin

- Endogenous hormone that activates smooth muscle V1 receptors.
- No β-adrenergic activity.
- Relatively greater skin, muscle, intestine, and fat vasoconstriction compared with coronary and renal vessels.
- Very potent agent with high efficacy. May be used in 'vasoplegia' where the circulation fails to respond to conventional vasoconstrictors.
- Unpleasant effects in conscious patients (pallor, nausea, abdominal cramps).
- Splanchnic blood flow may be compromised. Increases in liver enzymes.
- Clinical use:
  - Vasodilatory shock, sepsis, vasoplegia.
  - Particularly useful in hypotensive patients who have received angiotensin-converting enzyme inhibitors.
  - Has been considered as an alternative to epinephrine in shock-refractory ventricular fibrillation in cardiac arrest protocols.
  - Dose: 4–6 units/hour.

Vasodilators
Direct vasodilators
Glyceryl trinitrate (GTN)

- Direct, mixed arterial and venous but predominantly venous dilation. It activates vascular cGMP production.
- Redistributed and metabolized in muscle and liver. Half-life is 1–3 minutes.
- Venodilation reduces preload and decreases myocardial oxygen consumption.
- High doses (>10 µg/kg/min) produce arteriolar dilatation.

- Coronary blood flow is increased to ischaemic myocardium.
  - Heart rate   reflex increase
  - Contractility   reflex increase
  - Cardiac output   variable depending on preload and afterload effects
  - Blood pressure   decrease
  - Preload   decrease
  - SVR   decrease at high doses
  - PVR   decrease
- Clinical use:
  - Myocardial ischaemia.
  - Acute heart failure – decrease preload and pulmonary venous congestion.
  - Useful in ischaemia or heart failure with pulmonary hypertension.
  - Higher doses will decrease blood pressure, and possibly reflex tachycardia.
  - Dose: bolus for acute control of hypertensive surges, 50–500 µg. Very short duration.
  - Infusion: 0.1–0.7 µg/kg/min. Commonly infused in 'mg/hr' – typically 1–10 mg/hr.

Nitroprusside

- Direct vasodilator.
- Balanced arterial and venous dilation. Also dilates pulmonary vasculature.
- Very short duration of between 1 and 2 minutes. This facilitates titration.
- At low doses arterial dilation predominates.
- Unstable in light, must be protected by cover.
- Cyanide and thiocyanate toxicity possible.
- Cyanide produces tissue hypoxia in presence of normal PaO_2.
- Toxicity is dose and duration dependent, i.e. greater than 1 mg/kg over 24 hours.
  - Heart rate   reflex increase
  - Contractility   reflex increase
  - Cardiac output   variable
  - Blood pressure   decrease
  - SVR   decrease
  - PVR   decrease
- Clinical use:
  - Dose: 0.1–2 µg/kg/min. Avoid higher doses. Above 10 µg/kg/min no longer than 10 minutes.
  - Protect with light-resistant covering.
  - Wean infusions gradually to avoid rebound hypertension.

Hydralazine

- Direct, predominantly arteriolar vasodilator.
- Metabolized in liver. Slow acetylators will have pronounced effect.

- 'Vital' organs (coronary, cerebral, renal, splanchnic) preferentially affected.
  - Heart rate   reflex increase
  - Contractility   reflex increase
  - Cardiac output   increase
  - Blood pressure   decrease
  - SVR   decrease
  - PVR   decrease
- Clinical use:
  - Slow onset – up to 15 minutes.
  - Dose: 2.5–5 mg boluses.

α-adrenergic blockers

Phentolamine

- $\alpha 1$, $\alpha 2$, 5-HT antagonist.
- Predominantly arterial vasodilation.
- Hepatic metabolism and renal excretion. Duration 10 to 15 minutes.
  - Heart rate   increase
  - Contractility   increase
  - Cardiac output   increase
  - Blood pressure   decrease
  - SVR   decrease
  - PVR   decrease
- Tachycardia both reflex indirect and direct effect of $\alpha 2$ blockade.
- Gastrointestinal motility increased.
- Clinical use:
  - With epinephrine can cause hypotension due to unopposed β-agonism.
  - β-blockade will attenuate tachycardia and arrhythmias.
  - Dose: bolus 1–5 mg. Infusion 1–20 µg/kg/min.

Phenoxybenzamine

- $\alpha 1$ and $\alpha 2$ antagonist.
- Predominantly arterial vasodilation.
- Hepatic and renal metabolism/excretion.
- Prolonged duration of action – 24 hours.
- Tachycardia reflex and direct $\alpha 2$ effect.
- Clinical use:
  - Used in some paediatric centres to reduce afterload.
  - Otherwise mainly used in high catecholamine states such as phaeochromocytoma.

Further reading

1. Devereaux PJ, Yang H, Guyatt GH, et al. POISE trial. β-blockers in patients having non-cardiac surgery: A meta-analysis. *Lancet* 2008 May 31; 371 (9627): 1839–1847.
2. Friedrich JO, Adhikari N, Herridge MS, et al. Meta-analysis: Low-dose dopamine increases urine output but does not prevent renal dysfunction or death. *Annals of Internal Medicine* 2005; 142: 510–524.
3. Masetti P, Murphy SF, Kouchoukos NT. Vasopressin therapy for vasoplegic syndrome following cardiopulmonary bypass. *Journal of Cardiac Surgery* 2002; 17: 485–489.
4. Nolan JP, Deakin CD, Soar J, Bottiger BW, Smith G. European Resuscitation Council guidelines for resuscitation 2005. *Resuscitation* 2005; 67S1: S39–S86.
5. Opie LH, Messerli FH. Nifedipine and mortality. Grave defects in the dossier. *Circulation* 1995; 92 (5): 1068–1073.

Chapter 4

Ischaemic heart disease, arrhythmias, and heart failure

Dr M Patrick

Ischaemic heart disease (IHD) *52*
Perioperative arrhythmias *60*
Heart failure (HF) *64*
Further reading *70*

Ischaemic heart disease (IHD) (📖 see also Chapter 11)

Pathology

The arterial wall contains three layers, the intima, media, and adventitia. The intima is lined by endothelium. The endothelium is unique in that blood does not coagulate on it despite prolonged contact. This is largely due to the expression of heparan sulphate on the surface of endothelial cells, which interacts with antithrombin III, inhibiting thrombin. Healthy endothelial cells also express fibrinolytic activity. IHD is caused by formation of atheromatous plaques in the coronary arteries, which cause progressive narrowing of the arterial lumen (atherogenesis).

Atherogenesis (📖 see also Chapter 11 p. 170)

Atherogenesis occurs slowly and plaques take years to develop. Plaque formation occurs throughout the arterial system but the coronary, cerebral, and lower limb circulations are most commonly affected. Atherogenesis shows features of inflammation. It begins with accumulation of monocytes and lipoproteins on the endothelium. The monocytes cross the endothelium, accumulate lipid, and change into foam cells. Smooth muscle cells migrate into the developing plaque under the influence of chemoattractant molecules including platelet-derived growth factor (PDGF), and these smooth muscle cells replicate. Plaques develop and internal microcirculation and rupture of these vessels leads to haemorrhage within the plaque. This promotes further smooth muscle proliferation and plaque growth. Plaques also contain non-cellular elements including collagen, elastin, lipoproteins, and proteoglycans, and calcification may occur.

Flow limitation in coronary arteries does not occur until the cross-sectional area is reduced by 60–70%. When flow demand is high such as during exercise, flow limitation occurs, leading to cellular hypoxia. The clinical result is angina pectoris. As plaque growth progresses, flow limitation increases and the workload at which angina develops becomes less. This gradual increase in symptom severity is typical of stable angina.

Plaque rupture and coronary thrombosis

Plaque rupture is the single event leading to coronary thrombosis, though not all plaque disruptions result in thrombosis. There is no relationship between the degree of luminal obstruction and the likelihood of plaque rupture, and coronary thromboses occuring on non-obstructive plaques.

Endothelial destabilization leads either to erosion of the intima over the plaque, or to rupture of the surface of the fibrous cap of the plaque. In both cases, there is exposure of its contents, which are thrombogenic. Thinning of the fibrous cap, which is thought to be due to the action of macrophage-derived metalloproteinases and cathepsins (which break down collagen and elastin respectively), appears to be a precursor to rupture. Platelets adhere to the surface of the disrupted plaque, become activated, and thrombosis occurs.

Inflammation plays an important role in plaque rupture. Circulating levels of C-reactive protein (CRP) predict cardiovascular risk, as do levels of the cytokines tumour necrosis factor-α (TNF-α) and interleukin-6 (IL-6). Drugs that stabilize plaques such as aspirin and statins also reduce CRP levels. The role of inflammation may explain why plaque rupture is a risk after non-cardiac surgery.

Plaque rupture and coronary thrombosis lead to a spectrum of conditions known as acute coronary syndromes.

Acute coronary syndromes (📖 see also acute coronary syndromes Chapter 11 p. 171)

These include:
- Unstable angina (UA).
- Non S-T elevation MI (NSTEMI).
- S-T elevation MI (STEMI).

The location, extent, and persistence of the intracoronary thrombus determine which of these occurs. UA and NSTEMI are approximately three times commoner than STEMI.

Unstable angina is characterized by new onset angina or worsening stable angina that increases in frequency and severity, occurs at rest or on minimal exertion, and lasts for more than 20 minutes. Myocardial necrosis does not occur and serum cardiac troponins (troponin T and I) are normal.

Prolonged episodes of pain may lead to myocardial necrosis with release of troponins and this is characteristic of NSTEMI. In both UA and NSTEMI the ECG shows S-T segment depression or deep symmetrical T wave inversion, but not persistent S-T elevation or Q waves. The outcome of UA and NSTEMI is usually better than that of STEMI.

STEMI

STEMI is usually caused by large, persistent, and often propagated thrombi that extend up or down the artery away from the site of plaque rupture. The patient often presents with severe persistent pain unrelieved by nitrates. The ECG shows S-T segment elevation. The area of myocardium supplied by the artery undergoes full or nearly full thickness necrosis (transmural infarction). Ventricular arrhythmias (primary VF) are common. Affected cardiac muscle immediately loses its ability to contract. If a large area is involved, global LV systolic function is impaired and there is clinical evidence of pump failure with tachycardia, hypotension, and elevated venous pressures. Diastolic function is also impaired, evidenced acutely by impaired myocardial relaxation, and later by reduced LV compliance. Chronic LV failure may ensue (ischaemic cardiomyopathy).

The ECG evolves following a STEMI. The initial S-T elevation recedes and T wave inversion occurs before returning to normal over weeks. Q wave or reduced R wave progression appear. There may be conduction abnormalities such as left bundle branch block. The myocardium usually heals by fibrosis leaving a scar, but following anterior infarction, apical true aneurysm formation may occur. This is associated with persistent S-T elevation. Rupture of a papillary muscle, the septum, or the LV free wall is a potential consequence. STEMI leads to a change in the size, shape, and thickness of both infarcted and healthy portions of the LV. This is termed remodelling, and it can be attenuated by treatment with ACE inhibitors (ACEIs) or angiotensin receptor blockers (ARBs).

Treatment of acute coronary syndromes (📖 see also Chapter 11)

Acute coronary syndromes are managed according to American College of Cardiology/American Heart Association (ACC/AHA) Practice Guidelines.

Treatment varies depending on the type of acute coronary syndrome, and includes:

- Oxygen.
- Analgesia and antiemetics.
- Aspirin and clopidogrel.
- Beta-blockade.
- Nitrates.
- Treatment of ventricular arrhythmias (lidocaine, amiodarone, defibrillation).
- Low molecular weight heparin.
- Thrombolysis – STEMI (especially if large thrombus on angiography).
- Platelet glycoprotein IIB/IIIA antagonists – if percutaneous coronary intervention (PCI) planned.
- Revascularization by primary PCI (angioplasty and stent insertion) – potentially all STEMI, and NSTEMI/UA if evidence of continuing ischaemia or elevated troponin, adverse haemodynamics, or sustained ventricular arrhythmias.

Risk factors for IHD

- Age.
- Gender – premenopausal females are less affected than males of the same age. After the menopause the genders are equally affected.
- Diabetes mellitus and insulin resistance.
- Hypertension.
- Dyslipidaemias.
- Obesity and lack of exercise.
- Smoking.

The combination of type II diabetes mellitus, dyslipidaemia, hypertension, and central obesity is known as the metabolic syndrome. This syndrome is strongly associated with resistance to endogenous insulin.

Current therapies

- Slowing of disease progression.
- Treatment of angina.

Slowing of disease progression and perioperative medication

Primary prevention refers to intervention in individuals who do not have the disease but are at risk of developing it. Secondary prevention refers to intervention in individuals with existing evidence of disease. In both cases intervention is aimed at reducing the impact of modifiable risk factors (Table 4.1).

There is debate as to what constitutes optimal preoperative management of antiplatelet medication, ACEI, and ARB, as there are different risks inherent in either continuing or stopping these medications. Both aspirin and clopidogrel irreversibly inhibit platelet aggregation and this effect lasts for about one week after cessation of either drug. Continuation of either aspirin or clopidogrel or both, up to the time of surgery, is associated with significantly greater perioperative blood loss and transfusion requirements. There is weaker evidence for an increased rate of reoperation for bleeding and no evidence that mortality is increased. Antiplatelet therapy should be continued up to surgery in patients with a recent acute coronary syndrome. Aspirin should be restarted as soon as possible after surgery, preferably within six hours if the patient is not bleeding. Evidence for early reintroduction of clopidogrel is uncertain.

Thromboelastography (TEG) using standard kaolin activation is unable to assess aspirin- or clopidogrel-induced platelet inhibition and significant inhibition can be present even if the TEG maximum amplitude (MA) value suggests normal platelet function. Platelet transfusion may be needed if there is excessive postoperative blood loss in a patient who has received platelet inhibitors within one week, even if the MA is normal.

Continuation of ACEI or ARB up to surgery is associated with an increased requirement for intraoperative vasoconstrictor therapy. There is no evidence that this translates into worsened outcome.

Table 4.1 Evidence for interventions in coronary heart disease

Intervention	Evidence in primary prevention	Evidence in secondary prevention
Lipid lowering therapy: statins, fibrates	Class 1	Class 1
Treatment of hypertension: ACEI and ARB, thiazides, calcium antagonists, beta-blockers, alpha-blockers	Class 1	Class 1
Smoking cessation	Class 1	Class 1
Antiplatelet drugs: aspirin, clopidogrel	Class 2	Class 1
Diabetes control	Class 2	Class 2
Increased physical activity	Class 2	Class 2
Dietary measures: weight reduction, improved diet, moderate alcohol consumption	Class 2/3	Class 2/3

Class 1: Clear causal relationship; intervention clearly beneficial and cost-effective.
Class 2: Causal relationship; trial data limited and cost-effectiveness uncertain.
Class 3: Causality not clear; interventions untested or unavailable.

Treatment of angina

The purpose of antianginal therapy is to reduce the level of disability. Disability is assessed using the Canadian Cardiovascular Society (CCS) criteria (Table 4.2).

Lifestyle risk factor modification (diet, weight reduction, exercise, and smoking cessation) is important. Antiplatelet and lipid lowering therapy are given. ACEI and ARB are not used to treat angina but are important in reducing future events. Treatment of symptoms relies on drugs and cardiological or surgical intervention. In general antianginal drugs do not alter mortality rates in IHD. Failed medical therapy is an indication for intervention.

Table 4.2 Abbreviated Canadian Cardiovascular Society criteria

Class	Symptom severity
I	Ordinary physical activity such as walking or climbing stairs does not cause angina. Angina occurs during strenuous or rapid or prolonged exertion at work or recreation.
II	Slight limitation of ordinary activity. Walking or climbing stairs rapidly, walking uphill, walking or stair climbing after meals, in cold or windy weather, or when under emotional stress induces anginal pain, or pain occurs only during the first few minutes after awakening. Walking more than two blocks on the level and climbing more than one flight of ordinary stairs at normal pace and in normal conditions induces anginal pain.
III	Marked limitation of ordinary physical activity. Walking one to two blocks on the level or climbing one flight in normal conditions induces anginal pain.
IV	Inability to carry on any physical activity without discomfort. Angina may be present at rest.

Interventions in IHD (📖 see also Chapter 11 p. 172)
- Percutaneous coronary intervention (PCI) with or without stent insertion using bare-metal or drug-eluting stents.
- Coronary artery bypass surgery (CABG and OPCAB).
- Chronic pain techniques: dorsal column stimulation (used when other therapy fails).

Perioperative ischaemia
Perioperative ischaemia is the occurrence of new myocardial ischaemia from the time of premedication to the end of the first postoperative week. The importance of perioperative ischaemia is that it is associated with myocardial infarction, which increases mortality and morbidity. Most pre-bypass perioperative ischaemia is caused by adverse haemodynamic conditions such as tachycardia, or blood pressure changes. Surgical coronary revascularization can be incomplete, and although surgery reduces the likelihood of an ischaemic event, it does not eliminate it, and post-bypass ischaemia may still occur if adverse haemodynamic conditions are present.

Risk factors for perioperative ischaemia
- Recent acute coronary syndrome.
- CCS class IV angina.
- Poor LV function (EF <30%).

Causes of perioperative ischaemia

Preoperative
- Hypoxaemia following premedication.
- Anxiety.

Intraoperative
- Pre-bypass hypertension or hypotension.
- Pre-bypass tachycardia.
- Volume overload with ventricular distension.
- Failed myocardial protection during cross-clamping.
- Technically inadequate graft placement.
- Post-bypass hypertension or hypotension.
- Post-bypass tachycardia.

Postoperative
- Hypertension (common at extubation).
- Hypotension.
- Tachycardia (common at extubation).
- Arrhythmias.

Diagnosis

The two methods used for diagnosis of ischaemia are 5-lead ECG S-T segment analysis and perioperative trans-oesophageal echocardiography (TOE). New S-T segment depression is specific for ischaemia but it is not sensitive, particularly to anterior ischaemia, because the ischaemic area may be remote from the precordial ECG electrode. TOE is a highly sensitive but not specific diagnostic modality. Ischaemia is seen as a new regional wall motion abnormality (RWMA) appearing within seconds of the onset of new ischaemia and reverting with rapid restoration of normal wall motion when the cause of ischaemia is reversed. RWMA is not specific to ischaemia and also occurs in myocardial stunning, hibernation, and infarction. Nevertheless, **a new RWMA occurring pre-bypass is almost always due to acute ischaemia**.

Myocardial stunning is sometimes seen after bypass. It is thought to be caused by free radical damage induced by cardioplegia and reperfusion, which leads to abnormal handling of calcium by the myocardial cell. Contractility of stunned myocardium is depressed for hours to days. It improves with inotropic agents and treatment with these may be needed for days. Hibernation is a myocardial response to prolonged ischaemia. Hibernating myocardium is non-contractile but remains viable and recovers its contractile function within weeks to months following revascularization. Like stunned myocardium, it also recovers contractile function with inotropic agents (Table 4.3).

There is some evidence that the use of inhalational anaesthetic agents is associated with better postoperative myocardial function but no evidence for reduced mortality or morbidity. Ischaemia detection is (at present) a level II indication for TOE.

Table 4.3 Causes and features of RWMA

Cause of RWMA	S-T segment change	Response to restoration of blood supply	Response to inotropic stimulation
Ischaemia	Depressed	Return of normal wall motion within seconds to minutes	Wall motion transiently improves then deteriorates
Stunning	Not specific	Return of normal wall motion within hours to days	Wall motion improves
Hibernation	Not specific	Return of normal wall motion within weeks to months	Wall motion improves
Infarction	Elevated if new, normal if old	No return of function	No change

Prevention of perioperative ischaemia

- Aim for low heart rate (55–75 bpm); use beta-blockers to achieve rate reduction.
- Prophylactic use of intra-aortic balloon pump (IABP) to augment coronary blood flow. Consider IABP insertion before induction of anaesthesia in patients undergoing coronary revascularization with recent acute coronary syndrome, decompensated heart failure, LVEF <30%, or in redo surgery.
- Thoracic epidural analgesia (TEA) – shown to reduce postoperative ischaemic events but not yet shown to improve overall outcome.

Treatment of perioperative ischaemia

- Treat tachycardia (HR >75 bpm) using beta-blockers.
- Treat hypotension with vasoconstrictors. Aim for mean arterial pressure 70–90 mmHg.
- Treat hypertension by deepening anaesthesia or (if anaesthesia already adequate) with IV glyceryl trinitrate.
- Reduce elevated venous pressure using glyceryl trinitrate.
- Treat arrhythmias where there is haemodynamic compromise.
- Return to bypass and complete de-airing if air indicated by TOE.
- Consider placement of an additional bypass graft if TOE evidence of a substantial new RWMA and further surgery deemed technically feasible.
- Consider placement of a bypass graft if a coronary artery has been damaged or obstructed during valve surgery and if TOE evidence of a substantial new RWMA.

Perioperative arrhythmias

Introduction
New arrhythmias are often significant and need treating if causing haemodynamic compromise. Hypoxaemia, hypercarbia, hypovolaemia, and electrolyte disturbances (hyperkalaemia, hypokalaemia, and hypo-magnesaemia) all promote arrhythmias.

Intraoperative arrhythmias
Before bypass
- Sinus bradycardia common during induction of anaesthesia using high dose opioids in patients receiving beta-blockers; if heart rate less than 55 bpm prior to induction, be ready to treat with anticholinergic agent.
- Stimulation of the heart with a Seldinger wire or PA catheter causes ectopic beats; sustained arrhythmias (AF, VT, or VF) requiring cardioversion or defibrillation are very rare.
- Insertion of a pulmonary artery flotation catheter (PAFC) can cause third degree heart block in patients with left bundle branch block. This is a relative contraindication to a PAFC.
- Pre-bypass manipulation of the atria commonly causes AF; if haemodynamics unsatisfactory or evidence of ischaemia on TOE or ECG, cardiovert or commence bypass.
- During off-pump coronary artery bypass surgery (OPCAB), bradycardia can occur during manipulation of the heart, often associated with hypotension. This requires treatment with appropriate anticholinergic drugs, vasoconstrictors, or possibly inotropes.

During and after bypass
- AF is common after cross-clamp release. If new then cardiovert; if not new, cardioversion may not work but rate control may be required.
- Except during and immediately after aortic cross-clamping, malignant ventricular arrhythmias (VF or sustained VT) are rare and usually indicate myocardial damage. Defibrillate and (if recurrent) use amiodarone 300 mg over 20 minutes followed by 900 mg over 24 hours.
- Sinus and junctional bradycardia are common; correct with anticholinergic agent and/or low dose beta-adrenergic agonist or pacing.
- Use temporary pacing for heart block and any bradycardia that does not respond to drug treatment; use ventricular pacing if A-V block, but atrial pacing when A-V conduction is normal.
- To prevent electromagnetic interference, use fixed rate pacing (AOO, VOO, or DOO) during surgery and convert to demand pacing (VVI, VDD, or DDD) at end of operation.
- A few patients develop permanent third degree A-V block and require permanent pacing; commonest after aortic valve replacement for calcific aortic stenosis (3%) and closure of perimembranous VSD.

Postoperative arrhythmias

Atrial fibrillation (AF) and flutter (📖 see also Chapter 13)

- AF is classified as paroxysmal, persistent, or permanent.
- Underlying electrophysiological mechanisms include focal ectopic activity, single circuit re-entry, and multiple circuit re-entry.
- AF is characterized by rapid chaotic atrial firing at a rate of 300–400 per minute.
- Not all impulses reach the ventricles and ventricular rate is determined by the degree of A-V nodal block.
- Rapid atrial firing causes down-regulation of L-type calcium channels. This shortens atrial repolarization time and reduces the wavelength of the AF re-entry circuits. Thus AF promotes itself and successful restoration of sinus rhythm becomes more difficult the longer AF persists.
- New paroxysmal AF is the commonest perioperative arrhythmia, with an incidence of 30–50%. It is commoner following valve surgery than revascularization.
- AF most often occurs between postoperative days one and five. It is usually self-limiting, lasting between hours and a few days.
- Ventricular rate is often rapid. This can cause impaired LV filling with low output, hypotension, myocardial ischaemia, and congestive heart failure.
- AF can lead to embolic stroke and 15% of all strokes have been attributed to this mechanism. Anticoagulation should be considered in any patient who is in AF postoperatively.
- Atrial flutter is much less common. It too is usually self-limiting over hours to days. It may require rate control.

Substrates for postoperative AF

- Increased atrial muscle mass (mitral valve disease, LV hypertrophy, LV failure).
- Increased ectopic activity (hypovolaemia, inotropic drugs, beta-blocker withdrawal, hyperthyroidism).
- Hypokalaemia or hypomagnesaemia.
- Inflammatory mediators.

Management of postoperative AF

Management has three aims: prevention of AF; rhythm control (i.e. restoration of sinus rhythm); and rate control (i.e. control of ventricular rate).

Prevention of AF

- Prophylaxis against postoperative AF should be given routinely.
- Maintain normovolaemia and normal electrolytes (K^+ and Mg^{2+}).
- If beta-blocked preoperatively, restart reduced dose of same beta-blocker or low dose bisoprolol or sotalol (40 mg bd) on day one (note: atenolol is best given twice daily).
- If not beta-blocked preoperatively and no contraindication (see below), start beta-blocker such as bisoprolol.
- If in AF preoperatively, but sinus rhythm on return from theatre, many start amiodarone 300 mg IV over 1 hour followed by 900 mg IV over 24 hours, followed by 200 mg tds orally for one week, then once daily for five weeks. The efficacy of this is disputed.

Rhythm control (for patients in sinus rhythm preoperatively)
- Maintain normovolaemia and normal electrolytes (K^+ and Mg^{2+})
- Patient should already be receiving beta-blockers if no contraindication (see below). If using sotalol, double the dose.
- If AF lasting more than one hour and rate >100 with systolic BP <100 or symptomatic, add amiodarone 300 mg IV over 1 hour followed by 900 mg IV over 24 hour, followed by 200 mg tds orally for one week then once daily for five weeks.
- Do not use amiodarone if patient receiving sotalol.
- If this fails to control rhythm, consider increasing dose of beta-blocker. If this fails, consider adding diltiazem 60 mg bd or cardioversion.

Rate control (for patients in AF preoperatively)
- Maintain normovolaemia and normal electrolytes (K^+ and Mg^{2+}).
- Restart preoperative rate control regime.
- If rate >100 bpm, and not beta-blocked, add beta-blocker, e.g. bisoprolol 2.5 mg increasing to 10 mg.
- If this fails to control rate, consider increasing dose of beta-blocker. If this fails and AF persists, consider adding diltiazem 60 mg bd.
- Note: Contraindications to beta-blockade include decompensated heart failure, asthma, hypovolaemia, known intolerance to beta-blockers, heart rate <50 bpm.

Ventricular arrhythmias
- Isolated ventricular ectopic beats are common postoperatively and usually need no treatment. Other ventricular arrhythmias are infrequent. If they occur they usually indicate ischaemia.

Management of ventricular arrhythmias (VF, VT, and frequent ectopic activity)
- Defibrillate if indicated.
- Check position of PAFC; ectopic activity is common if catheter touching right ventricular outflow tract. Check correct position by confirming successful balloon occlusion ('wedge') before giving any other therapy.
- Maintain normovolaemia and normal electrolytes (K^+ and Mg^{2+}).
- Start amiodarone 300 mg IV over 1 hour followed by 900 mg IV over 24 hours, followed by 200 mg tds orally for one week then once daily for five weeks.

Heart failure (HF)

Heart failure (📖 see also Chapter 32) may be chronic or acute. Ischaemic heart disease is the commonest cause. It is defined as inability of the heart to generate an output appropriate to supply the body's oxygen consumption, or an ability only to do so at the expense of elevated filling pressures. Chronic HF is a condition characterized by the triad of elevated LV and RV filling pressures, elevated systemic vascular resistance (SVR), and low cardiac output (CO). This triad is diagnostic of decompensated chronic HF. With treatment, all three may return to normal, at least at rest, resulting in compensated HF. Even when HF is decompensated, arterial pressure is often normal.

HF is usually due to myocardial failure, but in mitral or tricuspid stenosis, heart failure can occur without myocardial failure. Myocardial failure is caused by systolic dysfunction (abnormal contractility), diastolic dysfunction (abnormal filling), or both, with roughly one third of patients falling into each category. Overt heart failure can occur in the presence of normal LV systolic function if diastolic dysfunction is severe.

Usually it is the left ventricle that fails (LVF). Right ventricular failure (RVF) can occur in response to chronic elevation of pulmonary vascular pressure secondary to LVF, but isolated RVF is rare (outside of congenital heart disease). RVF in conjunction with LVF is termed congestive heart failure (CHF).

Chronic HF is common and is a major cause of mortality and hospital admission. The prevalence is 1–2% in the sixth decade rising to 10% in the eighth decade of life. Increasing life expectancy means the incidence of HF continues to rise. In hospital mortality is about 5% and approximately one third of patients die within a year of diagnosis.

Disability is classified according to the New York Heart Association (NYHA) criteria (Table 4.4).

Table 4.4 Abbreviated New York Heart Association criteria

Class	Symptom severity
I	Patients with cardiac disease without resulting limitations of physical activity. Ordinary physical activity does not cause undue fatigue, palpitation, dyspnoea, or anginal pain.
II	Patients with cardiac disease resulting in slight limitation of physical activity. They are comfortable at rest. Ordinary physical activity results in fatigue, palpitation, dyspnoea, or anginal pain.
III	Patients with cardiac disease resulting in marked limitation of physical activity. They are comfortable at rest. Less than ordinary physical activity results in fatigue, dyspnoea, palpitation, or anginal pain.
IV	Patients with cardiac disease resulting in inability to carry on any physical activity without discomfort. Symptoms may be present at rest. If any physical activity is undertaken, discomfort is increased.

Causes of LVF and CHF

- Ischaemic heart disease (ischaemic cardiomyopathy).
- Hypertensive heart disease.
- Valvular heart disease.
- Congenital heart disease.
- Primary cardiomyopathies (obstructive, dilated, and restrictive).
- Uncontrolled tachyarrhythmias and bradyarrhythmias.
- Viral myocarditis.
- Drugs and toxins.
- Myocardial injury following heart surgery or interventional cardiology.

Causes of isolated RVF

- Elevated pulmonary vascular resistance (PVR).
- Chronic obstructive pulmonary disease (COPD).
- Pulmonary thromboembolic disease.
- Isolated right heart valvular disease.
- Congenital heart disease.
- Following orthotopic heart transplantation in recipients with elevated PVR.
- Ischaemic heart disease (following occlusion of a non-dominant right coronary artery).

Chronic HF

Pathophysiology

The heart is able to adapt to increased load or depressed intrinsic myocardial function. These short-term adaptive mechanisms are the Frank-Starling relationship, in which increased preload maintains stroke volume, and increased adrenomedullary secretion of catecholamines, which helps restore depressed contractility but at the expense of increased heart rate and SVR.

Longer-term adaptation, which takes weeks to months, is by ventricular remodelling. In valvular and hypertensive heart disease, the overloaded LV remodels to compensate for increased wall stress. Pressure overload causes concentric hypertrophy with myocardial thickening. Volume overload causes eccentric hypertrophy with increased cavity dimensions, but myocardial thickening is only sufficient to maintain a normal relationship between wall thickness and cavity size. The coronary circulation does not enlarge in proportion to muscle growth. There is an increase in interstitial collagen, which results in increased myocardial stiffness and diastolic dysfunction.

HF supervenes when adaptive mechanisms have reached their limit and a further increase in load can no longer be met. Myocardial norepinephrine stores and beta-adrenoreceptor density are reduced (ß-receptor down-regulation).

Low CO and stretching of cardiac myocytes lead to neurohumoral changes, which further worsen myocardial performance. Up-regulation of the renin-angiotensin-aldosterone system increases SVR and leads to sodium and water retention with oedema formation. Levels of circulating B-type natriuretic peptide (BNP) and endothelin 1 are elevated. High filling pressures, low systolic arterial pressure (<115 mmHg), and elevated serum urea, creatinine, or BNP are all associated with poor outcome.

Clinical features
Many of the symptoms and signs of HF, including dyspnoea, orthopnoea, ankle oedema, elevated jugular venous pressure, basal crepitations, and gallop rhythm are due to elevated cardiac filling pressures.

Symptoms
- Dyspnoea, orthopnoea, and paroxysmal nocturnal dyspnoea.
- Nocturnal cough.
- Fatigue.
- Dependent oedema.*

Signs
- Sinus tachycardia (if sinus rhythm).
- Elevated jugular venous pressure.*
- Displaced apex beat.
- Third heart sound (S3 gallop).
- Basal crepitations.
- Acute pulmonary oedema.
- Pleural effusion.*
- Hepatomegaly.*
- Elevated serum urea and creatinine.

Features marked * are only present in congestive heart failure.

Treatment
Drug treatment is used mainly to reduce elevated venous pressure and SVR. Cardiac output increases as a result of SVR reduction. Angiotensin-converting enzyme inhibitors (ACEIs) and angiotensin receptor blockers (ARBs) help reverse LV remodelling, and in so doing help maintain sinus rhythm. Beta-blockade improves outcome by reducing the incidence of arrhythmias and by up-regulation of ß-adrenergic receptors.

In patients with bundle branch block and HF, left ventricular or biventricular pacing (resynchronization therapy) can produce a major improvement in NYHA functional status. Suitability for resynchronization therapy is determined with a dyssynchrony study, using transthoracic echo with tissue Doppler velocity imaging to quantify timing variation of regional myocardial contraction. Greatest benefit appears to occur in patients with a non-ischaemic origin of HF, mitral regurgitation, and QRS duration >130 ms.

Many patients with chronic HF also have ventricular arrhythmias or paroxysmal AF. In this subgroup, insertion of an automated implantable cardioverter-defibrillator (AICD) improves survival (☐ see also Chapter 13).

The positive inotropic effects of digoxin may be useful in chronic HF and its use is not associated with increased mortality. Catecholamines and phosphodiesterase III inhibitors (PDEIs) are contraindicated because their use is associated with increased mortality and these drugs are only used as a temporary measure in cardiogenic shock or acute heart failure. Cardiac transplantation is reserved for patients with HF refractory to other therapies. New therapies, notably nesiritide (recombinant B-natriuretic peptide) and levosimendan (a calcium sensitizer and lusitropic agent), may prove useful.

In summary, treatments include:
- Diuretics (mainly loop diuretics and spironolactone).
- ACEI or ARB.
- Nitrates.
- Calcium antagonists.
- Potassium channel activators.
- Beta-blockers.
- Digoxin.
- Cardiac resynchronization.
- AICD implantation.
- Cardiac transplantation.

Acute HF

Pathophysiology

Acute HF following heart surgery is different to chronic HF. It is characterized primarily by low CO and low arterial pressure. Filling pressures are
elevated but SVR may be low, normal, or high. Treatment is also different
to chronic HF and relies heavily on inotropic agents (see below). Acute
HF may follow any cardiac surgical procedure if the myocardium of either
ventricle is damaged, such as by technically inadequate revascularization or
failed myocardial preservation. Postoperative acute HF is much commoner
if preoperative myocardial function is poor.

Diagnosis and quantification of low CO and monitoring of therapy
is best achieved with echocardiography, usually TOE in the intubated
patient. Although PAFCs are widely used to measure cardiac output and
vascular resistances in acute heart failure, they give no information about
intracardiac volume and there is little evidence that their use improves
outcome, indeed largely the opposite.

Differential diagnosis

It is vital to distinguish between low CO due to true myocardial failure and
low CO due to the conditions below, which mimic it but which require
different treatments. These are:
- Hypovolaemia.
- Cardiac tamponade.
- LV intracavity or outflow tract obstruction.

Central venous and wedge pressures often do not correlate with cardiac
filling and hypovolaemia can occur with elevated filling pressures.

Clinical features

- Sinus tachycardia (if sinus rhythm).
- Arterial hypotension.
- Elevated venous pressures.
- Low CO.
- Oliguria.
- Cool peripheries.

Echocardiographic diagnosis

The following echocardiographic features allow distinction of true heart failure from other causes of low cardiac output:

- Evidence of poor systolic LV function either with large regional wall motion abnormality or global hypokinesia. Overall fractional area change markedly reduced to 30% or less.
- Evidence of restrictive LV filling such as E wave deceleration time less than 150 ms and mitral annular tissue Doppler E wave velocity less than 8 cm/s.
- Evidence of poor systolic right ventricular function, usually associated with obvious marked right ventricular dilatation.
- Absence of cardiac tamponade. Effusion is common but only significant if there is evidence of tamponade physiology. Tamponade is seen as right ventricular systolic collapse or right atrial diastolic collapse. Transmitral E wave deceleration time is less than 150 ms but mitral annular velocities are normal in tamponade.
- Absence of hypovolaemia. Hypovolaemia is likely when LV end diastolic diameter is less than 3.5 cm in the transgastric mid-papillary short axis view.
- Absence of LV intracavitary systolic obstruction (hourglass ventricle), which occurs when a hypertrophied LV is underfilled. This is best seen in transgastric two-chamber view.
- Absence of LV outflow tract obstruction (LVOTO). LVOTO is due either to systolic anterior motion (SAM) of the anterior mitral valve leaflet, or narrowing of the LVOT due to septal hypertrophy. These do not occur when systolic function is poor.

Treatment of acute heart failure (📖 see aslo Chapter 3)

Treatment of acute HF is aimed at increasing cardiac output. Both catecholamines and phosphodiesterase III inhibitors (PDEIs) have powerful inotropic actions. All catecholamines have half-lives of a few minutes and have to be infused. PDEIs have half-lives of a few hours and can be given as a slow bolus or infusion, or both. Use of catecholamines is sometimes limited by excessive increase in heart rate, necessitating dose reduction. PDEIs also have a lusitropic action, which improves LV relaxation and filling. Thus PDEIs are useful when diastolic function is poor, and this can be assessed with TOE using Doppler indices of diastolic function. Calcium chloride can be used to correct hypocalcaemia, but overdosage causes hypercalcaemia, which is deleterious to myocardial mitochondrial integrity.

The effectiveness of treatment is assessed clinically using arterial pressure, peripheral temperature, and urine output. Serial or continuous cardiac output measurement or repeated echo assessment can be used to quantify effectiveness of therapy. Tolerance to all these agents develops over time.

In summary, treatments include:

- Beta-adrenergic agonists (usually dobutamine 2–20 g/kg/min).
- Phosphodiesterase III inhibitors (usually milrinone 50 µg/kg bolus followed by infusion at 0.5 µg/kg/min).
- Norepinephrine or phenylephrine (if SVR low).
- Correction of hypocalcaemia.
- Intra-aortic balloon pump (to maximize coronary blood flow).

- Inhaled nitric oxide or other pulmonary vasodilator (if predominant right ventricular failure).
- Ventricular assist devices (especially following heart transplantation).

Treatment of conditions mimicking heart failure
- Hypovolaemia: colloid or blood infusion depending on haematocrit; reduction of inotropic and vasoconstrictor therapy.
- Cardiac tamponade: surgical exploration and removal of the effusion or clot.
- LV intracavity or outflow tract obstruction:
  - Cessation of all inotropic and vasodilator therapy.
  - Removal of intra-aortic balloon pump.
  - Volume administration to increase LV and LVOT diameter.
  - Vasoconstrictors to increase SVR.
  - Consideration of beta-blockade.

Further reading

1. Hansson G. Inflammation, atherosclerosis, and coronary artery disease. *New England Journal of Medicine* 2005; 352: 1685–1695.
2. Hunt SA, Abraham WT, Chin MH, et al. 2009 Focused Update: ACCF/AHA Guidelines for the diagnosis and management of heart failure in adults: A report of the American College of Cardiology Foundation/American Heart Association Task Force on Practice Guidelines. *Circulation* 2009; 119: 1977–2016. http://circ.ahajournals.org/cgi/content/full/119/14/1977
3. Libby P, Theroux P. Pathophysiology of coronary artery disease. *Circulation* 2005; 111: 3481–3488.
4. Owan T, Hodge D, Herges R, Jacobsen S, Roger V, Redfield M. Trends in prevalence and outcome of heart failure with preserved ejection fraction. *New England Journal of Medicine* 2006; 355: 251–259.
5. The Task Force for the diagnosis and treatment of chronic heart failure of the European Society of Cardiology. Guidelines for the diagnosis and treatment of chronic heart failure (update 2005). *European Heart Journal* 2005; 26: 2472.

Part 2

Organ system implications of cardiac surgery

5	Central nervous system	**73**
6	Haematology	**91**
7	The inflammatory response	**109**
8	Renal	**125**
9	Respiratory implications of cardiac surgery	**137**
10	Infection	**149**

Central nervous system

Dr J Arrowsmith

Introduction *74*
General considerations *76*
Incidence and etiology *78*
Prevention *82*
Management of established neurological complications *86*
Further reading *89*

Introduction

Injury to the brain and spinal cord after cardiac surgery represents a significant cause of morbidity and disability. Neurological complications increase the length of ICU and hospital stay, and reduce the likelihood of return to independent living. Minor neurological complications are very common and often go undiagnosed. It is now recognized that transient and early postoperative problems such as confusion, agitation, and delirium – previously considered self-limiting nuisances – are associated with significant morbidity and mortality. Furthermore, a decline in cognitive function in the early postoperative period is predictive of late (five-year) cognitive decline.

General considerations

Clinical spectrum

The spectrum of central nervous system injury during and after cardiac surgery encompasses a wide range of clinical entities ranging from death or persistent vegetative state to subtle changes in memory and concentration:

- Fatal brain injury – the intracranial 'catastrophe'.
- Focal brain injury:
  - Stroke/cerebrovascular accident (CVA).
  - Reversible ischaemic neurological deficit (RIND).
  - Transient ischaemic attack (TIA).
- Diffuse non-fatal encephalopathy:
  - Impaired consciousness (e.g. coma, stupor, delirium).
  - Behavioural disturbance (e.g. agitation).
  - Impaired cognitive function (e.g. confusion, disorientation).
- Other:
  - Seizures/choreoathetosis (especially infants and children).
  - Ophthalmological – visual field defect/reduced visual acuity.
  - Emergence of primitive reflexes.
  - Spinal cord injury (e.g. anterior spinal artery syndrome).

Neurological injury may be: *immediate* – apparent soon after the patient recovers from anaesthesia; or *delayed* – with onset after a 'lucid' interval of apparently normal neurological recovery.

Stroke refers to irreversible cerebral injury due to partial or complete obstruction of a cerebral artery by thrombosis, embolism, dissection, or vasospasm (secondary to intracerebral or subarachnoid haemorrhage) or (rarely) venous obstruction. Symptoms and physical signs are dependent upon the site and extent of injury as well as hemispheric dominance (Box 5.1). Incomplete recovery may occur over weeks to months. It should be borne in mind that the left hemisphere is dominant for speech and language in 95% of right-handed patients.

The term reversible ischaemic neurological deficit (RIND) refers to the recovery of neurological function following a stroke within three weeks – typically 24–72 hours.

The term transient ischaemic attack (TIA) is used when there is complete recovery of neurological function within 24 hours.

Box 5.1 Symptoms and signs of stroke
- Depressed conscious level – coma, delirium, confusion.
- Contralateral (body) hemiparesis and hemiplegia, myotonia, myoclonus.
- Ipsilateral (cranial nerve) distribution motor/sensory impairment.
- Hemibody (thalamic) pain.
- Cortical blindness, quadrantopia, hemianopia, gaze palsy.
- Neglect, extinction, impersistence, allaesthesia.
- Cognitive impairment, disinhibition.
- Dysphasia – conductive, confabulation, agnosia, Broca's, Wernicke's.
- Dyspraxia – ideomotor, constructional, dressing, callosal.
- Dysphagia.
- Ataxia, dysmetria, intention tremor.
- Autonomic dysfunction, Horner syndrome, hyperhydrosis, incontinence.
- Vertigo, nystagmus, nausea, vomiting, hoarseness, hiccups.
- Primitive reflexes: grasp, plantar, snout, pout, corneomandibular, glabella tap.
- Rarely – athetosis, chorea, dystonia.

Cognitive dysfunction implies interference with intellectual and higher mental functions such as memory (verbal, non-verbal), attention, concentration, psychomotor function, verbal fluency, executive function (abstract reasoning, problem solving, judgement, planning), perception, and visuospatial skills. Whilst cognitive function is not directly linked to intelligence, a higher premorbid level of educational attainment does appear to 'protect' patients from cognitive impairment.

Delirium can be defined as a transient mental syndrome of acute onset characterized by global cognitive impairment, reduced conscious level, abnormalities of attention, increased or decreased psychomotor activity, and disordered pattern of sleep.

Patients with delirium are more likely to: have postoperative respiratory insufficiency; require reinstitution of mechanical ventilation; develop sternal instability or require sternal wound debridement; and have prolonged duration of ICU and hospital stay. Delirium following cardiac surgery is associated with a five-fold increase in mortality.

Incidence and etiology

The reported incidence of neurological injury after cardiac surgery is dependent upon the type of surgery performed, the clinical endpoint chosen (i.e. stroke, encephalopathy, cognitive dysfunction), and study design (i.e. retrospective or prospective). In retrospective studies the incidence of stroke after CABG has been reported as 0.8–3.2%, whereas in prospective studies the reported incidence is higher: 1.5–5.2% (Table 5.1).

Table 5.1 Incidence of stroke by cardiac surgical procedure at Johns Hopkins University (2001–2004)

Procedure	Stroke rate	Days 1–2
Isolated CABG (primary or redo)	4.1%	84%
Isolated valve surgery	3.1%	65%
CABG + valve surgery	7.9%	76%
CABG + other* surgery	7.2%	80%
Aortic repair	8.7%	83%
Other* surgery	3.6%	59%

Right-hand column indicates proportion of strokes identified within two days of surgery.
* Other procedures include: patent foramen ovale; surgical ventricular reconstruction; carotid endarterectomy; maze procedure; and ventricular assist device.

Reproduced with permission from McKhann GM, Grega MA, Borowicz LM, Jr, Baumgartner WA, and Selnes OA. Stroke and encephalopathy after cardiac surgery: An update. *Stroke* 2006; 37: 562–571, originally published online Dec 22, 2005. Published by the American Heart Association. Copyright Lippencott Williams and Wilkins © 2006.

The reported incidence of cognitive dysfunction following cardiac surgery varies considerably (8%–80%) and is dependent on: the type of surgery performed; the type, number, and timing of cognitive function tests; and the statistical definition of cognitive impairment used.

Preoperative (patient), intraoperative, and postoperative factors contribute to the overall risk of neurological injury (Table 5.2). The risk factors for focal (type I) and non-focal (type II) neurological injury are similar but not identical.

Table 5.2 Risk factors for neurological injury after cardiac surgery

Preoperative	Age, female gender, genotype, education level, aortic atheroma, carotid atheroma, previous stroke/TIA, diabetes mellitus, cardiac function, previous CABG, use of IABP, ethanol intake, pulmonary disease, hypertension, dysrhythmia, dyslipidaemia, diuretic use
Intraoperative	Surgery type, combined procedures, aortic clamp site, aortic clamp duration, macroemboli, microemboli, arterial pressure, CPB pump flow, temperature, haematocrit, use of DHCA, rapid rewarming
Postoperative	Hypotension, long ICU stay, renal dysfunction, atrial fibrillation, cardiac arrest, temperature

The incidence of delirium after cardiac surgery is largely dictated by patient age, the type of surgical procedure undertaken, and the presence or absence of a number of independent predictors. In a retrospective study of 16,184 patients undergoing cardiac surgery between 1996 and 2001, the overall prevalence of delirium was 8.4%. Factors associated with the development of delirium (in decreasing order of importance) were:

- Age.
- Diabetes mellitus.
- Urgent surgery.
- Operating time >180 minutes.
- Peripheral vascular disease.
- Preoperative cardiogenic shock.
- Intraoperative haemofiltration.
- Red cell transfusion >2000 ml.
- Left ventricular ejection fraction <30%.
- Atrial fibrillation.
- History of cerebrovascular disease.

Fewer patients undergoing off-pump surgery had postoperative delirium, although the prevalence of risk factors was lower in this group. The very low incidence of delirium in patients undergoing minimally invasive direct coronary artery bypass (MIDCAB) suggests that surgical manipulation and instrumentation of the proximal aorta – avoided during MIDCAB – contributes to the genesis of delirium. This finding lends weight to the notion that off-pump surgery combined with 'no touch' aortic techniques eliminates a number of the risk factors for stroke during conventional surgery.

Pathophysiology

A number of distinct but as yet incompletely understood mechanisms underlie the spectrum of adverse neurological injuries. Clinical outcome is more related to anatomical location of the injury, inherent reparative mechanisms, and central nervous system plasticity, rather than the amount of lost neuronal tissue.

Global injury results from cessation of cerebral blood flow or from prolonged cerebral hypoperfusion. This pattern of injury typically follows prolonged cardiac arrest, profound cerebral hypoperfusion, or gross hypoglycaemia.

Watershed injury occurs in the regions supplied by the terminal branches of two neighbouring cerebral arteries. Areas such as the parietotemporal cortices, which are supplied by the middle and posterior cerebral arteries, are thus particularly vulnerable to prolonged periods of cerebral hypoperfusion.

Focal injury (stroke, RIND, TIA) typically follows total or subtotal occlusion of a cerebral artery by embolic material. This yields a zone of irreversible injury (*umbra*) surrounded by an area of potentially reversible injury (*penumbra*). The eventual extent of recovery of tissue in the ischaemic penumbra is dependent upon a number of local and systemic factors: ischaemic susceptibility, collateral circulation, time to reperfusion, temperature, haematocrit, and blood glucose.

Diffuse-microfocal injury typically follows widespread cerebral microembolism and appears to occur in virtually all patients undergoing cardiac surgery and a significant proportion of patients undergoing percutaneous intervention.

Regardless of the mechanism of injury the fate of individual neurons is dependent upon the so-called 'ischaemic cascade'.

- Hypoxia, hypoglycaemia, and various toxins induce neuronal energy failure and the release of excitotoxic amino acid neurotransmitters (e.g. glutamate).
- Activation of ligand-gated ion channels leads to an influx of Na^+, Ca^{2+}, and water, which eventually overwhelms energy-dependent sequestration and extrusion mechanisms.
- The rise in cytosolic Ca^{2+} activates protein kinases and phospholipases, and a series of cascades that liberate compounds with vasoactive, lipolytic, chemotactic, and other properties.
- Worsening acidosis hampers cellular recovery mechanisms.
- Release of oxygen free radicals and metabolites of arachidonic acid result in loss of cell membrane integrity and irreversible damage to the cytoskeleton.
- In non-lethal injury, the rise in Ca^{2+} may induce gene up-regulation and expression of neurotrophic and growth factors.

Determining risk

The risk of neurological injury following cardiac surgery parallels that of mortality. Indeed, many of the risk factors for neurological injury can be found in risk models such as the Parsonnet score, Tu score, and EuroSCORE. A study of 2000 patients undergoing CABG surgery at 24 US centres revealed an overall incidence of neurological injury of 6.1% and identified 13 independent predictors of adverse neurological outcome (Table 5.3). Data from this study were subsequently used to develop and validate a predictive model – the *stroke risk index* (Figure 5.1).

Table 5.3 Adjusted odds ratios [95% confidence intervals] for adverse neurological outcomes after CABG surgery associated with independent risk factors

Risk factors	Outcomes	
	Type I	Type II
Proximal aortic atherosclerosis	4.52 [2.52–8.09]	
History of neurological disease	3.19 [1.65–6.15]	
Use of IABP	2.60 [1.21–5.58]	
Diabetes mellitus	2.59 [1.46–4.60]	
History of hypertension	2.31 [1.20–4.47]	
History of pulmonary disease	2.09 [1.14–3.85]	2.37 [1.34–4.18]
History of unstable angina	1.83 [1.03–3.27]	
Age (per additional decade)	1.75 [1.27–2.43]	2.20 [1.60–3.02]
Admission systolic BP >180 mmHg		3.47 [1.41–8.55]
History of excessive alcohol intake		2.64 [1.27–5.47]
History of CABG		2.18 [1.14–4.17]
Dysrhythmia on day of surgery		1.97 [1.12–3.46]
Antihypertensive therapy		1.78 [1.02–3.10]

Type I = non-fatal stroke, transient ischaemic attack, stupor or coma at discharge, death caused by stroke, or hypoxic encephalopathy. Type II = new deterioration in intellectual function, confusion, agitation, disorientation, memory deficit, or seizure without evidence of focal injury.

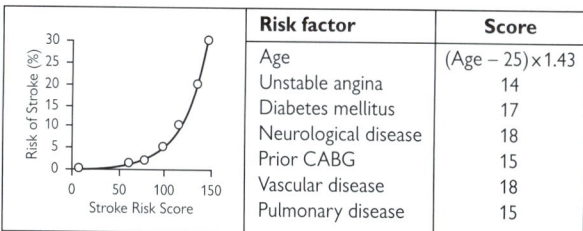

Risk factor	Score
Age	(Age − 25) × 1.43
Unstable angina	14
Diabetes mellitus	17
Neurological disease	18
Prior CABG	15
Vascular disease	18
Pulmonary disease	15

Figure 5.1 Preoperative stroke risk index for CABG patients.

Prevention

Routine clinical monitoring

Continuous monitoring of arterial pressure, central venous pressure, and temperature combined with intermittent measurement of blood glucose and arterial blood gas analysis should be undertaken in all cases. Gross hypoglycaemia or prolonged periods of profound cerebral hypoperfusion may result in irreversible cerebral injury. It should be borne in mind that cerebral perfusion pressure (CPP) is dependent upon mean arterial pressure (MAP), intracranial pressure (ICP), and central venous pressure (CVP), i.e. CPP = MAP − (ICP + CVP). In the presence of seemingly adequate MAP, a sustained increase in CVP associated with elevation of the heart or external compression of the superior vena cava may cause a reduction in CPP.

Conduct of cardiopulmonary bypass

Despite considerable research, the characteristics of 'optimal' CPB perfusion remain to be defined. Within the bounds of usual CPB conduct, however, perfusion pressure, pump flow rate, and flow character appear to have little influence on neurological outcome. By contrast, the rate and extent of rewarming – measured by cerebral arteriovenous DO_2 – does appear to influence cognitive outcomes. The impact of CPB management on neurological outcome has been reviewed by Hogue et al. (Table 5.4).

Table 5.4 Evidence for neuroprotective CPB interventions

Class	Intervention
I	None
IIa	None
IIb	Change in surgical approach guided by epiaortic ultrasound
	Maintaining 'higher' MAP (>50 mmHg) in high-risk patients
	Non-pulsatile (vs. pulsatile) perfusion – Class Indeterminate in high-risk patients
	α-stat (vs. pH-stat) acid base management – Class Indeterminate in high-risk patients
Indeterminate	Heparin-bonded CPB circuits
	Modified aortic cannula
	Leucocyte-depleting filters
	Cell-saver processing of cardiotomy blood
	Insufflation of operative site with CO_2
	Maintenance of 'high' (e.g. >27%) haematocrit
	'Tight' intraoperative control of serum glucose
	Hypothermia
	Drugs: remacemide, lidocaine, aprotinin, pexelizumab, allopurinol
III	Drugs: thiopental, propofol, nimodipine, epoprostenol, GM1-ganglioside, pegorgotein, clomethiazole

Class I: Always acceptable, proven safe, and definitely useful. **Class IIa**: Acceptable, safe, and useful. Standard of care. Considered prudent. Intervention of choice by majority of experts. **Class IIb**: Acceptable, safe, and useful. Within standard of care. Reasonably prudent. Considered optional or alternative intervention by majority of experts. **Class Indeterminate**: Used, but insufficient evidence of efficacy. **Class III**: No evidence of efficacy or evidence of harm.

Reproduced with permission from Hogue CW Jr, Palin CA, Arrowsmith JE. Cardiopulmonary bypass management and neurologic outcomes: An evidence-based appraisal of current practices. *Anesthesia and Analgesia* 2006; 103 (1): 21–37. Copyright Lippincott Williams and Wilkins © 2006.

Off-pump coronary artery bypass (OPCAB) surgery (📖 see also Chapter 24)

A reduction in the risk of neurological injury – particularly in high-risk, elderly, female, and 'redo' patients – is one of the many proposed benefits of cardiac surgery without CPB. Despite confounding factors such as surgeon experience and predilection, as well as patient preference, the weight of currently available evidence suggests that OPCAB *reduces* but does not *eliminate* the risk of neurological injury. Off-pump total arterial revascularization using 'Y' or 'T' grafts and an aortic 'no touch' technique appears to confer the greatest degree of neuroprotection.

Neurological monitoring

Emerging evidence suggests that neurological monitoring during cardiac output permits both outcome prediction and outcome modification. Despite this, routine neurological monitoring during cardiac surgery remains largely in the hands of enthusiasts and researchers. Monitors of neurological function can be considered in three categories: clinical, non-invasive, and invasive (Table 5.5).

Table 5.5 Types of neurological monitoring

Clinical	Detection of aortic cannula misplacement/migration
	Detection of venous air entrainment
	Detection of hypoxia, hypoglycaemia, acidosis, cerebral hypoperfusion, and cerebral hyperthermia
Non-invasive	Electroencephalography (EEG), CFAM
	Cerebral near infra-red spectroscopy (NIRS)
	Transcranial Doppler (TCD) ultrasound
	Evoked (visual, auditory, somatosensory, motor) potentials
Invasive	Jugular venous oxygen saturation ($S_{JV}O_2$)

CFAM, cerebral function analysing monitor.

Pharmacological neuroprotection

Despite numerous preclinical and clinical studies using a wide diversity of promising compounds, no drug is yet licensed for neuroprotection during cardiac surgery. Despite encouraging findings in animal models, most human studies have failed to demonstrate efficacy or have resulted in harm. Many clinical studies have suffered from poor experimental design and have been inadequately powered.

Management of established neurological complications

Diagnosis

Neurological injury after cardiac surgery is usually a clinical diagnosis. The degree of disability can be recorded using the National Institutes of Health (NIH) Stroke Index (Table 5.6).

Cranial computed tomography (CT) or magnetic resonance imaging (MRI) is invariably undertaken to document the presence or absence of cerebral pathology, but rarely influences management – other than to guide withdrawal of treatment. Diffusion-weighted MRI can be used to detect extracellular water (i.e. cerebral oedema) long before any abnormality is apparent on CT or conventional MRI.

Cognitive dysfunction may only become apparent after formal cognitive function testing. It is generally accepted that the patient's subjective opinion of their cognitive impairment is inaccurate.

Table 5.6 National Institutes of Health (NIH) Stroke Index

1A: **Level of consciousness**
0 alert; 1 drowsy; 2 obtunded; 3 coma/unresponsive
1B: **Orientation** (replies to two questions)
0 both correct; 1 one correct; 2 neither correct
1C: **Response to commands** (two commands)
0 both tasks correct; 1 one task correct; 2 neither task correct

2: **Gaze**
0 normal horizontal movements; 1 partial gaze palsy; 2 complete gaze palsy

3: **Visual fields** (hemianopia)
0 no defect; 1 partial; 2 complete; 3 bilateral

4: **Facial movement** (degree of weakness)
0 normal; 1 minor; 2 partial; 3 complete

5: **Motor function**: **arm** (a: left; b: right)
0 no drift; 1 drift before 5 seconds; 2 falls before 10 seconds; 3 no effort against gravity; 4 no movement

6: **Motor function**: **leg** (a: left; b: right)
0 no drift; 1 drift before 5 seconds; 2 falls before 10 seconds; 3 no effort against gravity; 4 no movement

7: **Limb ataxia**
0 none; 1 one limb; 2 two limbs

8: **Sensory loss**
0 none; 1 mild; 2 severe

9: **Language** (degree of aphasia)
0 normal; 1 mild; 2 severe; 3 mute/global aphasia

10: **Articulation** (degree of dysarthria)
0 normal; 1 mild; 2 severe

11: **Extinction or inattention**
0 absent; 1 mild (one sensory modality); 2 severe (two sensory modalities)

The inclusion of findings in the unaffected (contralateral) limbs emphasizes the need for recording observations *without* neuroanatomical interpretation.

Management

- Prevention of secondary brain injury:
  - Maintenance of cerebral oxygenation.
  - Treatment of low cardiac output states (e.g. dysrhythmia).
  - Aggressive treatment of hyperthermia and hyperglycaemia.
  - Treatment of brain oedema/raised intracranial pressure – hyperventilation, mannitol, dexamethasone, deliberate hypothermia.

- Surgical intervention – only applicable in a minority of cases:
  - Evacuation of subdural or intracerebral haemorrhage.
  - Repair of proximal aortic dissection.
  - Intracranial aneurysm clipping, carotid/cerebral artery angioplasty, ventriculo-atrial shunt.
- Supportive measures:
  - Hydration and nutrition.
  - Avoidance of pressure sores.
  - Antimicrobial therapy.
  - Thromboprophylaxis – anticoagulants, antiplatelet drugs.
- Physical therapy:
  - Avoidance of contractures.
  - Rehabilitation – speech and language therapy.
- Specific drug therapy:
  - Seizures – phenytoin, benzodiazepines.
  - Muscle spasm – baclofen, tizanidine.
  - Myoclonus – clonazepam, piracetam.
  - Depression – fluoxetine, citalopram, paroxetine, sertraline.
  - Agitation – haloperidol, clonidine.
  - Chronic pain syndromes – amitriptyline, gabapentin.

Prognosis

A quarter of patients sustaining a stroke after cardiac surgery will suffer significant long-term disability. A proportion of this group will succumb to the complications of prolonged intensive care (sepsis, multi-organ failure, etc.) or pneumonia secondary to pulmonary aspiration. Prolonged depression of conscious level, coma, and persistent vegetative state are associated with significant (i.e. >90%) mortality.

The eventual extent of recovery of neurological function in survivors is largely determined by the speed/extent of recovery of function within the first few days.

While delirium is often a short-lived and self-limiting phenomenon, it is associated with significant morbidity and increased risk of death from other complications.

Most studies have shown that the prevalence and severity of cognitive dysfunction following cardiac surgery tends to decline in the first few months after surgery. Long-term follow-up studies, however, suggest that early postoperative cognitive decline is a significant predictor of long-term cognitive impairment.

Further reading

1. Hogue CW Jr, Palin CA, Arrowsmith JE. Cardiopulmonary bypass management and neurologic outcomes: An evidence-based appraisal of current practices. *Anesthesia and Analgesia* 2006; 103: 21–37.
2. Kapatanakis EI, Stamou SC, Dullum MKC, et al. The impact of aortic manipulation on neurologic outcomes after coronary artery bypass surgery: A risk-adjusted study. *The Annals of Thoracic Surgery* 2004; 78: 1564–1571.
3. McKhann GM, Grega MA, Borowicz LM Jr, et al. Stroke and encephalopathy after cardiac surgery: An update. *Stroke* 2006; 37: 562–571.
4. Selnes OA, Royall RM, Grega MA, Borowicz LM, Quaskey S, McKhann GM. Cognitive changes 5 years after coronary artery bypass grafting. Is there evidence of late decline? *Archives of Neurology* 2001; 58: 598–604.
5. Stygall J, Fitzgerald G, Steed L, et al. Cognitive change 5 years after coronary artery bypass surgery. *Health Psychology* 2003; 22: 579–586.

Chapter 6

Haematology

Dr A Cohen and Dr D Farran

Heparin and protamine 92
Preoperative antithrombotic drugs 94
Bleeding and transfusion 96
The postoperative bleeding patient 102
Management of patients requiring postoperative
    anticoagulation 106
Further reading 107

Heparin and protamine

To understand the use of pharmacological interventions, a broad overview of coagulation pathways is required.

Coagulation pathways

Classically coagulation is described as extrinsic and intrinsic systems with a final common pathway. The extrinsic system involves exposed tissue factor which activates factor VII, and the intrinsic system is initiated by exposure of blood to collagen leading to activation of factors XII, XI, and IX. Both pathways generate active factor X, which in turn leads to thrombin and fibrin formation. In fact there is a more complicated and finely balanced system with cross-over of the two pathways.

Heparin and protamine management

Careful management of anticoagulation and its reversal can contribute to avoidance of bleeding following cardiac surgery.

Heparin management

Heparin binds with and accelerates the action of antithrombin III (AT-III), inhibiting the activated factors XII, XI, IX, and thrombin. Increasing evidence suggests that higher doses of heparin can contribute to avoidance of postoperative coagulopathy. The mechanism for this involves reduction of thrombin generation, which in turn leads to reduced platelet activation and consumption, particularly when CPB is used, so that platelets are preserved for the postoperative period. Proponents of this theory advocate direct monitoring of heparin levels (e.g. using the Hepcon analyser), since these have been shown to drop during CPB; or alternatively administering additional heparin at fixed intervals, regardless of the activated clotting time (ACT).

Protamine management

Administration of an adequate dose of protamine is necessary to avoid residual heparinization in the postoperative period; however, excessive amounts of protamine cause platelet inhibition and contribute to postoperative bleeding. Furthermore, monitoring of adequate heparin reversal is difficult. Although the ACT is commonly used for this purpose, it is known to be a poor guide in low level heparinization, so that incomplete reversal may not be identified. Paired tests (either ACT or TEG) on the same sample using heparinase may give a better indication of the presence of heparin.

When choosing the dose of protamine:
- Significant amounts of additional heparin may have been given during CPB by the perfusionist.
- Elimination of heparin occurs throughout CPB.
- The half-life of protamine unbound to heparin is short (less than 30 minutes); additional protamine may need to be given with any heparin containing 'pump blood' given later in the post-CPB period.
- Although it is often recommended to give protamine on a 'ml for ml' basis with the initial heparin dose, some studies report that the optimal protamine dose is 0.5 to 0.7 (mg protamine/1000 IU heparin) of the total heparin dose.

Problems with heparinization

Heparin resistance

Heparin resistance is an inability to reach adequate heparinization with conventional heparin doses. It is sometimes seen with preoperative heparin use, which leads to reduced AT-III levels. Predisposing factors include infective endocarditis, ventricular aneurysm with thrombus, hepatic failure, and also congenital AT-III reduction. Most cases respond to increased doses of heparin. Otherwise supplementation of AT-III in the form of recombinant human AT-III or using fresh frozen plasma (FFP) is required.

Heparin-induced thrombocytopaenia (HIT) syndrome

HIT (sometimes referred to as HITT if thrombosis is present) typically develops after 5 to 14 days of heparin therapy but can occur after a day if there is previous exposure to heparin. HIT is caused by IgG antibodies to the heparin/platelet factor 4 complex. These result in a marked drop in platelet count. The risk for the patient is thrombosis rather than bleeding because platelets are activated and thrombus is formed. HIT is likely to be under-diagnosed as many differential diagnoses exist, such as sepsis and platelet clumping.

Diagnosis begins with clinical suspicion and is confirmed using enzyme-linked immunosorbent assay (ELISA). The laboratory diagnosis is confirmed by adding platelets and serum with heparin and detecting serotonin release (a sign of platelet activation).

Management involves imaging aimed at the detection of possible thrombosis and discontinuing all heparin. A heparin alternative (see below) should be used as ongoing protection against thrombus.

Alternatives to heparin

In the presence of HITS or heparin allergy, alternatives may be required. Hirudin (isolated from leech salivary glands) and lepirudin are agents that bind tightly to thrombin and block all thrombin-catalysed reactions, including activation of protein C, so AT-III is bypassed. Their actions are short-lasting, so they are administered by continuous infusion and require monitoring using ecarin clotting time (ECT). They are not reversed by protamine; the infusion is ceased following termination of CPB and the action wears off. Clinical experience of these drugs for patients requiring CPB is limited, underlying the importance of accurate diagnosis (or exclusion) of HITS.

Danaparoid, a heparinoid/factor Xa inhibitor, is more widely used in ITU patients with HITS. It has a longer half-life.

Preoperative antithrombotic drugs

Patients presenting for cardiac surgery may have been managed with antithrombotic drugs.

Warfarin

An inhibitor of vitamin K-dependent coagulation. If possible, warfarin should be discontinued 3–4 days before surgery, aiming for an INR <2. Heparin infusion may be started if necessary. In more urgent situations, it can be reversed with Prothrombin Complex Concentrate (PCC). Fresh frozen plasma or vitamin K can also be used and have a longer duration of action.

Aspirin

A cyclooxygenase inhibitor is used in patients with coronary or cerebro-vascular disease. The benefit of continuing aspirin for graft patency must be weighed against the detrimental effect on platelet function post-surgery.

Clopidogrel

Clopidogrel is a non-competitive antagonist at platelet ADP receptors. Blockade induces profound inhibition of platelet aggregation, which continues for as long as the platelet survives. Clopidogrel and aspirin together are synergistic and a common combination in cardiac surgical patients with previous coronary interventions.

Glycoprotein IIb/IIIa receptor antagonists (abciximab; ReoPro)

GPIIb/IIIa receptors are platelet fibrinogen receptors that cause fibrinogen bridging and platelet aggregation. Abciximab inhibits platelet aggregation, and reduces mortality and morbidity during percutaneous coronary intervention (PCI). If emergency surgery becomes necessary there is potential for severe bleeding.

Bleeding and transfusion

Cardiac surgery is a major user of blood and blood components (FFP and platelets). Cardiac anaesthetists and surgeons should strive to ensure appropriate use. (The term 'blood product' more accurately refers to substances that have been manufactured from whole blood.)

There are two important types of transfusion in the cardiac surgical patient:
- Avoidance of unnecessary transfusion.
- Management of the severely bleeding patient.

Blood conservation in cardiac surgery

This is a multidisciplinary exercise involving anaesthetists, surgeons, perfusionists, and nurses.

Factors that increase the risk of perioperative blood transfusion include:
- Increased age.
- Low red cell volume (preop anaemia or low body size).
- Preop antiplatelet (especially clopidogrel) or anticoagulant therapy.
- Reoperation or complex procedures.
- Emergency surgery.
- Non-cardiac comorbidity.

This allows a targeted approach for blood conservation measures (antifibrinolytics, cell salvage).

There are three ways of avoiding unnecessary transfusion:

Start with higher red cell mass
- Preoperative autologous donation – rarely used in UK, especially in patients with coronary artery disease.
- Erythropoietin – safe and effective in increasing preoperative Hb in patients with anaemia (in combination with iron supplements); rarely used in the UK, because of expense.

Minimize blood loss
- Preoperative measures – e.g. planned cessation of antiplatelet and anticoagulant treatment.
- Intraoperative measures:
  - Meticulous surgical haemostasis.
  - Appropriate heparin/protamine management.
  - Additional pharmacological interventions (☐ see also antifibrinolytics p. 97).
  - Intraoperative cell salvage (☐ see also p. 99).
  - Avoidance of CPB.
  - Use of specialized CPB techniques, e.g. heparin-bonded circuits.
  - Appropriate use of blood components.
  - Topical sealants (☐ see also Bioglue, Tisseel, FloSeal, p. 99).
  - Acute normovolaemic haemodilution.

- Postoperative measures:
  - Avoidance of hypertension.
  - Appropriate use of haemostatic therapy.
  - Postoperative cell salvage.
  - Tamponade using PEEP.

Appropriate transfusion
- Red cells:
  - Trigger-based management.
  - Although centres vary, most UK units use a postoperative haematocrit threshold of approximately 24% (Hb 8 g/dl) measured by point of care photometry (Haemocue). Conductance measurement by modern blood gas analysers is acceptable, although less accurate.
  - Each unit of red cells should only be given following a current measurement of haematocrit/haemoglobin, unless the patient is bleeding severely, or the haematocrit is low (e.g. less than 18%; Hb 6 g/dl). On this basis, single unit transfusions are acceptable and can be viewed as a unit saved rather than a unit wasted.
  - Judgement should be exercised for individual patients.
  - During cardiopulmonary bypass with moderate hypothermia, a haematocrit threshold of 18% (Hb 6 g/dl) is acceptable, although higher levels are appropriate for patients at risk of ischaemia or end-organ injury, or during normothermic CPB.

Antifibrinolytics

Antifibrinolytics are commonly used to reduce blood loss occurring as a result of fibrinolysis caused by contact of blood with the CPB circuit. They limit the breakdown of clot by plasmin and can be classified as serine protease inhibitors (such as aprotinin) and lysine analogues (such as tranexamic acid and aminocaproic acid).

Choice of antifibrinolytics is based on the following factors:
- Efficacy.
- Expense.
- Side effects.

Aprotinin

Aprotinin is a polypeptide (6500 Daltons) that inhibits a number of enzymes, including plasmin (resulting in its antifibrinolytic effect) and kallikrein. It has been widely used in cardiac surgery since the late 1980s when a significant reduction in bleeding was observed following cardiac surgery in patients given high doses of the drug. More recently, its use has been associated with concerns about postoperative cardiovascular complications including renal failure, stroke, and myocardial infarction, as well as mortality. Its use in the United Kingdom has declined substantially. It remains available on a named patient basis.

The dose of aprotinin varies. The high dose 'Hammersmith regimen' consists of 2 MU (100 ml) of aprotinin pre-CPB; 2 MU of aprotinin added to the CPB prime; and a perioperative infusion of 0.5 MU aprotinin continued into the early postoperative period. In addition, it is usual to give an intravenous 'test dose' of 2–3 ml of the drug before giving the full loading dose (and before adding any aprotinin to the CPB prime). Due to its peptide nature, aprotinin has the potential to cause hypersensitivity reactions, including anaphylaxis (most commonly on repeat exposure within six months of previous administration of the drug). The effectiveness of the test dose has been questioned.

Aprotinin is a mild anticoagulant and it interferes with the celite ACT, although not the kaolin ACT. If using celite ACT, a threshold of 750 seconds is required before commencing CPB.

Lysine analogues

The lysine analogues, tranexamic acid and epsilon-aminocaproic acid, are also used to reduce surgical blood loss due to fibrinolysis. They both act by binding to the lysine binding site on the plasminogen molecule, inhibiting its activity.

The lysine analogues are less expensive than aprotinin and have minimal side effects but are also less efficacious at reducing blood loss. Different dosage regimens have been described; the dose range in the literature and in clinical practice for tranexamic acid varies between 30 mg/kg and 100 mg/kg.

Desmopressin

Desmopressin acts by releasing von Willebrand factor, tissue plasminogen activator, and endogenous factor VIII precursors from vascular endothelium. It is not used routinely but may be effective in patients with uraemic platelet dysfunction or those with acquired or inherited von Willebrand's disease.

Recombinant factor VIIa (rFVIIa: Novoseven®)

Recombinant factor VIIa is reserved for life-threatening perioperative non-surgical bleeding refractory to other measures.

It acts by initiating an early and massive 'thrombin burst' in areas where there are activated platelets, causing a massive stimulus to coagulation. The mechanism of this effect is the direct stimulation of factor X on activated platelets to initiate the production of large amounts of thrombin (the 'thrombin burst'). This is in contrast to the effect of endogenous FVIIa, which is responsible for the initiation of the coagulation process by binding to tissue factor.

The use of rFVIIa is controversial for the following reasons:
- Most evidence supporting its use is anecdotal.
- Meta-analyses from randomized studies have failed to confirm the reports of immediate clinical improvement following administration of rFVIIa.
- It is very expensive.
- Concern over the possibility of systemic thrombotic complications.

Nevertheless, it has been increasingly used in severe intractable bleeding resistant to all other measures.

Use – practical aspects
- Use of rFVIIa should not replace other measures (attention to surgical haemostasis and standard treatment of coagulopathy).
- Dose: 70–90 µg/kg given over several minutes (repeated after two hours, if necessary).
- Cardiac units will benefit from written guidelines for use of rFVIIa.

Topical sealants

- A variety of topical sealants are becoming increasingly used in refractory bleeding, particularly where there is a 'surgical' origin.
- Tisseel is an aprotinin-containing fibrin glue, which may be applied to areas not actively bleeding (e.g. before restoration of blood flow).
- FloSeal, a thrombin/gelatine-based combination, may be used when there is active blood loss.
- Bioglue is a glutaraldehyde/albumin combination that appears to have a stronger adhesive effect than the other sealants and is becoming popular.
- The evidence base for all of these products is mainly case reports/ series but their clinical effectiveness is accepted. There are some concerns about long-term sequelae of products such as Bioglue.

Choice of surgery, e.g. OPCAB

'Off-pump' coronary surgery is associated with a lower transfusion rate, partly because of avoidance of CPB-related coagulopathy, but also because of avoidance of haemodilution related to the CPB prime.

Cell salvage

- Intraoperative cell salvage (IOCS) is commonly used during cardiac surgery for patients at high risk for bleeding. In routine patients it may not be cost-effective. Costs can be minimized by not opening processing disposables until sufficient volumes of blood have been collected. The use of thrombin-containing topical sealants may be a contraindication to the use of IOCS.
- Preoperative plateletpheresis with post-CPB administration of collected platelets has not been shown to be effective, despite theoretical advantages.
- Postoperative reinfusion of shed mediastinal blood may be beneficial provided the blood is washed in a cell saver. Its routine use on postoperative ICUs presents logistical difficulties (e.g. training, expense, workload) and it is currently not widely used. Infusion of unwashed shed mediastinal blood contains high levels of inflammatory cytokines, complement, endotoxin, and fibrinolytic substances.

Predonation

Although popular in other countries, preoperative autologous donation is not widely used in the UK because of practical constraints.

PEEP

Although PEEP has not been found to be useful in preventing excessive postoperative bleeding, it may be useful in treating it.

Choice of CPB equipment – reservoirs, bonded circuits

- Heparin-bonded CPB circuits and 'mini-CPB' circuits (creating less haemodilution) may reduce coagulopathic blood loss and transfusion. They are not yet widely used because of cost and complexity. The mini-CPB circuit requires understanding of the implications of having no reservoir, but has been associated with a reduction in red cell transfusion.

- Careful use of cardiotomy suction avoiding aspiration of air has reduced platelet activation during prolonged CPB.
- Retrograde autologous CPB priming involves release of the arterial return clamp immediately prior to CPB in order to partially fill the CPB reservoir ('backbleeding'). This minimizes the prime volume and reduces haemodilution. The technique lowers transfusion rates but is not widely used, primarily because of unfamiliarity and concerns about safety.

Surgical Blood Ordering Schedule (SBOS)

Consideration of the routine cross-match is an important means of avoiding unnecessary wastage, laboratory time, and expense. The advent of 'electronic issue' has allowed single unit and even zero unit cross-matches for routine coronary and valve surgery. More complex or redo cases should usually have at least three units of blood cross-matched.

Non-red cell haemostatic blood components
- In general, these should be given only:
  - To patients who are bleeding.
  - When guided by tests of haemostasis.

The two most important factors in blood conservation are surgical attention and avoidance of unnecessary transfusion by appropriate trigger-based transfusion practice.

The postoperative bleeding patient

Excessive postoperative bleeding is an important and frequent complication of cardiac surgery.

Chest tube drainage should be measured at least hourly after cardiac surgery; haemoglobin or haematocrit should initially be measured at least two-hourly. Blood loss usually diminishes over the course of the first 12 to 18 hours.

The causes of bleeding following cardiac surgery are multiple, and include:
- 'Surgical' bleeding (from anastomoses, sternal wires, and grafts).
- Residual heparinization (either inadequate reversal or heparin rebound).
- CPB-related coagulopathy and/or fibrinolysis.
- Drug-induced platelet dysfunction (e.g. clopidogrel).

Excessive bleeding perioperatively should be managed aggressively with:
- Appropriate haemostatic tests to assess for non-surgical bleeding.
- Prescription of drugs and/or blood components (platelets and/or FFP) as necessary.
- Transfusion of red cells to maintain haemoglobin/haematocrit.
- Surgical re-exploration if necessary.

Investigation of the cause

The cause of bleeding may be apparent from careful review of the patient's preoperative status and knowledge of the intraoperative course. The total heparin dose (including by the perfusionist) and the protamine dose should be reviewed.

Blood should be sent for a full blood count and clotting screen and thromboelastography (TEG). A chest X-ray in the bleeding patient is performed to assess for pleural collections.

Thromboelastography (TEG)

TEG is now used in the majority of UK cardiac surgical units. It is a 'visco-elastic' test of haemostasis, which measures the strength of a developing blood clot over a period of 60–90 minutes, at 37°C. The result is a computerized trace, which has a characteristic cigar shape, where the width of the trace represents the strength of the clot. The test is usually carried out following the addition of a coagulation activator such as kaolin, which speeds up the clotting process and increases the utility of the test.

The parameters of the trace are measured automatically. The two most important ones are:
- **Maximum amplitude (MA):** The width of the trace at its widest point. It represents the strength of the clot, and is mainly a function of platelet activity (number and function), but also fibrinogen cross-linkage.
- **The 'r' (reaction) time:** This is the time from the start of the test until the trace starts to split (width 2 mm). Initiation of coagulation measured by the TEG depends on contact activation; therefore the r time is analogous to standard tests of coagulation such as PT and aPTT. It is prolonged by clotting factor depletion or heparinization. These can be distinguished by carrying out paired tests from the same sample. One of the tests is carried out in the presence of heparinase, which

inactivates heparin, and comparison of the r times indicates whether the sample contains heparin. This is a useful test for detecting low level residual heparinization following protamine administration.

- Other parameters (k time; alpha angle) are less useful. Fibrinolysis is easily recognized by simple observation of the trace but can be quantified by the TEG software.

The TEG has several advantages over traditional clotting tests:

- It is quick. Useful information about haemostasis can be obtained within 20 minutes of sampling. This means that empirical treatment of presumed coagulopathy is less frequently justified.
- It is a 'point of care' test, carried out in the surgical unit.
- It has also been shown to be superior to the PT and aPTT as a predictor of bleeding; this may be because it is a whole blood test in which the platelet surface is available for coagulation reactions, as *in vivo*. The r time is often normal when the INR is mildly elevated (<1.5) and it may be reasonable to withhold FFP in this situation.

The major disadvantage of the traditional TEG in cardiac surgical practice is its insensitivity to aspirin and clopidogrel. Patients taking these drugs, particularly clopidogrel, who have significant bleeding are often given platelets, regardless of results from the TEG. The platelet mapping assay overcomes these problems.

Routine use of the TEG allows protocolized management of postoperative bleeding. An example is given below:

- MA <48 mm: Give 1 platelet pool.
- MA <40 mm: Give 2 platelet pools.

Plain trace	Heparinase trace	
r >14 mm <21 mm	Identical	Give 1 FFP
r >21 mm <28 mm	Identical	Give 2 FFP
r >28 mm	Identical	Give 4 FFP
r >14 mm <21 mm	Normal	Give 25 mg protamine
r >21 mm	Normal	Give 50 mg protamine

Treatment options for non-surgical bleeding

These include:

- Haemodynamic control: It is important to control blood pressure with adequate sedation and vasodilators. The systolic blood pressure should usually be limited to 100–120 mmHg in bleeding patients.
- Further protamine (25–50 mg): This can be given over 2–3 minutes.
- Restoration of normothermia: Hypothermic-related platelet dysfunction will aggravate postoperative bleeding. It is not detected by tests such as the TEG, which are carried out at 37°C. Ideally fluid warmers should be used for patients who are bleeding, particularly when infusion of recently thawed FFP is given.

- PEEP has been shown to be useful in post-cardiotomy bleeding but it is important to be wary of the possibility of a drop in venous return in a patient who may already be hypovolaemic.
- Aprotinin (1 MU over 10 minutes, followed by 0.5 MU per hour): (📖 see also p. 97) Postoperative aprotinin has been shown to be useful in postoperative bleeding where fibrinolysis is suspected, and is a useful empirical option. Renal function should be taken into consideration.
- Platelet infusion for:
  - A low platelet count (less than 50,000).
  - A narrow TEG maximum amplitude (<50 mm).
  - A history of recent clopidogrel administration, regardless of the TEG appearance (as this does not detect clopidogrel effect). Platelet infusion may also be considered in patients who have a history of recent aspirin administration, although this is more controversial since aspirin is a weaker antiplatelet agent.
  - Administration of platelets to patients with suspected surgical blood loss is not recommended and should not be allowed to delay re-exploration.
- FFP is often transfused unnecessarily following cardiac surgery. Significant depletion of clotting factors is uncommon, except in patients with pre-existing coagulopathy (usually due to hepatic dysfunction or treatment with warfarin) or those with particularly long bypass times. FFP should not be given empirically, particularly if the TEG is available. In this respect it is more useful than the INR and aPTT.
- Factor VIIa: Recombinant factor VIIa (rFVIIa) is reserved for patients with refractory life-threatening bleeding (see above).

Red cell transfusion

It is important to measure haematocrit or haemoglobin frequently in patients who are bleeding heavily, using 'near patient' devices. Spectrophotometric (Haemocue) measurement is ideal for this purpose, although the conductivity-based measurements made by blood gas analysers are also acceptable.

It is usual to maintain the postoperative haematocrit above 23–24% (Hb 8 g/dl). A higher threshold of 28–30% (Hb 9–10 g/l) may be prudent in patients with postoperative concerns regarding coronary anatomy (e.g. incomplete revascularization; small vessel coronary disease in patients with diabetes). Autologous products should be given first. In patients who are bleeding heavily it is sensible to maintain an availability of at least three units of bank blood.

Surgical re-exploration

Approximately 2–5% of patients require surgical re-exploration. As a general rule, the following chest tube losses should trigger consideration of reopening the chest:

- >400 ml/hr in the first hour.
- >200 ml/hr in two consecutive hours.
- >100 ml/hr in four consecutive hours.

It is usual to exclude or treat non-surgical bleeding before considering return to theatre for resternotomy, particularly since re-exploration is associated with increased postoperative mortality. Brisk life-threatening bleeding may need early re-exploration before the results of haemostatic tests are available.

Management of patients requiring postoperative anticoagulation

Following cardiac surgery, certain groups of patients require formal anticoagulation. Other groups of patients will need to restart warfarin for an indication other than their recent surgery, such as atrial fibrillation. In general, low molecular weight heparin commences on the day following surgery. Patients requiring ongoing coagulation are then commenced on warfarin, although care must be taken with timing of removal of temporary pacing wires (INR <2.5).

Further reading

1. Karkouti K, Scott Beattie W, Crowther M, et al. The role of recombinant factor VIIa in on-pump cardiac surgery: Proceedings of the Canadian Consensus Conference. *Canadian Journal of Anesthesia* 2007; 54: 573–582.
2. Karkouti K, Yau T, van Rensburg A, et al. The effects of a treatment protocol for cardiac surgical patients with excessive blood loss. *Vox Sanguinis* 2006; 91: 148–156.
3. Murphy G, Reeves B, Rogers C, Rizvi S, Culliford L, Angelini G. Increased mortality, postoperative morbidity and cost after red blood cell transfusion in patients having cardiac surgery. *Circulation* 2007; 116: 2544–2552.
4. Pouplard C, May M, Regina S, Marchand M, Fusciardi J, Gruel Y. Changes in platelet count after cardiac surgery can effectively predict the development of pathogenic heparin-dependent antibodies. *British Journal of Haematology* 2005; 128: 837–841.
5. Welsby I, Podgoreanu M, Phillips-Bute B, et al. Genetic factors contribute to bleeding after cardiac surgery. *Journal of Thrombosis and Haemostasis* 2005; 3: 1206–1212.

The editors are grateful to Andrew Mumford, Gavin Murphy, Murli Krishna and Edwin Massy for contributions to this chapter.

The inflammatory response

Dr L Kevin

The inflammatory response *110*
Activation of the inflammatory response *112*
Components of the inflammatory response *114*
Organ effects *118*
Modulation of the inflammatory response *120*
Further reading *123*

The inflammatory response

Patients undergoing cardiac surgery exhibit activation of inflammatory cells including leucocytes, monocytes, basophils, and mast cells. These cells release a variety of active substances including cytokines, chemokines, and reactive oxygen species. Inflammation is a protective response to prevent infection and ultimately to restore organ homeostasis and promote wound healing. In the majority of patients undergoing cardiac surgery, activation of inflammatory pathways is mild, self-limited, and sub-clinical. However, a significant minority exhibit more extreme and prolonged inflammation similar to the systemic inflammatory response syndrome (SIRS) seen in critical care patients.

There is evidence that inflammatory activation contributes to organ dysfunction and adverse outcomes. Inflammation is implicated in coagulopathy, respiratory failure, cardiac failure, renal failure, and neurocognitive deficits. It is not clear why some patients follow an uncomplicated recovery pattern whereas others enter uncontrolled SIRS. Host factors, including genetic polymorphisms and organ comorbidities, probably interact with intraoperative factors (duration of bypass, haemodynamic instability) to determine the severity of the response.

Diagnosis

Conventional definition criteria (pyrexia, tachypnoea, tachycardia, and leucocytosis) are not useful since:
- Temperature may be abnormal due to CPB and surgery.
- Respiratory rate is controlled by mechanical ventilation.
- Heart rate is frequently controlled by pacemakers or beta-blockers.
- Leucocytosis is common in many patients.

Serum markers may therefore be used, including:
- Cytokines, such as tumour necrosis factor-alpha (TNF-α) and interleukins (ILs).
- Complement system components, such as C3.
- Acute phase reactants, such as C-reactive protein (CRP).
- Products of tissue injury, including peroxidation products of free-radical mediated injury.

Activation of the inflammatory response

Surgical trauma

Tissue trauma activates inflammation and coagulation. Complement activation occurs even without CPB. Denuded endothelium exposes tissue factor leading to activation of the coagulation cascade. Activated coagulation factors interact with inflammatory cascades causing further inflammation.

Contact with the extracorporeal circuit

Healthy vascular endothelium suppresses inflammation and coagulation by releasing inhibitors such nitric oxide (NO), prostacyclin, and tissue factor pathway inhibitor. These protective mechanisms are lost when blood makes contact with the extracorporeal circuit. Two important pathways become activated:

• The complement system.
• The kallikrein-kininogen-kinin system.

Air-blood mixing

Blood-gas interfaces in the venous reservoir and cardiotomy suction activate cellular immunity.

Ischaemia-reperfusion injury

Reperfusion of ischaemic tissue causes generation of free radicals. Ischaemia-reperfusion also activates cellular immunity. Neutrophils accumulate in reperfused tissue and cause tissue injury by generating further free radicals and through release of cytotoxic enzymes such as elastase and myeloperoxidase.

Heparin and protamine

Heparin has weak anti-inflammatory effects. In contrast, heparin-protamine complexes activate the complement system. This has several important downstream effects (see below).

Coagulation-fibrinolytic system activation

The coagulation-fibrinolytic and inflammatory systems are linked. Thrombin, factor Xa, and fibrin directly activate mononuclear cells causing the synthesis of cytokines. Activated platelets also contribute by releasing a pro-inflammatory mediator, CD40 ligand.

Acute phase reaction

Cytokines, including IL-1β and IL-6, induce hepatic synthesis of a broad range of proteins, termed acute phase reactants (APRs). APRs, including CRP, serum amyloid A, and fibrinogen, function in host defence, tissue repair, and control of response duration. CRP has attracted interest as a serum marker. More recently evidence has emerged for an active biologic role for CRP; it is believed to contribute to myocardial ischaemia/reperfusion injury and atrial fibrillation.

Blood transfusion

Blood transfusion alone can promote inflammation. Leucocytes are activated and cytokine levels increase. A worse outcome for patients who receive multiple units of allogenic blood has been documented despite multiple confounding factors. There is also concern about autotransfusion of shed blood suctioned from the thoracic cavity. Blood retrieved in this manner makes contact with non-endothelial surfaces and undergoes trauma and blood-air interfacing. Elevated levels of pro-inflammatory cytokines and activated leucocytes are found in cardiotomy suction and cell-saved blood.

Endotoxin

Endotoxin is a component of the cell wall of gram-negative bacteria. Plasma levels have been shown to rise during cardiopulmonary bypass. The origin of this endotoxin is uncertain but the presumed source is gut bacteria that translocate to the circulation during splanchnic hypoperfusion. Endotoxin has the following effects:

- Activation of the cellular immune response.
- Activation of complement via the alternate pathway.
- Activation of inducible nitric oxide synthase (iNOS).
- Enhanced expression of tissue factor on macrophages leading to extrinsic coagulation pathway activation.

There is evidence that natural immunity to endotoxin protects against organ dysfunction following cardiac surgery. Nonetheless, the magnitude of endotoxaemia during cardiac surgery is variable and its significance is controversial.

Genetic predisposition

There is marked inter-patient variability in the extent of inflammatory response to cardiac surgery. Certain patients may have a genetic predisposition to an exaggerated response and adverse outcomes:

- A polymorphism in the TNF-α locus is associated with increased TNF-α and increased rates of postoperative ventricular dysfunction and respiratory complications.
- An IL-6 polymorphism is associated with increased IL-6 levels and a greater incidence of postoperative atrial fibrillation.
- A polymorphism for complement C4 activation is linked to increased capillary permeability.

Components of the inflammatory response

Complement

The complement system comprises in excess of 20 proteins involved in multiple aspects of inflammation and coagulation/fibrinolysis. Activation of complement occurs through two pathways, classical and alternate. During and after cardiac surgery there are several triggers to activate complement:

- Contact of blood with the extracorporeal circuit (alternate pathway).
- Ischaemia-reperfusion (classical pathway).
- An immune reaction to protamine-heparin complexes (classical pathway).
- Endotoxin exposure (alternate pathway).
- During the days after cardiac surgery the classical pathway is triggered as part of the acute phase response (CRP-triggered).

Classical and alternate pathways ultimately lead to generation of the anaphylatoxins C3a and C5a, and the 'terminal membrane attack complex', C5b-9. C3a and C5a cause release of histamine from mast cells, increased vascular permeability, and activation of leucocytes. C3a triggers platelet activation. C5b-9 is proteolytic and causes direct cellular injury. Levels of complement activation have been shown to correlate with pulmonary, renal, cardiac, and CNS dysfunction.

Cellular response

Cellular components of inflammation are central to tissue injury:

- Neutrophils are activated by complement (C5a), cytokines, and ischaemia-reperfusion. When activated they express adhesion molecules causing them to adhere to endothelium via corresponding endothelial adhesion molecules, and then to transmigrate to the interstitium. Neutrophils generate cytokines and reactive oxygen species (ROS). Degranulation of neutrophils leads to release of the cytotoxic enzymes elastase and myeloperoxidase. These substances cause lipid peroxidation of cell membranes, proteolysis, cellular oedema, and cellular death. Neutrophil-mediated injury is widespread but is especially severe in ischaemia-reperfused tissue. Furthermore, leucocyte-platelet aggregates cause microvascular obstruction.
- Mast cells, monocytes, macrophages, and basophils are also activated. They release mediators including histamine and leukotrienes that cause vasodilation, pulmonary vasoconstriction, and increased vascular permeability. Monocytes produce pro-inflammatory cytokines. Monocytes and macrophages express tissue factor causing activation of coagulation pathways.

Cytokines

Cytokines are signalling proteins released by multiple cell types including activated lymphocytes, macrophages, monocytes, and endothelial cells.

They are responsible for modulation of the immune response. The cytokines most important to the inflammatory response to cardiac surgery include:

- IL-1β: Initiation of cell-mediated immune response, activation of T-cells and macrophages, iNOS expression, production of acute phase reactants.
- TNF-α: Neutrophil activation, adhesion molecule expression, iNOS expression, myocardial dysfunction.
- IL-6: Endogenous pyrogen, production of acute phase reactants, myocardial dysfunction.
- IL-8: Neutrophil chemotaxis and activation.

A characteristic temporal profile is seen with IL-1β and TNF-α peaking early and IL-6 and IL-8 peaking later. Other cytokines are *anti-inflammatory*, serving to counteract the above effects. In addition, soluble cytokine receptors 'mop up' circulating pro-inflammatory cytokines. As the inflammatory response progresses, there is a shift in production of pro- to anti-inflammatory substances, thus the process is self-limiting. Patients who fail to adequately achieve this shift enter uncontrolled SIRS. Important anti-inflammatory cytokines and soluble receptors are:

- IL-10: Inhibition of neutrophil-endothelial interactions, inhibition of TNF-α and IL-1β.
- IL-1 receptor antagonist (IL-1ra): Binds to IL-1β.
- TNF soluble receptors 1 and 2 (TNFSR): Bind to TNF-α.

Kallikrein-kininogen-kinin system

Contact with artificial surfaces causes factor XII activation with subsequent conversion of prekallikrein to kallikrein and generation of bradykinin from high molecular weight kininogen. Bradykinin causes vasodilation, pain sensitization, and increased endothelial permeability. Kallikrein activates the intrinsic coagulation cascade causing formation of thrombin.

Coagulation-fibrinolysis

Coagulation and fibrinolytic cascades are activated by surgical trauma and by contact with the extracorporeal circuit. There is a complex interaction between coagulation and inflammation: factor Xa, thrombin, and fibrin cause direct activation of the cellular response, induce expression of adhesion molecules on endothelial cells, and promote cytokine release. Conversely, activated inflammatory systems activate coagulation: activated macrophages express tissue factor, which activates the extrinsic pathway of coagulation. Fibrinogen is an acute phase reactant with a prothrombotic effect.

Nitric oxide (NO)

Endotoxin and pro-inflammatory cytokines activate the inducible form of NO synthase (iNOS). iNOS produces much larger quantities of NO than the constitutive form (cNOS). While small quantities of NO are essential for regulation of vascular tone, large excesses of NO cause vasodilation and increased pulmonary vascular permeability. Excess NO is also implicated in reversible myocardial dysfunction ('myocardial stunning') and in neurocognitive dysfunction after CPB.

Reactive oxygen species (ROS)

Oxygen-containing free radicals or reactive oxygen species (ROS) are generated by neutrophils in a reaction catalysed by the enzyme NADPH oxidase. This is the so-called 'respiratory burst', an important component of host defence. Reperfusion of ischaemic tissues causes generation of ROS in a reaction catalysed by xanthine oxidase. In the heart the main source of ROS is the mitochondria. ROS attack multiple cell substituents, particularly lipid membranes. ROS-mediated injury has been implicated in post-ischaemic ventricular failure, vascular dysfunction, arrhythmias, necrosis, and apoptosis.

Elastase and myeloperoxidase

These proteolytic enzymes are released from neutrophil granules. Damage is inflicted on endothelial cells and subendothelial structures.

Organ effects

Pulmonary (📖 see also Chapter 9)

Cardiac surgery is associated with post-operative increased extravascular lung water, decreased pulmonary compliance, and increased work of breathing. There may be acute lung injury in the most severely affected patients. Serum levels of TNF-α, IL-6, and IL-8 correlate with postoperative pulmonary dysfunction and duration of ventilation. Furthermore, high levels of cytokines are detected in serum and bronchoalveolar lavage specimens of affected patients. Histologic studies show extensive neutrophil sequestration in the lungs.

Renal (📖 see also Chapter 8)

The incidence of renal failure complicating cardiac surgery is 2–5%. Aetiology is multifactorial. CPB-associated factors, including embolism of plaque from the ascending aorta and non-pulsatile flow, are believed to contribute. Some trials have found an association between duration of CPB and risk of renal failure. Acute renal failure is associated with SIRS in critically ill patients.

CNS (📖 see also Chapter 5)

CNS injury after cardiac surgery ranges from stroke (incidence 1–8%) to subtle neurocognitive deficits (incidence up to 80%). Evidence implicating the inflammatory response includes an association between duration of CPB and elevation of serum S100β, a marker of neuronal cell death. In addition, several trials utilizing therapies to suppress the inflammatory response have reported improved neurologic outcome.

Cardiac

Cardiac dysfunction after cardiac surgery can be attributed to multiple factors including incomplete myocardial preservation and revascularization. The contribution of the inflammatory response is uncertain. Biopsies of cardiac muscle show accumulation of neutrophils after ischaemia/ reperfusion. Cytokines IL-1β, IL-6, and TNF-α depress contractility. Particular interest has focused on atrial fibrillation. The incidence of atrial fibrillation is higher in patients that show increased monocyte activation, increased IL-6 levels, or CRP after cardiac surgery.

Modulation of the inflammatory response

Off-pump coronary bypass

Off-pump coronary bypass grafting raised expectations of reduced inflammation and improved outcomes. Trials have demonstrated decreased levels of complement, cytokines, and reactive oxygen species compared to on-pump. Although some investigators have reported improved renal and neurologic outcomes, others have found no difference. Despite avoidance of CPB, several potential triggers of the inflammatory response remain, including surgical trauma and formation of heparin-protamine complexes. Additional factors associated, such as haemodynamic instability, may mitigate the beneficial effects of reduced inflammation.

The Drew-Anderson technique

Arterial cannulation of both the aorta and the pulmonary artery, double venous cannulation of both atria, and continued ventilation of the lungs throughout CPB, provides a technique in which the patient's lungs are used as the gas exchange interface despite arrest of the heart. An extracorporeal oxygenator is avoided, thereby eliminating a major source of inflammatory activation. Small trials have shown decreased IL-6 and IL-8 and increased anti-inflammatory IL-10, along with decreased blood loss and duration of postoperative ventilation. The complexity of this technique has limited its popularity.

Design of the extracorporeal circuit

Heparin-coated circuits

Heparin molecules bound to the surface of the extracorporeal circuit reduce direct contact of blood with foreign material. Complement activation, leucocyte activation, and cytokine generation are reduced. Some clinical trials show improved outcomes, including reduced respiratory and renal dysfunction and shorter ICU stays. Whether the dose of systemic heparin should be reduced is controversial.

Pulsatile flow

Physiologic blood flow is pulsatile, a feature lost with conventional CPB. Non-pulsatile flow was suggested to be a contributor to inflammatory activation and has been specifically linked to renal injury. Technologies that create pulsatile flow have been assessed but have failed to provide evidence of improved outcomes.

Leucocyte depletion

Activated leucocytes are central to inflammation and contribute to ischaemia/reperfusion injury. Filtration of leucocytes during CPB has shown benefits in small clinical trials but this has not been widely adopted.

Ultrafiltration

Convection removes water and small molecules, including cytokines, from plasma. Removal of water is useful to overcome excess haemodilution during CPB. Clinical trials of ultrafiltration during CPB have confirmed reduced levels of cytokines. However, anti-inflammatory cytokines such as IL-10 are also removed, thus potentially countering beneficial effects. Benefits have been shown in paediatric cardiac surgery, where blood loss and duration of mechanical ventilation are reduced. In adult patients ultrafiltration has not been demonstrated to show significant benefit.

Corticosteroids

Multiple studies have used corticosteroids to attenuate the inflammatory response to cardiac surgery. Complement activation is reduced and the balance of pro- vs. anti-inflammatory cytokines is shifted favourably. Neutrophil sequestration and ROS release are also decreased, and iNOS expression is inhibited. Some studies show attenuated organ injury based on serum markers. Randomized controlled trials, however, have generally failed to show convincing outcome benefits. An additional consideration is the potential for hyperglycaemia, known to be associated with adverse outcomes such as wound infections, electrolyte abnormalities, and exacerbation of cerebral ischaemic injury. Corticosteroids have become standard therapy in some institutions but the practice is controversial.

Aprotinin

Aprotinin was widely used in cardiac surgery because of its haemostatic effects, related to inhibition of serine proteases including plasmin and plasminogen, central to the fibrinolytic cascade. Aprotinin also inhibits the serine protease kallikrein, required for contact activation. This effect is believed to account, at least in part, for decreases in pro-inflammatory cytokines with aprotinin. Other effects include decreases in complement activation and cytokine-induced iNOS expression. Protective effects of aprotinin have been shown on myocardial injury in animal models. Small clinical trials in high-risk patients show reductions in lung injury and stroke incidence. Doses required to elicit anti-inflammatory effects are higher than those required for the haemostatic effect.

A recent observational study and a prospective randomized trial have raised concerns over aprotinin's safety. The role of aprotinin is currently being re-evaluated in light of these concerns and some regulatory authorities have withdrawn its marketing authorization.

Antioxidants

Agents that inhibit the formation of ROS (allopurinol), or scavenge ROS (superoxide dismutase, vitamins C and E), or increase the supply of endogenously-produced antioxidants (N-acetylcysteine) have been used to attenuate radical-mediated tissue injury. Whilst laboratory studies have conclusively shown that antioxidant therapies reduce cardiac ischaemia-reperfusion injury, clinical trials in the setting of cardiac surgery have produced conflicting results.

Complement inhibitors

Small clinical trials using antibodies to complement C5 have shown decreases in CK-MB, blood loss, and adverse neurologic outcomes. A recent multicentre trial showed a reduction in mortality in high-risk patients although no benefit in low-risk patients, perhaps because in the latter the inflammatory response is self-limited.

Further reading

1. Carrier M, Menasche P, Levy JH, et al. Inhibition of complement activation by pexelizumab reduces death in patients undergoing combined aortic valve replacement and coronary artery bypass surgery. *Journal of Thoracic Cardiovascular Surgery* 2006; 131: 352–356.
2. Levi M, Cromheecke ME, de Jonge E, et al. Pharmacological strategies to decrease excessive blood loss in cardiac surgery: A meta-analysis of clinically relevant endpoints. *Lancet* 1999; 354: 1940–1947.
3. Mangano DT, Tudor IC, Dietzel C, et al. The risk associated with aprotinin in cardiac surgery. *New England Journal of Medicine* 2006; 354: 353–365

Further reading

Renal

*Dr A Smith, Dr S Webb, and
Dr S Allen*

Acute renal failure *126*
Prevention *130*
A practical approach to perioperative renal protection *134*
Key points *135*
Further reading *136*

Acute renal failure

Acute renal failure (ARF) is a serious complication associated with considerable morbidity and mortality. Renal dysfunction after surgery is often associated with multiple organ dysfunction syndrome and may result in a mortality of up to 60%. It is also associated with a high risk of infection, prolonged intensive care unit (ICU) and hospital stay, progression to chronic renal failure (CRF), and dialysis-dependent end-stage renal disease (ESRD). The chance of full recovery from an episode of ARF in the surgical setting is low – many patients progress to develop varying degrees of chronic renal dysfunction. A large multicentre cohort study demonstrated that ARF requiring dialysis occurred in 1.1% of cardiac surgical patients and was associated with an operative mortality of 63.7%. This confirmed that ARF was an independent predictor of mortality, resulting in a 7.9-fold increase in risk of death.

Definition of acute renal failure

The term acute renal failure is a non-specific description of an acute, sustained decrease in renal function. There is a spectrum of severity of acute renal injury ranging from mild reversible impairment to severe dysfunction necessitating renal replacement therapy (RRT). An international collaborative group, the Acute Dialysis Quality Initiative (ADQI), has formulated a standard grading system for acute renal dysfunction and has defined cardiac surgery-associated kidney injury (CSA-AKI). The term acute renal dysfunction encompasses the full range of abnormalities of renal function. The acronym RIFLE defines three grades of increasing severity of acute renal dysfunction (R, risk; I, injury; F, failure) and two outcome variables (L, loss; E, end-stage) that are based on the change in serum creatinine or urine output (Table 8.1). The RIFLE criteria have undergone evaluation in cardiac surgical patients and in ICU patients, and have been shown to appropriately define acute renal dysfunction. The acute kidney injury network (AKIN) has defined acute kidney injury as an abrupt increase in creatinine > 26μmol/l, 50% increase in creatinine or oliguria <0.5ml/kg/hr.

Table 8.1 RIFLE grading system for renal dysfunction

Grade	GFR criteria	Urine output criteria
R, Risk	Serum creatinine increase: 1.5-fold; GFR decrease: >25%	UO <0.5 ml/kg/hr for 6 hrs
I, Injury	Serum creatinine increase: 2-fold; GFR decrease: >50%	UO <0.5 ml/kg/hr for 12 hrs
F, Failure	Serum creatinine increase: 3-fold; GFR decrease: >75%; serum creatinine decrease: >350 μmol/l (4 mg/dl) with acute increase >44 μmol/l (0.5 mg/dl)	UO <0.3 ml/kg/hr for 24 hrs or anuria for 12 hrs
L, Loss	Persistent ARF = complete loss of renal function for >4 weeks	
E, End-stage	ESRD = complete loss of renal function for 3 months	

Pathophysiology

The aetiology of ARF is classically divided into pre-renal, renal, and post-renal causes. The majority of cases of ARF in surgical and critically ill patients are because of intrinsic renal causes; acute tubular necrosis (ATN), which is typically caused by ischaemic or toxic processes, is the most common of these.

Acute tubular necrosis

A combination of microvascular and tubular injury contributes to the development of ATN. Intra-renal vasoconstriction because of local vasoactive mediators, activation of tubuloglomerular feedback, structural endothelial damage, and leucocyte activation all lead to microvascular damage. Mechanisms of tubular injury include epithelial apoptosis and necrosis, tubular obstruction, and transtubular leak of glomerular filtrate. Inflammatory responses induced by renal ischaemia–reperfusion injury also play a significant role in the development of ATN.

Nephrotoxic agents

Nephrotoxic agents commonly used in perioperative patients include non-steroidal anti-inflammatory drugs, angiotensin-converting enzyme inhibitors, aldosterone-receptor antagonists, IV radio-contrast agents, aminoglycoside and beta-lactam antibiotics, amphotericin B, and ciclosporin (cyclosporine).

Cardiac and vascular surgery

Specific factors involved in the development of ARF related to cardiac surgery include:

- Renal hypo-perfusion outside the limits of auto-regulatory reserve, particularly during cardiopulmonary bypass (CPB), is a major determinant of ATN.
- The systemic inflammatory response syndrome (SIRS) triggered by major surgery results in cell-mediated and cytotoxic injury.
- ATN may also be exacerbated by renal embolic injury: aortic atheroma disrupted by operative manipulation and thrombus, air, lipid, and tissue may contribute to embolic load.
- Prolonged surgery produces haemolysis: renal excretion of haem-derivatives may result in renal tubular injury.
- Toxic injury from the administration of nephrotoxic drugs may also contribute to postoperative ARF. Patients who present for non-elective cardiac surgery shortly after preoperative cardiac catheterization are at increased risk related to both the radio-contrast load and surgery itself.

Risk factors

Evidence from epidemiological studies has established major risk factors for perioperative ARF (Table 8.2). Two risk stratification tools for ARF after cardiac surgery have been tested and validated. The incidence is increasing because of the increasing age of the surgical population and the performance of more complex surgery.

Table 8.2 Risk factors for perioperative acute renal failure

Preoperative factors	Intraoperative factors	Postoperative factors
Chronic disease	Type of surgery:	Acute conditions:
Advanced age	Cardiac	Acute cardiac dysfunction
Female sex	Aortic	Haemorrhage
Chronic renal disease	Peripheral vascular	Hypovolaemia
Diabetes mellitus	Non-renal solid organ transplantation	Sepsis
Chronic cardiac failure		Rhabdomyolysis
Aortic and peripheral vascular disease	Cardiac surgery:	Intra-abdominal hypertension
	Prolonged CPB time	Multiple organ dysfunction syndrome
Chronic liver disease	Combined procedures	
Genetic predisposition	Emergency surgery	Drug nephrotoxicity
Acute conditions:	Previous cardiac surgery	
Hypovolaemia	Aortic surgery	
Sepsis		
Preoperative IABP	Aortic clamp placement	
Multiple organ dysfunction syndrome	Aortic clamp placement	
	Intraoperative radiocontrast	

Prevention

The identification of high-risk patients and the implementation of prophylactic measures are the goals of perioperative renal protection. Strategies to reduce the occurrence of renal injury in patients without evidence of acute renal dysfunction are referred to as primary prevention. The avoidance of additional renal injury in the setting of established acute renal dysfunction is termed secondary prevention. Both non-pharmacological and pharmacological interventions may be considered.

Non-pharmacological strategies

These include intravascular volume expansion, maintenance of renal blood flow and renal perfusion pressure, avoidance of nephrotoxic agents, strict glycaemic control, and appropriate management of postoperative complications.

Intravascular volume expansion

Perioperative hypovolaemia should be rapidly corrected. The role of crystalloids compared with colloids for intravascular volume expansion remains unclear. Although not a primary outcome measure, a large multicentre trial of fluid resuscitation in critically ill patients found no difference between albumin and 0.9% sodium chloride in terms of the risk of ARF. The renal effects of different colloids have not yet been fully elucidated. Albumin and gelatin appear to be safe in patients with normal renal function. The safety of hydroxyethyl starch solutions in the setting of established renal impairment is unclear. Recent evidence suggests that hydroxyethyl starch is associated with a higher incidence of ARF than Ringer's lactate in critically ill patients with severe sepsis. Surgical patients receiving radiological contrast will benefit from the use of the lowest possible volume of non-ionic, iso-osmolar contrast in conjunction with isotonic IV fluids.

Maintenance of renal blood flow and renal perfusion pressure

Maintenance of adequate renal blood flow and perfusion pressure involves maintenance of both cardiac output and systemic arterial pressure. The initial approach should be intravascular volume expansion to reverse hypovolaemia. Inotropic and vasopressor therapy may then be initiated for the management of low cardiac output and systemic arterial hypotension, respectively. Despite historic concerns, norepinephrine is an excellent first-line vasopressor agent. There is no firm evidence to suggest that it compromises renal, hepatic, or gastrointestinal blood flow when used to treat arterial hypotension. Vasopressin and terlipressin may be useful agents in the treatment of postoperative catecholamine-resistant vasodilatory shock. The optimal therapeutic target for systemic arterial pressure for renal protection has not been established. A minimum mean arterial pressure of 65–75 mmHg is often targeted in clinical practice; however, a higher target may be necessary in patients with pre-existing hypertension.

Avoidance of nephrotoxic drugs

Minimizing perioperative exposure to nephrotoxic drugs is important. The use of once-daily aminoglycoside dosing and the use of lipid formulations of amphotericin B have been demonstrated to lower the risk of nephrotoxicity associated with these drugs. There are specific concerns regarding the risk of renal injury associated with the antifibrinolytic agent aprotinin.

Glycaemic control

Strict glycaemic control using intensive insulin therapy improved survival and reduced the incidence of ARF requiring RRT in a trial in mechanically-ventilated surgical ICU patients. Although some evidence suggests that strict normoglycaemia is required for optimum benefit, this approach increases the risk of hypoglycaemia.

Cardiac surgery

The conduct of CPB during cardiac surgery may affect the incidence of postoperative ARF. Limiting the duration of CPB and maintaining adequate flow and perfusion pressure are of primary importance. Several other strategies may also reduce renal injury, including avoidance of excessive haemodilution, avoidance of red cell transfusion, extracorporeal leuco-depletion, and haemofiltration during CPB. The evidence that off-pump CABG (OPCAB) surgery reduces renal morbidity is conflicting. New developments in minimally invasive surgical techniques that avoid ascending aortic manipulation may result in a reduction in renal morbidity.

Postoperative complications

A number of postoperative complications are known to be associated with renal dysfunction. Prompt diagnosis and management of acute cardiac dysfunction, haemorrhage, sepsis, rhabdomyolysis, and intra-abdominal hypertension are essential to prevent the development of ARF.

Pharmacological strategies

The postulated pathophysiology of ATN suggests that perioperative interventions that optimize renal oxygen delivery may prevent ARF. However, pharmacological strategies (Box 8.1) that increase renal blood flow or decrease renal oxygen consumption have not proved successful. Despite extensive investigation, few drug interventions have been demonstrated to provide clinical benefit and some have been clearly shown to be ineffective. A recent systematic review examined 37 randomized, controlled trials and concluded that there is no evidence that pharmacological interventions are effective in protecting renal function during surgery.

Box 8.1 Postulated pharmacological perioperative renal protection strategies

- Vasodilators:
  - Dopamine agonists.
  - Adenosine antagonists.
  - Calcium-channel antagonists.
  - Angiotensin-converting enzyme inhibitors.
  - Sodium nitroprusside.
- Diuretics:
  - Loop diuretics.
  - Osmotic diuretics.
- Natriuretic peptides:
  - Atrial natriuretic peptide.
  - Urodilatin B-type natriuretic peptide.
- Antioxidants:
  - N-acetylcysteine.
  - Corticosteroids.
- Other agents:
  - Volatile anaesthetic agents.
  - Insulin-like growth factor-1.
  - Erythropoietin.
  - Mesenchymal stem cells.

Dopamine agonists

- Dopamine acts on a number of different types of receptor. Renal blood flow is increased by dopaminergic receptor-mediated renal vasodilation, beta-adrenoreceptor stimulation increases cardiac output, and alpha-adrenoreceptor stimulation increases renal perfusion pressure. A large multicentre trial has demonstrated that low-dose dopamine does not prevent ARF, avert the need for RRT, or reduce the mortality in critically ill patients with early acute renal dysfunction in the ICU. In the perioperative setting, dopamine increases postoperative urine output but does not improve outcome. A number of systematic reviews have concluded that there is no role for low-dose dopamine for clinically significant renal protection.
- Dopexamine is a synthetic dopamine analogue with beta-adrenergic and dopaminergic effects. Perioperative use of dopexamine does not provide renal protection for cardiac or vascular surgical patients.
- Fenoldopam increases renal blood flow by its selective action on dopamine-1 receptors. At present, there is conflicting evidence regarding its usefulness as a potential renal protective agent. Recent trials suggest that the drug does not prevent radio-contrast-induced nephropathy in patients with pre-existing renal impairment, does not improve outcome in critically ill ICU patients with early acute renal dysfunction, and does not protect perioperative renal function in high-risk cardiac surgical patients. However, a meta-analysis of 16 randomized, controlled trials suggested a beneficial impact in critically ill patients.

Other renal vasodilator agents

Theophylline, an adenosine antagonist, reverses adenosine-mediated renal arterial vasoconstriction, but does not appear to prevent perioperative ARF during CABG. Similarly, calcium channel antagonists and angiotensin-converting enzyme inhibitors have not been shown to produce renal protection. A recent single-centre trial demonstrated that sodium nitroprusside administration during the rewarming phase of CPB in patients undergoing CABG decreases the incidence of postoperative ARF.

Diuretics

In the setting of acute renal dysfunction, diuretics increase urine output by decreasing tubular reabsorption through several mechanisms. Increasing tubular flow maintains patency and prevents obstruction and back-leak. Loop diuretics inhibit tubular reabsorption in the loop of Henle, whereas mannitol acts primarily as an osmotic diuretic. The available evidence for the use of diuretics in surgical and critically ill patients is scarce. The perioperative use of neither loop diuretics nor mannitol demonstrates significant renal protection in patients undergoing cardiac surgery. However, a recent meta-analysis of five randomized, controlled trials demonstrated that loop diuretics did not increase mortality in patients with ARF.

Natriuretic peptides

Natriuretic peptides induce a natriuretic and diuretic effect by increasing glomerular perfusion pressure and filtration. These peptides have shown conflicting results in the prevention of ARF. Large multicentre trials have demonstrated that atrial natriuretic peptide (ANP) does not prevent death or dialysis in critically ill patients with ARF. However, in a small single-centre trial, recombinant human ANP has been shown to reduce the need for dialysis in postoperative cardiac surgical patients with early acute renal dysfunction.

N-acetylcysteine

Substantial evidence supports the prophylactic use of the antioxidant N-acetylcysteine (NAC) along with intravascular volume expansion for the prevention of radio-contrast nephropathy. Disappointingly, recent trials in the perioperative and ICU settings have shown a lack of renal protective benefit of NAC. These trials have been performed in high-risk patients undergoing cardiac surgery, open abdominal aortic aneurysm repair and abdominal aortic EVAR.

Future strategies

Several experimental strategies are currently undergoing investigation including volatile anaesthetic agents, insulin-like growth factor-1, erythropoietin, and mesenchymal stem cells.

A practical approach to perioperative renal protection

Cardiopulmonary bypass

Preoperative
- Optimize volume status, cardiac output, and systemic arterial pressure.
- Withhold nephrotoxic drugs.
- Maintain glycaemic control in diabetic patients.
- Correct metabolic and electrolyte disturbances.
- Delay surgery until recovery of acute renal dysfunction if possible.
- Arrange preoperative dialysis for dialysis-dependent patients.
- Administer isotonic IV fluids and N-acetylcysteine for prevention of radio-contrast-induced nephropathy.

Intraoperative
- Optimize volume status, cardiac output, and systemic arterial pressure.
- Avoid nephrotoxic drugs.
- Consider maintaining glycaemic control in all patients.
- Maintain adequate flow and mean systemic arterial pressure during CPB.
- Limit the duration of CPB.
- Avoid excessive haemodilution.
- Avoid red cell transfusion.
- Consider extra-corporeal leucodepletion.
- Consider haemofiltration during CPB.
- Consider off-pump coronary artery bypass surgery.
- Provide appropriate organ support for multiple organ dysfunction syndrome.
- Institute renal replacement therapy for RIFLE grade F acute renal dysfunction.

Key points

- Perioperative acute renal failure is a common complication of major surgery and is associated with increased morbidity and mortality.
- Ischaemia- or toxin-mediated acute tubular necrosis is the primary cause of perioperative acute renal failure.
- The key non-pharmacological strategies are intravascular volume expansion, maintenance of renal blood flow and renal perfusion pressure, avoidance of nephrotoxic agents, careful glycaemic control, and the appropriate management of postoperative complications.
- At present, there is no firm evidence to suggest that the use of any specific pharmacological intervention is clinically beneficial.
- Dopamine infusion has not been shown to prevent acute renal failure, avert the need for renal replacement therapy, or reduce mortality, and should not be administered solely for renal protection.
- The RIFLE classification of acute renal dysfunction (📖 see also Acute renal failure, p. 126).

Further reading

1. Aronson S, Fonte ML, Miao Y, et al. Risk index for perioperative renal dysfunction/failure: critical dependence on pulse pressure hypertension. *Circulation* 2007; 115: 733–742.
2. Bellomo R, Ronco C, Kellum JA, et al. Acute renal failure – definition, outcome measures, animal models, fluid therapy and information technology needs: The Second International Consensus Conference of the Acute Dialysis Quality Initiative (ADQI) Group. *Critical Care* 2004; 8: R204–R212.
3. Friedrich JO, Adhikari N, Herridge MS, et al. Meta-analysis: Low-dose dopamine increases urine output but does not prevent renal dysfunction or death. *Annals of Internal Medicine* 2005; 142: 510–524.
4. Kellum JA. Acute kidney injury. *Critical Care Medicine* 2008; 36: S141–S145.
5. Thakar CV, Arrigain S, Worley S, et al. A clinical score to predict acute renal failure after cardiac surgery. *Journal of the American Society of Nephrology* 2005; 16: 162–168.
6. Zacharias M, Gilmore IC, Herbison GP, et al. Interventions for protecting renal function in the perioperative period. *Cochrane Database Systematic Reviews* 2005; 3: CD003590.

Respiratory implications of cardiac surgery

Dr B Woodcock

Introduction *138*
Preoperative assessment *140*
Intraoperative management of mechanical ventilation *141*
Postoperative respiratory function *142*
Further reading *147*

Introduction

Respiratory complications remain a leading cause of post-cardiac surgical morbidity. Preoperative assessment can help predict which patients are more likely to suffer respiratory complications. Factors associated with atelectasis and pneumonia can be identified. Methods can be employed to minimize and manage pulmonary complications. Recent advances in surgical and anaesthetic techniques have reduced the physiological insult of cardiac surgery. These include minimally invasive and off-pump procedures, and the movement towards streamlined postoperative care (early extubation).

Preoperative assessment

Preoperative respiratory function

Pulmonary function tests (PFTs)

- Spirometry.
- Gas transfer.
- V/Q scanning.

Most studies of routine spirometry in otherwise healthy patients have not shown any predictive value. PFTs may give information on the pulmonary status of patients with known respiratory disease and smokers. A Veterans Affairs study of preoperative pulmonary function showed that FEV1 of less than 1.25 litres was associated with an increased mortality of 11% compared with 3.8%.

Predictors of postoperative respiratory dysfunction

- Congestive heart failure.
- Old age.
- Obesity.
- Smoking within eight weeks.
- Chronic obstructive pulmonary disease (COPD).
- Asthma.
- Re-exploration for bleeding.
- Diabetes mellitus.
- Emergency surgery.
- Previous cardiac surgery.

Although these predictors identify those at higher risk of pulmonary complications they may still benefit from cardiac surgery. For example, although patients with significant COPD have a higher risk after CABG compared to patients without COPD, they still benefit from operation when the long-term natural history of their course is followed.

Intraoperative management of mechanical ventilation

Methods employed intraoperatively to minimize pulmonary complications include:
- Reduced FiO_2.
- Continuous positive airway pressure (CPAP) on cardiopulmonary bypass (CPB).
- Intermittent positive pressure ventilation (IPPV) during CPB.
- Positive end-expiratory pressure (PEEP) post-bypass.
- Vital capacity manoeuvre after CPB.
- Open lung ventilation (OLV).

Most of these techniques have not been demonstrated to influence postoperative pulmonary outcomes. There is little evidence that the effect of nitrogen splinting when using a reduced FiO_2 improves postoperative lung function. A vital capacity manoeuvre (pressure of 40 cm H_2O maintained for 15 seconds) can abolish atelectasis. This should be confirmed by direct visualization of lung expansion at the end of bypass. Postoperative recruitment manoeuvres have a short-lived effect unless elevated levels of PEEP (14 cm H_2O) are employed.

Postoperative respiratory function

Causes of postoperative respiratory dysfunction include:
- Altered lung mechanics following median sternotomy.
- Cardiac dysfunction.
- Pulmonary oedema/congestive heart failure.
- Intrinsic pulmonary pathology.
- Pneumonia.
- Atelectasis.
- Phrenic paralysis.
- Pleural effusion.
- Acute lung injury (ALI).
- 'Pump lung' – due to inflammatory response following CPB.
- Pneumothorax/barotrauma.

VC and FEV_1 may be reduced more than 50% following sternotomy and may persist for several months. These changes are due to altered chest wall and rib cage mechanics, pain, and pleural effusions, and are worse if an internal mammary artery (IMA) graft is used. These effects are not significantly ameliorated if coronary artery bypass is performed off-pump. Minimally invasive surgery using mini-sternotomy or limited anterior or posterior thoracotomy may reduce changes in pulmonary mechanics.

Radiological evidence for atelectasis may be present in as many as 70% of CABG patients with IMA graft and 50% with vein grafts. Clinically significant pulmonary complications are less common.

It is uncertain how much cardiopulmonary bypass contributes to postoperative pulmonary dysfunction. Studies comparing on- and off-pump CABG have shown that the duration of ventilatory support may be reduced in high-risk patients undergoing repeat CABG, but not in those patients undergoing primary CABG off-pump.

A meta-analysis of trials comparing pain management with perioperative epidural anaesthesia against other parenteral analgesia demonstrated a reduction in pulmonary complications with an odds ratio of 0.41. The issue of anticoagulation and postoperative coagulopathy leading to a risk of epidural haematoma generally precludes this technique.

Atelectasis

Causes of atelectasis
- Manual compression of the lung during:
  - Elevation of the heart to view the posterior surface.
  - IMA dissection.
  - Cannulation of the inferior vena cava.
  - One lung ventilation in thoracotomy or mini-thoracotomy.
- Functional residual capacity (FRC) decreases due to:
  - General anaesthesia.
  - Apnoea during CPB.
- Postoperative poor inspiratory effort and coughing.
- Pleural effusions.
- Gastric distension.
- Phrenic paralysis.

- Retention of secretions due to:
  - Pain.
  - Weakness.
  - Neurological complications.
- Immobilization and bedrest.
- Aspiration due to:
  - Postoperative swallowing difficulties.
  - Neurological and cognitive impairment.
- Trans-oesophageal echocardiography (TOE).

Increased incidence of atelectasis after TOE may be related to postoperative swallowing difficulties or oesophageal dysmotility and aspiration.

Techniques to minimize atelectasis
- Reverse Trendelenburg position.
- Incentive spirometry.
- Chest physiotherapy:
  - Deep-breathing exercises.
  - Percussion.
  - Postural drainage.
- CPAP/BiPAP.

Reverse Trendelenburg position improves oxygenation and lung mechanics in morbidly obese patients.

Because of the low incidence of postoperative pulmonary complications, in spite of the frequency of radiological atelectasis, it is difficult to demonstrate that the routine use of these techniques improves respiratory outcome following cardiac surgery. Deep breathing exercises using a positive expiratory pressure 'blow-bottle' device may reduce atelectasis and improve postoperative pulmonary function.

CPAP by facemask or nasal mask can be used to treat atelectasis. There is some evidence that non-invasive pressure support ventilation may have a greater effect in resolving radiological atelectasis than CPAP.

Phrenic paralysis
Phrenic paralysis may occur due to cold trauma. The incidence is increased with lower body temperatures. The incidence also increases if an insulating pad is not used to protect the phrenic nerve when surface cooling of the heart is used with slush.

Pneumonia
Factors associated with pneumonia
- COPD.
- Blood transfusion.
- H_2-blocking agents.
- Smoking.
- Low cardiac output.
- Ventilator-associated pneumonia (VAP).
- Prolonged intubation and ventilation.

Pneumonia is more frequent in patients with pre-existing lung disease. Some (but not all) studies have suggested that H_2 blockade, by decreasing stomach acidity, allows bacterial overgrowth, which can lead to pneumonia following micro-aspiration. Prolonged intubation can lead to ventilator-associated pneumonia. Anaesthetic techniques utilizing lower doses of opioids and early extubation protocols (fast-tracking) have decreased the duration of positive pressure ventilation and have improved pulmonary outcomes and reduced the incidence of atelectasis and nosocomial pneumonia.

Methods used to reduce the incidence of VAP
- Bed head up, position 30°.
- Oral decontamination.
- Continuous subglottic suction.
- Sucralfate for stress ulcer prophylaxis.
- Kinetic beds.
- Orotracheal intubation.
- Closed ET suction system.
- Avoid circuit changes unless soiled.
- Intensive insulin therapy.

Late onset VAP with gram-negative organisms is thought to be due to micro-aspiration of oropharyngeal secretions. Some of these techniques aim to reduce the risk of this, but there is conflicting evidence as to whether many actually have a beneficial effect.

Management of pneumonia
- Collect lower respiratory tract culture before antibiotic therapy.
- 'Semi-quantitative' or 'quantitative' culture data can be used.
- Early broad-spectrum antibiotic.
- Cultures should be used to narrow antibiotic coverage.
- Negative cultures can be used to stop antibiotic therapy.

Early broad spectrum antibiotic treatment is key to the management of pneumonia. Knowledge of the local susceptibilities of organisms will influence the choice of drug. Management of respiratory failure due to pneumonia is similar to that of hypoxia due to ALI/ARDS (see below).

Pulmonary oedema

Cardiogenic pulmonary oedema
Cardiogenic oedema results from increased hydrostatic forces in the lung. These most commonly occur due to decreased left ventricular function. Residual mitral regurgitation following the operation should also be considered.

Management depends on the severity of the condition and may consist of diuresis, inotropic support of the heart, positive pressure ventilation and mechanical assist devices such as an intra-aortic balloon pump (IABP) or a left ventricular assist device (LVAD).

Non-cardiogenic pulmonary oedema
Non-cardiogenic pulmonary oedema results from a breakdown in the integrity of the capillary basement membrane, leading to the accumulation of protein-rich alveolar oedema fluid, even in the face of low hydrostatic pressures.

ARDS/ALI

Possible causes of ARDS/ALI

- Systemic inflammatory response to cardiopulmonary bypass.
- Reaction to protamine.
- Hypothermia.
- Lung deflation during CPB.
- Blood transfusion.
- Shock.
- Aspiration.
- Lung infection.
- Sepsis.

Steroids have been used to try to minimize the inflammatory response but have not been effective in reducing the incidence of postoperative pulmonary complications. Patients treated with steroids had similar or higher postoperative P(A-a)O$_2$ levels and pulmonary shunt function, as well as longer duration of intubation.

Management of hypoxia due to ALI/ARDS

- CPAP/BiPAP.
- Intubation and positive pressure ventilation.
- PEEP – level based on severity of oxygenation deficit.
- Lung protective ventilation:
  - Low tidal volume – 6 ml/kg ideal body weight.
  - End-inspiratory plateau pressures <30 cm H$_2$O.
- Pressure control ventilation.
- Inverse ratio ventilation.
- Hypercapnia can be tolerated.
- Pronation.
- High-frequency oscillatory ventilation.
- ECMO.
- Steroids.

The management of ARDS is similar whether it follows cardiac surgery or occurs in other circumstances. Some of these techniques may improve oxygenation but have not been demonstrated to improve outcomes. The use of corticosteroids in ARDS remains controversial; administration after 14 days increases mortality and the benefit of earlier administration has not been clearly established.

Pulmonary embolism

Full systemic anticoagulation during CPB and the postoperative coagulopathy seen following cardiac surgery may explain why deep vein thrombosis (DVT) and pulmonary embolism are relatively unusual compared to incidence in major non-cardiac surgery.

Recommended prophylaxis is aspirin and elastic gradient compression stockings for CABG patients and heparin or low molecular weight heparin and sequential compression stockings for those who are bedridden and not ambulating by 2–3 days postop. Off-pump CABG may be associated with a relatively hypercoagulable state and anticoagulant prophylaxis has been recommended.

Pneumothorax/barotrauma

Causes of barotrauma
- Surgical trauma.
- Central line cannulation.
- Spontaneous rupture of lung bullae.
- Barotrauma from mechanical ventilation.
- High inflation pressures or volumes.
- PEEP.

Central line cannulation may cause pneumothorax, but the most common cause of perioperative pneumothorax is breach of the pleura during surgery. Pleural chest drains are routinely inserted intraoperatively when this occurs. Barotrauma from mechanical ventilation is more likely to occur in the setting of increased inflation pressures and volumes. Barotrauma may cause pneumothorax, pneumopericardium, pneumoperitoneum, and subcutaneous emphysema.

Tracheostomy

Patients requiring prolonged ventilatory support may benefit from early tracheostomy. Benefits include reduced pulmonary dead space, improved pulmonary toilet and increased patient comfort. Weaning from the ventilator is facilitated by tracheostomy mask trials, which can be terminated if the patient fatigues by reattachment to the ventilator without requiring re-intubation.

Some surgeons prefer to wait 14 days before tracheostomy because of a risk of mediastinitis due to the closer proximity of secretions to the fresh sternotomy wound.

Traditionally an open tracheostomy has been performed but the development of percutaneous dilational tracheostomy has allowed bedside insertion on the intensive care unit.

Further reading

1. Cohen AJ, Katz MG, Frenkel G, Medalion B, Geva D, Schachner A. Morbid results of prolonged intubation after coronary artery bypass surgery. *Chest* 2000; 118 (6): 1724–1731.
2. Gale GD, Teasdale SJ, Sanders DE, et al. Pulmonary atelectasis and other respiratory complications after cardiopulmonary bypass and investigation of aetiological factors. *Canadian Anaesthetists Society Journal* 1979; 26 (1): 15–21.
3. Grover FL, Hammermeister KE, Burchfield C. Initial report of the Veterans Administration Preoperative Risk Assessment Study for Cardiac Surgery. *Annals of Thoracic Surgery* 1990; 50 (1): 12–26; Discussion 27–28.
4. Pasquina P, Tramer MR, Walder B. Prophylactic respiratory physiotherapy after cardiac surgery: Systematic review. *BMJ* 2003; 327 (7428): 1379.
5. Ranes JL, Gordon S, Arroliga AC. Guidelines for the management of adults with hospital-acquired, ventilator-associated, and healthcare-associated pneumonia. *American Journal of Respiratory Critical Care Medicine* 2005; 171 (4): 388–416.
6. Weissman C. Pulmonary complications after cardiac surgery. *Seminars in Cardiothoracic and Vascular Anesthesia* 2004; 8 (3): 185–211.

Infection

Dr P Wilson

Infection risks *150*
Infection prophylaxis in cardiac surgery *152*
Infective endocarditis *154*
Sternal wound infections *160*
Further reading *162*

Infection risks

Cardiac surgery is generally regarded as clean surgery with the most common pathogens being *Staphylococci*, which can be coagulase negative or positive. Coagulase negative species are the most common cause of postoperative infections while *Staphylococcus aureus* is the most important coagulase positive species.

Gram negative bacteria can colonize wounds that are discharging or contain necrotic material. Many risk factors have been identified as contributing to the development of infections after cardiothoracic surgery (Box 10.1).

Box 10.1 Risk factors for cardiac wound infection

- Extremes of age.
- Diabetes mellitus.
- Malnutrition.
- Chronic liver disease.
- Chronic respiratory disease.
- Renal failure.
- Smoking.
- Immunosuppressive states:
  - AIDS/HIV.
  - Steroids.
  - Cytotoxics.
- Obesity.
- Previous cardiac surgery.
- Blood transfusions.
- Prolonged intubation.
- Bacterial colonization of catheters.
- Duration of cardiothoracic surgery.
- Insertion of catheters and balloon pumps.
- Technical errors.
- Omission of prophylactic antibiotics perioperatively.
- Carriage of MRSA.
- Peripheral occlusive arterial disease.

Wound contamination

- Obesity is most closely linked to wound infection. Close apposition of the wound edges is more difficult in the obese patient. Accumulation of tissue fluid within the wound provides a good medium for the growth of contaminating bacteria. Antibiotic penetration into fat is often poor, especially if a patient is not given a weight-related dose. The area of tissue exposed during surgery is large and the contaminating load of bacteria both from air and surrounding tissue is high.
- Prolonged surgery increases the bacterial load in the wound, predominantly seeded from the air. Usually such surgery is more complicated and there is a larger area of tissue damage and haematoma formation. Further doses of prophylactic antibiotics may be necessary if a procedure lasts more than six hours.

- The risk of sternal wound infection in coronary artery surgery is greater than in valvular surgery. Harvest of veins from the leg can result in Gram negative and other flora contaminating the wound, especially if the wound extends into the groin.

Impaired local immune response

- Use of the internal mammary arteries has been found in some cases to result in ischaemia of the parasternal area and increased wound infection.
- Diabetes is associated with poor microvasculature and relative ischaemia of the tissues such that local immune defence is impaired.

Colonization and establishment of infection

- Sutures and dead tissue following the use of diathermy form a nidus for infection. The inoculum of bacteria needed to establish infection is 100-fold lower when foreign material is present in the wound. The volume of foreign material is exponentially related to the risk of infection.
- The care and expertise of the surgeon in closing a wound is important.
- Carriage of *Staphylococcus aureus* (coagulase positive) in the general population is 30% and significantly increases the risk of wound infection with that organism. Topical decontamination can be used to prevent skin *Staphylococci* being inoculated into the wound.
- More problematic is carriage of methicillin-resistant *Staphylococcus aureus* (MRSA), which is difficult to treat and more likely to be invasive. Screening for MRSA and topical decontamination is standard in most hospitals. Infecting strains vary in their ability to cause infection.
- Different strains of *Staphylococcus aureus* express different levels of protein A, coagulase, aggressins, lipase, hyaluronidase, haemolytic toxins, leucocidins, and epidermolytic toxins.
- Coagulase negative *Staphylococci* are particularly associated with infection on metal sutures or indwelling devices and produce a number of virulence factors: haemolysins, phosphatase, lipase, galactosidase, decarboxylase, adhesions, and slime.

Infections in the early postoperative period

- If the wound continues to leak in the early postoperative period it is easy for skin flora or contaminating pathogens to gain entry to the wound during dressing changes.
- Approximately half of the coagulase negative *Staphylococci* causing sternal wound infection are derived from flora circulating in the ward environment.
- Respiratory or urinary infection present before operation can cause serious complication unless treated. If possible surgery should be delayed until treatment has been completed.

Infection prophylaxis in cardiac surgery

Preoperative preparation and screening

- All patients having cardiac surgery should be screened for MRSA.
- MRSA may be more invasive than methicillin-sensitive *S. aureus* and doubles the mortality risk.
- MRSA infection is associated with preoperative carriage of the organism and the risks of infection can be substantially reduced by appropriate topical decontamination with intranasal mupirocin and body wash with chlorhexidine.
- Screening is best performed at a pre-assessment clinic 1–2 weeks before the planned date of surgery but can be achieved within two hours with rapid PCR test.
- Topical decontamination should be administered in the five days before surgery and not earlier, as MRSA can return in up to one third of cases.
- General prophylactic measures should be addressed to the infection risk factors already described, for example, treatment of pre-existent infections, loss of excessive weight, cessation of smoking, and careful control of diabetes.

Antibiotic prophylaxis

- Although cardiac surgery has a relatively low rate of infection, antibiotic prophylaxis is mandatory because the consequences of infection are severe and costly.
- Antibiotics used for surgical prophylaxis should be rational, safe, and effective. Usually the microbiologist will have prepared a local antibiotic prophylaxis policy based on the antibiotic susceptibility of local flora, cost, safety, and published trial evidence.
- Antibiotic prophylaxis is usually with standard agents such as cefuroxime, flucloxacillin plus gentamicin, or where there is allergy or a greater than 10% prevalence of MRSA, vancomycin or teicoplanin. Vancomycin is associated with an increased inotrope requirement in the early postoperative period. Agents should be administered intravenously to achieve peak blood levels at the time of skin incision, when *Staphylococci* are dispersed through the bloodstream.
- Although there is some evidence that a single dose may be adequate, most authorities use a 24-hour course. Although some guidelines suggest longer courses, clinical trials and experimental evidence do not suggest any additional benefit. Prolonged courses increase the risk of adverse effects and the emergence of bacterial resistance.
- Senior clinicians need to be involved with the choice and implementation of antibiotic policy. Do not forget to document antibiotic administration by time and person.
- High doses of antibiotics are required to ensure tissue levels are adequate to inhibit and kill bacteria contaminating the wound during surgery. Weight-related doses should be used, especially for the obese patient. Antibiotic should be administered with induction of anaesthesia and **not** with the premedication. They are most effective when given *before* skin incision.

Operative procedures

- Skin preparation with 2% chlorhexidine or povidone iodine is effective but should be allowed to dry before application of protective drapes. In the case of alcohol-based preparations, bacterial killing is achieved when the alcohol evaporates.
- Beware of pooling around the patient when using alcohol solutions; fire can be ignited by the diathermy causing severe burns!
- The minimum number of personnel should be present in the operating theatre.
- During surgery, care should be taken with aseptic technique and haemostasis. Haematoma formation should be prevented but use of diathermy should not be so excessive as to create islands of necrotic tissue.
- The minimum of suture material should be used.
- Tissue perfusion should be maintained in as optimal a state as possible.
- The wound should be thoroughly irrigated before closure to remove as many contaminating bacteria as possible.
- Closed-style non-woven clothing is recommended as it reduces aerial counts of bacteria over open-style non-woven or cotton clothing.

Postoperative procedure

- Many wound infections develop in the early postoperative period while the wound is discharging.
- Pathogens circulating in the intensive care unit have been associated with infections. Maintenance of an occlusive dressing and replacement of any dressing that shows breakthrough of discharge will reduce the risk of bacteria entering the wound.
- Dressings generally should not be removed earlier than 48 hours after operation. When dressings are changed attention to aseptic technique must be scrupulous and rapid inspections during ward rounds without proper aseptic procedures should not be permitted.

Infective endocarditis

Definition
An infection of the endocardial surface of the heart by a microorganism.

Epidemiology
Endocarditis was previously classified as acute or subacute based upon the pathogenic organism and clinical presentation. The distinction has become less useful and the specific term infective endocarditis is now used. The incidence is 1.8–6 cases per 100,000 person years in Europe and USA, with men more commonly affected than women. Prosthetic valve endocarditis accounts for up to 25% of cases in Europe and USA.

Pathogenesis
Endocarditis can affect native valves and prosthetic valves. Normal cardiac tissue is resistant to infection. Transient bacteraemia is very common and the immune system plays an effective role in preventing endocarditis. Damaged endothelium due to trauma, congenital defects, turbulent flow, valvular heart disease, or atherosclerosis results in platelet and fibrin deposition resulting in biofilm and vegetation formation. Bacteraemia from any potential source, e.g. intravascular catheter, wound infections, or urinary and respiratory tract infections can colonize these vegetations. Endocarditis promotes monocyte adhesion and triggering of the coagulation cascade. Common causes of endocarditis are post-dental work, septicaemia (from any cause), and bacteraemia from the use of contaminated needles in intravenous drug abusers (usually right-sided endocarditis).

Types of endocarditis
Sites:
- Native valve versus prosthetic valve.
- Predominantly left-sided endocarditis (95%).
- Mitral valve (85%), aortic valve (55%), tricuspid valve (20%).
- Pulmonary valve endocarditis is rare (1%).
- Jet lesions: atrial surface of the mitral valve in MR, or ventricular surface of the aortic valve in AR.

Aetiology
There is a wide variety of microorganisms that can cause endocarditis (Box 10.2). Polymicrobial infections are uncommon and are normally associated with intravenous drug abuse.

Box 10.2 Microbial causes of endocarditis

Bacteria
- *Staphylococcus* spp. (*S. aureus*, coagulase-negative *Staphylococci*).
- *Streptococcus* spp. (e.g. *Strep. sanguis*, *Strep. bovis*, *Strep. mutans*, and *Strep. mitis*).
- *Enterococcus* spp.
- HACEK group:
  - *Haemophilus aphrophilus.*
  - *Actinobacillus actinomycetemcomitans.*
  - *Cardiobacterium hominis.*
  - *Eikenella corrodens.*
  - *Kingella kingae.*
- *Brucella* spp.
- *Bartonella* spp.
- *Chlamydia* spp.
- *Mycoplasma* spp.
- *Coxiella* spp.
- Polymicrobial.

Fungi
- *Candida* spp.
- *Aspergillus* spp.

Protozoa
- Chagas disease.
- *Entamoeba histolytica.*

Sterile
- Others.

Clinical features

Diagnosis of infective endocarditis is based on a combination of clinical, microbiological, and echocardiographic manifestations of the disease called the Duke diagnostic criteria (Box 10.3). The main echocardiographic features are vegetations, valve dehiscence, and abscess formation.

Box 10.3 Duke diagnostic criteria for infective endocarditis

Major criteria
- Positive blood culture (two separate cultures) for microorganism.
- Echocardiographic evidence of: oscillating intracardiac mass (in absence of other explanation); abscess; new regurgitant lesion; new partial dehiscence of prosthetic valve.

Minor criteria
- Fever (>38°C), embolic phenomena, one positive blood culture, other ECHO evidence.

Definite endocarditis:
Two major, or one major + three minor, or five minor.

Possible endocarditis:
One major + one minor, or three minor.

Symptoms and signs
- **Bacteraemia/septicaemia** – fever, rigors, chills, malaise, anorexia, confusion, arthralgia.
- **Tissue destruction** – valvular incompetence, root and myocardial abscess, prosthetic valve dehiscence, heart block, cardiac failure.
- **Embolic phenomena** – occur in 50% of cases of infective endocarditis resulting in: neurological events, acute peripheral limb ischaemia, myocardial infarction, spleen and kidney infarction, pulmonary embolism, mycotic aneurysms.
- **Circulating immune complexes** – splinter haemorrhages, Osler's nodes (tender nodes in pulp of fingertips), Janeway lesions (macules on palms or wrists), vasculitis rash, Roth spots (flame-shaped haemorrhages in the retina), arthralgia, nephritis, splenomegaly.

Mortality rates
- The overall mortality rate is up to 25% and is dependent on the organism and the valvular pathology. Late prosthetic valve endocarditis has a mortality of up to 60%.
- *Staphylococcal* and fungal infections have up to 50% mortality, *Enterococci* 25%, and α-haemolytic *Streptococci* 15%.

Investigations
- Blood cultures (90% yield positive culture; 10% are sterile).
- FBC, differential, ESR, and CRP.
- Chest X-ray and ECG.
- Echocardiography.
- Special cultures for *Coxiella*, *Bartonella*, and *Mycoplasma* if initial cultures are negative.
- Preoperative MRSA screen.

Treatment

Patients with infective endocarditis are frequently extremely unwell and may deteriorate rapidly, thus the possibility of eradicating the infection with antibiotics versus surgical intervention must be evaluated carefully. Timing of surgical intervention can be one of the most difficult decisions in medicine.

Empirical medical treatment

- Acute onset: flucloxacillin (8–12 g IV daily in 4–6 divided doses) plus gentamicin (1 mg/kg body weight IV 8-hourly, modified according to renal function).
- Gradual presentation: penicillin (7.2 g IV daily in six divided doses) or ampicillin/amoxicillin (2 g IV 6-hourly) plus gentamicin (1 mg/kg body weight 8-hourly IV, modified according to renal function).
- Penicillin allergy, intracardiac prosthesis, or suspected MRSA: vancomycin (1 g 12 hourly IV, modified according to renal function) plus rifampicin (300–600 mg 12-hourly by mouth) plus gentamicin (1 mg/kg body weight 8-hourly IV, modified according to renal function).
- Treatment is continued for four weeks or up to six weeks if disease present for three months. Oral follow-on antibiotics are not recommended.

Staphylococcal endocarditis

- Meticillin (methicillin) sensitive: flucloxacillin (2 g 4–6 hourly IV).
- Meticillin (methicillin) resistant/penicillin allergy: vancomycin (1 g IV 12-hourly, modified according to renal function) plus rifampicin (300–600 mg 12-hourly by mouth) or gentamicin (1 mg/kg body weight 8-hourly, modified according to renal function) or sodium fusidate (500 mg 8-hourly by mouth).

Streptococcal endocarditis

Benzyl penicillin is recommended for four weeks for a susceptible strain with a minimal inhibitory concentration (MIC) <0.5 mg/l, and penicillin or vancomycin plus gentamicin for 4–6 weeks for less sensitive strains. Teicoplanin is less nephrotoxic than vancomycin, especially in the presence of gentamicin.

Enterococcal disease

Should be treated with ampicillin (2 g 4-hourly IV) plus gentamicin (1 mg/kg 8–12-hourly IV) or vancomycin/teicoplanin plus gentamicin.

Surgical treatment

Indications for surgical intervention are listed in Box 10.4. The aims of surgery are to:

- Remove infected tissue and drain abscesses.
- Restore the cardiac and vascular architecture.

Box 10.4 Indications for surgery in infective endocarditis

For those with native valve endocarditis
- Acute mitral regurgitation with heart failure.
- Acute mitral regurgitation with aortic regurgitation.
- Evidence of aortic abscess or annular abscess, sinus or aneurysm.
- Failure of antibiotic treatment after 7–10 days (e.g. evidence of sepsis or persistent valve dysfunction).
- Recurrent emboli after antibiotic therapy.
- Fungal endocarditis.

For those with prosthetic valve endocarditis
- Prosthetic valve dysfunction with heart failure.
- Endocarditis within two months of replacement.
- Endocarditis not responding to antibiotics.
- Gram-negative organism endocarditis.
- Vegetations on prosthesis.
- Fungal endocarditis.

Prevention of infective endocarditis

Recent guidelines from the National Institute for Health and Clinical Excellence no longer include antibiotic cover for routine dental, respiratory tract, genitourinary, or gastrointestinal tract procedures in high-risk patients, unless the actual surgical procedure is at an infected site. This is based on the lack of evidence that any bacteraemia from these procedures is associated with development of endocarditis, as well as a desire to avoid adverse effects of antibiotics. These guidelines have proved controversial.

High-risk patients
- Prosthetic heart valves.
- Previous bacterial endocarditis.
- Congenital heart disease.
- Rheumatic valve dysfunction.
- Hypertrophic cardiomyopathy.
- Mitral valve prolapse with regurgitation.

Recommendations change and it is wise to consult a national formulary.

Current prophylaxis for high-risk patients when surgical site infected
- Dental surgery: 3 g PO amoxicillin, clindamycin 600 mg PO, azithromycin 500 mg PO, or amoxicillin 1 g IV.
- Genitourinary, gastrointestinal, respiratory, or obstetric/gynaecological procedures: a single dose of 1 g amoxicillin plus gentamicin 1.5 mg/kg IV given just before the procedure or at induction of anaesthesia.
- Allergic to penicillin: teicoplanin 400 mg IV plus gentamicin 1.5 mg/kg IV is given.

Sternal wound infections

Predisposing factors

- Wound infection is a serious cause of morbidity and prolonged hospital stay following cardiac surgery. As it is clean surgery the rate of infection would be expected to be less than 2% but there are additional risks that can increase this proportion:
  - Length of operation.
  - Number of staff present.
  - Contamination of blood during recirculation.
  - Depressed function of most components of the immune system.
- Diabetes and the use of internal mammary grafts are recognized risk factors, probably because of devascularization of the wound edges.
- Obesity is probably the most important predisposing factor because of the difficulty with wound apposition and the prevention of fluid accumulation within the wound.

Incidence and signs

- The incidence of severe sternal sepsis varies with the definition used and whether aspiration or debridement has been used to confirm the diagnosis. Some studies include only the most severe, for example mediastinitis.
- Usually between 0.2 and 4.5% of patients develop severe infection, compared with another 4–7% who develop more minor infections. Around 5–13% of patients having coronary artery surgery develop leg wound infection, which can itself predispose to sternal infection.
- Most studies include pus and all include isolation of bacteria in their definition of infection but smaller proportions additionally require combinations of erythema, serous exudate, wound dehiscence, prolonged stay, reoperation, antibiotic treatment, or fever.
- Some studies rely entirely on clinical diagnosis without defining their criteria, while the widely used Center for Disease Control (CDC, USA) definition includes the clinical opinion of the surgeon. Periods of observation vary between 10 and 30 days.
- Many infections are missed if the patient is not followed after discharge. Wounds may heal initially only to discharge later at home.
- Prolonged fever after the first week is a good predictor of severe wound breakdown. It is less likely in minor infections.
- 40% of severe infections are accompanied by bacteraemia and most demonstrate pus.
- Some discharge only serous fluid or show only erythema.
- Associated wound discharge delays the patient leaving hospital and significantly increases hospital costs.

Causes

- *Staphylococcus aureus* is the most common cause of infection and is reported in over 20% of infections. Antibiotic prophylaxis is effective in reducing the incidence of infection.
- *Staphylococcus epidermidis* causes a similar proportion of infections but is sometimes dismissed by laboratories as a skin contaminant. The organism is highly adapted to adhere to prosthetic material including metal sutures, and pure repeated growth from swabs should be considered diagnostic. Presentation is often indistinguishable from *S. aureus* infection. Many infections show sensitivity patterns that suggest they were acquired in the postoperative ward rather than from the patient's normal flora at surgery. Over 90% are resistant to flucloxacillin and many are resistant to common prophylactic antibiotics. Of a series of 22,180 operations in one series, coagulase-negative *Staphylococci* caused 100 of 436 sternal wound infections, 56% being superficial, 27% deep, and 17% mediastinitis. However, the average delay from surgery to diagnosis was 24 days.
- Coliforms (*Klebsiella* spp, *Escherichia coli*, *Enterobacter* spp, *Proteus* spp, and *Pseudomonas aeruginosa*) are the third most common cause. Most are associated with necrotic or sloughy open wounds and may represent colonization and secondary infection. They tend to be more common in coronary artery surgery where there is a leg wound and often appear within one week of surgery.

Treatment

- Most minor sternal infections can be managed with local dressings.
- Major infection may need debridement, antibiotics, and irrigation.
- Mediastinitis is the most difficult to manage and requires evacuation of all exudate and necrotic material plus radical debridement. Irrigation with saline is preferable to chlorhexidine or antibiotic solutions as serious toxic reactions can occur, as well as emergence of resistance or fungal infection. Hospital stay may be prolonged to 26–46 days and there is a mortality of 7–24%. Haemorrhage from exposed mediastinal vessels is a potentially fatal complication. Plastic surgeons are often involved in the treatment and reconstruction of sternal defects.

Further reading

1. Ashrafian H, Bogle R. Antimicrobial prophylaxis for endocarditis: Emotion or science? *Heart* 2007; 93: 5–6.
2. Gould FK, Elliott TS, Foweraker J, et al. Guidelines for the prevention of endocarditis: Report of the Working Party of the British Society for Antimicrobial Chemotherapy. *Journal of Antimicrobial Chemotherapy* 2006; 57 (6): 1035–1042.
3. National Institute for Health and Clinical Excellence. *NICE Guidelines: Antimicrobial prophylaxis against infective endocarditis in adults and children undergoing interventional procedures*. London, NICE March 2008. http://www.nice.org.uk/Guidance/CG64/Guidance/pdf/English
4. Paul M, Raz A, Leibovici L, Madar H, Holinger R, Rubinovitch B. Sternal wound infection after coronary bypass graft surgery: Validation of existing risk scores. *The Journal of Thoracic and Cardiovascular Surgery* 2007; 133: 397–403.
5. Weaver W, Nishimura R, Warnes C. Antimicrobial prophylaxis to prevent infective endocarditis: Why did the recommendations change? *JACC* 2008; 52: 495–497.
6. Wilson AP. Post Operative Surveillance, registration and classification of wound infection in cardiac surgery – experiences from Great Britain. APMIS 2007; 115: 996–1000.

Part 3

Clinical practice of cardiac anaesthesia

Cardiac interventions

11	Interventional cardiology and coronary artery disease	**165**
12	Interventions in congenital heart disease	**179**
13	Electrophysiological procedures	**189**
14	Cardiac surgery	**195**

Anaesthesia for cardiac surgery and interventions

15	Preoperative assessment and investigations	**207**
16	Monitoring	**223**
17	Trans-oesophageal echocardiography	**241**
18	Cardiopulmonary bypass	**261**
19	Deep hypothermic circulatory arrest	**273**
20	Intra-aortic balloon counter-pulsation	**287**
21	Ventricular assist devices	**297**
22	Postoperative care	**307**
23	Anaesthesia for coronary artery disease	**331**

24 Off-pump surgery 34

25 Aortic valve surgery 35

26 Surgery of the thoracic aorta 37

27 Mitral valve surgery 39

28 Other valve disease 41

29 Paediatric congenital heart disease 42

30 Adult congenital heart disease 46

31 Hypertrophic cardiomyopathy 49

32 Anaesthesia for heart failure and
transplantation 50

33 Urgent cardiac procedures 52

34 Anaesthesia for electrophysiology
procedures 54

35 Cardiac disease in pregnancy 5

Interventional cardiology and coronary artery disease

Dr M Westwood and Dr C Dollery

What is coronary intervention? *166*
Pathophysiology of coronary artery disease *170*
The clinical spectrum of coronary heart disease *171*
Percutaneous coronary intervention *172*
PCI and non-cardiac surgery *176*
Anaesthetic support during a PCI *177*
Further reading *178*

What is coronary intervention?

Percutaneous coronary intervention is one of the three key options for treatment of atherosclerotic narrowing of the coronary arteries – the others being medical therapy and coronary artery bypass grafting. In the UK, despite decreasing mortality rates, approximately 260,000 people have an acute MI and 340,000 new cases of angina occur each year.

The umbrella term **percutaneous coronary intervention** (PCI) describes percutaneous transluminal coronary angioplasty (PTCA) with or without adjunctive stenting. PTCA describes percutaneous access to the coronary arteries using wires and catheters and the inflation of a balloon threaded over a guidewire across a coronary stenosis. The balloon is inflated and expands to widen the inner dimensions of the artery, thus increasing downstream blood flow. A **stent** is a metal mesh tube that is deployed by inflating an angioplasty balloon, and it eventually becomes part of the vessel wall coated in endothelial cells. Various anticoagulants and antiplatelet agents are employed during and after coronary intervention and are essential to suppressing the thrombotic response to vascular injury, which would otherwise occlude the vessel with thrombus.

The development of coronary intervention

PTCA

Andreas Grundzig carried out the first PTCA in Switzerland in 1977. Initially used only to treat proximal coronary lesions, PTCA rapidly developed as an alternative to coronary artery bypass grafting (CABG). PTCA had two major limitations – coronary artery dissection and restenosis. Restenosis is more common in small vessels, vein grafts, long lesions, or totally blocked vessels, and in diabetics.

Stents

Coronary artery stents addressed some of the problems of PTCA (Figure 11.1). A stent could be inserted at a dissection, controlling the flap. The clinical impact of stenting on restenosis was significant, although the exact impact varied between studies. Stent usage rose steeply from <10% in 1993 to 80% in 1999.

Although better than PTCA, in-stent restenosis was still recognized to cause further symptoms in 10–20% of patients. Drug-eluting stents (DES) addressed this – they gradually elute drugs such as rapamycin (sirolimus) or paclitaxel to reduce or arrest cell proliferation. DES reduce the need for repeat revascularization after stenting. A National Institute for Clinical excellence (NICE) meta-analysis demonstrated an odds ratio of 0.42 for target vessel revascularization at two years compared with bare metal stents. By 2004 DES were in use in 80% of angioplasty cases in the United States. In 2003 DES were used in 17% of UK stent procedures but this rose to 62% by 2005.

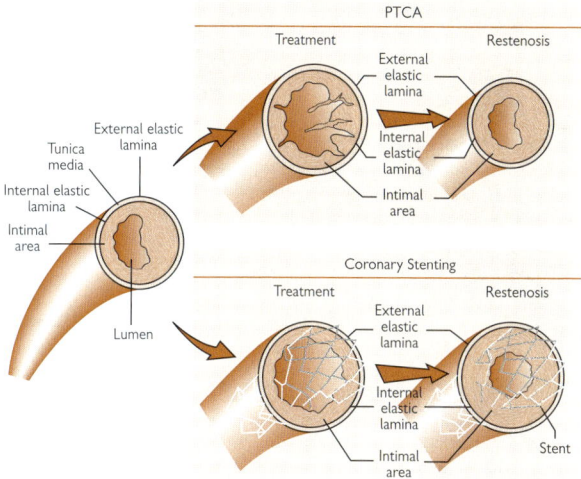

Figure 11.1 PTCA and coronary stenting.

Stent thrombosis

Case reports of acute stent thrombosis in DES began to emerge and two studies in 2006 showed a small but significant increase in death or MI after DES procedures, with 0.6% acute stent thrombosis rates per year (Figure 11.2). A particular concern has been the occurrence of stent thrombosis late (>1 month) or very late (>1 year) after implantation of DES. This is probably due to inflammation or failure of endothelialization of DES because of the anti-proliferative drugs or stent malposition. This is a rare event but may carry a mortality of up to 50% and questions remain about when, if ever, this risk abates. The United States Food and Drug Administration (FDA) reviewed the use of drug-eluting stents and concluded that 'on-label' use, i.e. within the original licences, should continue as the substantial benefit in the need for revascularization outweighed the risk of stent thrombosis. They also warned that 'off-label' use (complex disease or major comorbidities) was a risk for stent thrombosis and stressed the importance of uninterrupted use of clopidogrel and aspirin. The risk of stent thrombosis may rise up to 80-fold if antiplatelet agents are stopped prematurely. The optimal duration of clopidogrel treatment after stenting is unknown. The FDA and the British Cardiac Interventional Society (BCIS) recommend that clopidogrel is used for 12 months after drug-eluting stent procedures. Further NICE technology appraisals of DES will follow.

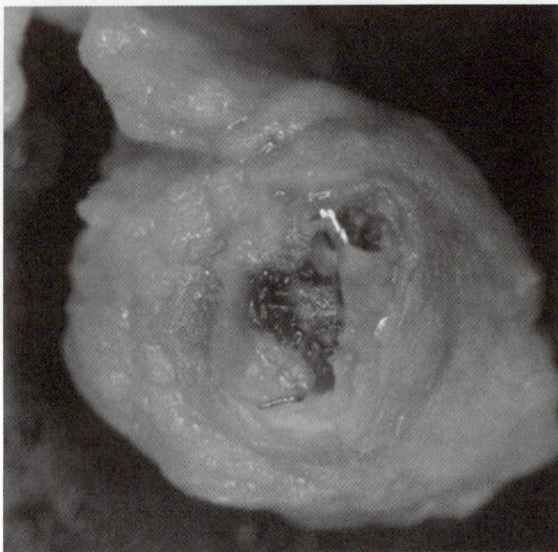

Figure 11.2 Acute stent thrombosis.

Pathophysiology of coronary artery disease

(📖 see also Chapter 4) Previously atherosclerosis was regarded as a disease of progressive cholesterol accumulation in atheromatous lesions that finally and inevitably lead to vascular stenosis or occlusion and symptoms of angina or myocardial infarction. This concept disregarded evidence from autopsy studies that only 25–33% of lethal coronary thrombi are associated with the most stenotic segments in the affected vessels. It is also clear that benefits of cholesterol-lowering therapies in altering cardiovascular event rates exceed the minimal change in severity of coronary stenoses following treatment.

We now accept atherosclerosis as a more complex interaction between cells and molecular messengers of the artery wall and the blood. Our expanding knowledge supports inflammation as the driving force behind initiation, progression, and catastrophic thrombotic complications in atherosclerosis. Acute revascularization may accomplish important damage limitation but does not address the underlying processes governing the condition.

The initial steps to atherogenesis involve accumulation of cholesterol in the intima, which mediates recruitment of inflammatory leucocytes, followed by development of a fibro-fatty plaque comprising a lipid core and macrophages that ultimately will evolve into lipid-rich foam cells. Recruitment of leucocytes into the atherosclerotic plaque provides the building blocks for intense local inflammation. Atheroma then progresses by gradual cellular accumulation punctuated by crises that are pivotal to lesion development. These crises might occur when a plaque erodes or ruptures as proteinases from inflammatory cells disrupt the fibrous cap, exposing the thrombogenic lesion core and causing luminal thrombosis. These plaque rupture events are probably frequent and often sub-clinical. Healing follows, which may stabilize but also enlarges the plaque burden. In this respect, a plaque is like an active volcano adding to its cinder cone by gradual small eruptions, but the size of the cinder cone itself does not help to predict the onset of a catastrophic explosive eruption. In the same way the severity of a coronary stenosis does not predict the onset of a myocardial infarction. In this context it is understandable that routine coronary intervention is effective at relieving symptoms and improving quality of life, but does not necessarily reduce mortality or subsequent myocardial infarction.

The clinical spectrum of coronary heart disease

Definitions and terminology

Angina

Angina encompasses chest, neck, arm, and upper abdominal pain or tightness often related to exertion, which originates from a lack of blood supply to the myocardium. 'Unstable' denotes angina that is increasing in frequency, occurring on less effort, or happening at rest, although this term is falling out of use as this definition allows all new cases of angina to be considered unstable.

Acute coronary syndromes

Most now prefer the term 'acute coronary syndromes' (ACS) to cover:

- STEMI – S-T elevation myocardial infarction.
- NSTEMI – non-S-T elevation myocardial infarction, where release of biomarkers of myocardial necrosis such as troponin T and I is detected in association with a presentation of severe angina, but there is no S-T elevation on 12-lead ECG.
- Unstable angina without any biochemically detectable myocardial damage.

These definitions broadly associate with intended treatment – STEMI requires immediate revascularization by thrombolysis or primary PCI; NSTEMI confers a high risk of further cardiovascular events and is usually followed by inpatient angiography to consider revascularization. Unstable angina may be further risk stratified by non-invasive testing (exercise tolerance test, ETT, and myocardial perfusion scanning, MPS).

Stable angina

This encompasses exertion-related chest pain or discomfort that is relieved by rest, and is caused by slow progression of lesions. The ECG may be normal or abnormal. Most patients have a non-invasive test (exercise ECG or MPS) to assess likelihood of future coronary events. Medical therapy may include use of antiplatelet agents such as aspirin, statins, beta-blockers, nitrates, and calcium antagonists.

Percutaneous coronary intervention

Traditionally PCI was only attempted on short discrete lesions clear of side branches (type A lesions). Technological developments now allow PCI on more complex lesions, longer segments of disease, and bifurcation lesions. It is also possible to reopen completely occluded arteries.

- The use of antiplatelet therapy before PCI is pivotal. Most patients will already be on low-dose aspirin. Patients also receive clopidogrel at the time of PCI, which is usually given as a loading dose (either 300 mg or 600 mg) six hours before the procedure. The use of this loading dose of clopidogrel significantly reduces the risk of stent thrombosis.
- A guide catheter is positioned in the relevant coronary ostium. Guide catheters have a larger lumen to allow passage of a guidewire, balloon, and stent but are less flexible than diagnostic catheters and may carry a higher risk of aortic or coronary ostial dissection.
- Before beginning the PCI, an angiographic road map is acquired including at least two orthogonal angiograms of the lesion to be attempted.
- A weight-adjusted bolus dose of unfractionated heparin or low molecular weight heparin is administered at the start of PCI. This prevents clots on the wires and catheters.
- A guidewire is passed across the lesion into the distal part of the relevant coronary artery using X-ray fluoroscopy to visualize the wire. A device called a torquer may be attached distally to the wire, facilitating manipulation.
- A balloon (with radio-opaque markers) is passed over the guidewire and positioned at the stenosis using fluoroscopy. The balloon is inflated using a pressure-regulating insufflator. Then the balloon is deflated and removed. An angiogram is acquired to check for coronary dissection.
- A stent is usually deployed across the lesion. Stents are deployed on a balloon to which they have been crimped, so positioning the stent is similar. When the balloon is inflated in the artery, the stent detaches from the balloon and is deployed, indenting the arterial wall. Sometimes it is not necessary to dilate the lesion with a balloon and a stent can be deployed directly. Stents come in various lengths and diameters, the smallest being 2.25 mm in diameter. If the artery is smaller than this then it can only be treated with balloon angioplasty.
- If the angiogram following stent deployment is satisfactory, the guidewire is removed and a final angiographic picture of the artery is acquired. The guide catheter is then removed and the access site is sealed as for an angiogram.
- No reflow refers to no or slow flow down the artery following balloon deflation. It usually responds to vasodilators. Abciximab, which is a monoclonal antibody to GpIIb/IIIa and a highly potent inhibitor of platelet aggregation, can be given. Abciximab may be routinely administered in primary angioplasty for myocardial infarction, in diabetic patients, and sometimes after complex intervention at the discretion of the operator. Minor haematuria or gum bleeding are common and there is a small risk of significant bleeding.

Complications of angiography/PCI

Peri-procedural complications

- Local arterial access complications:
  - Arterial dissection – usually self-limiting and treated by manual pressure and removing the sheath. The dissection will usually have been caused by the retrograde insertion of the catheter so the antegrade blood flow will promote sealing of the tear.
  - Arterial bleeding – it is important to apply manual pressure at the site of puncture into the artery and not at the site of the skin incision. Even with the use of antiplatelet therapy and GpIIb/IIIa inhibitors, haemostasis will eventually be attained.
  - Arterial occlusion – this is more common with the radial and brachial approach. With the brachial artery the arterial puncture site is closed with a small suture and this can lead to brachial artery occlusion. If limb ischaemia develops, an urgent vascular surgical opinion should be sought.
  - A variety of closure devices based on plugs or sutures are available to achieve haemostasis of the femoral artery. On occasion these can fail to deploy properly. Manual pressure of the femoral access site is then required.
  - Use of a Femostop – the Femostop is a device including a belt and pressurized dome that can be used to apply pressure to the femoral access site. A Femostop can apply a more uniform pressure for longer periods than manual compression. It is important that the device is applied not at the site of the skin incision but where the puncture into the femoral artery was made (usually 1–2 cm higher up). If bleeding continues the device should be checked and possibly replaced with manual compression, and a vascular surgical opinion considered.
  - Retroperitoneal bleeding from femoral access – this is rare (<1%) but should be suspected where there is gross haemodynamic instability and other causes of hypotension and shock have been excluded. Emergency assistance from vascular intervention teams may be required, as concealed bleeding into the retroperitoneum can be fatal either due to primary blood loss or tamponade of retroperitoneal organs.
  - Severe bradycardia can occur with removal of the femoral sheath, especially in young males. This generally self-terminates, although atropine can be given if it persists.
- Arrhythmic complications:
  - VT/VF. There are several causes of this:
    - Injection of air into the coronary arteries due to incorrect manifold setup.
    - Contrast injection directly into the small conus branch of the RCA.
    - Catheter entry into the left ventricle. This is usually self-limiting.
    - In primary PCI due to either the infarction itself or so-called reperfusion arrhythmias, where the re-establishment of flow down the occluded coronary artery results in arrhythmia.
    - Coronary artery dissection or tamponade can provoke VT/VF.

- Management is usually aimed at rectification of the underlying cause followed by rapid DC shock.
- Atrial arrhythmias:
  - PCI to the right coronary artery.
  - In primary PCI due to infarction or reperfusion arrhythmias.
  - If not causing haemodynamic problems no specific treatment is required and they often resolve. If they persist, chemical or electrical cardioversion can be carried out after the PCI.
- Bradycardia:
  - Occasionally occurs on injection of dye into the coronary arteries but it is usually self-limiting. More frequent in those with any degree of heart block.
  - Can occur on catheter entry into the left ventricle. This may need atropine but asking the patient to cough often restores sinus rhythm.
- Coronary artery dissection:
  - Localized dissection – this most often occurs after balloon inflation or stent deployment but may follow passage of a guidewire. Treated by deployment of a stent across the dissected portion. It is critical to maintain the position of the original guidewire to ensure that the correct lumen is re-established by stenting with that wire. If the guidewire is displaced, e.g. if the patient moves, it may not be possible to re-establish the guidewire across the dissection, potentially necessitating emergent coronary artery surgery.
  - Ostial coronary artery dissection by the guide catheter – treated by stent deployment as long as the dissection is localized and does not extend into the aorta. The alternative is CABG.
  - Severe coronary dissection leading to dissection of the aorta. This is an emergency and the patient is likely to become critically unstable. If the left main stem is involved the patient may suffer extensive acute ischaemia/infarction and arrest. In general all guide catheters and wires are left in place and urgent arrangements are made for surgical intervention.
  - Diagnostic catheters can also cause ostial coronary artery dissection if they are moved too vigorously.
- Hypotension during the procedure:
  - Administration of intracoronary nitrates. Typically 100–200 µg is given as an intra-arterial bolus dose. The hypotension is short lived (about 20–30 seconds).
  - Pre-procedural dehydration is usually remedied by giving intravenous fluids.
  - Cardiac tamponade due to coronary perforation or rupture will lead to worsening hypotension and should always be suspected during PCI where no other readily identifiable cause can be found.
  - Severe contrast reactions. These are rare with modern contrast agents, but can still occur. The patient should be inspected for signs of an urticarial rash and oxygen saturations noted. Note: A rash can be missed if the sterile drapes are not lifted to inspect the skin.
  - Arterial bleeding and retroperitoneal bleeding (see above).

- Cardiac tamponade during PCI:
  - Guidewire perforation at the lesion site.
  - Guidewire perforation through the distal arterial wall, having passed too far down the vessel.
  - A balloon or stent has caused arterial rupture (invariably fatal but rare).
  - A guidewire perforating the coronary artery can usually be removed without precipitating tamponade as long as no balloon or stent has passed through the perforation. This is true even in the presence of antiplatelet therapy and GpIIb/IIIA inhibitors. Where a stent strut or calcium spicule cause coronary rupture by perforation during balloon inflation, it may be possible to plug the hole by very rapid deployment of a covered stent (a stent entirely covered by an impermeable membrane).
  - Tamponade is diagnosed without the need for echocardiography when there is residual dye-staining in the pericardium following arterial dye injection. Drainage of the tamponade using the subxiphoid approach follows. If tamponade is suspected but there is no dye-staining of the pericardium then urgent transthoracic echocardiography should be performed.

Post-procedural complications

- Pulmonary oedema is precipitated by the combination of an osmotic contrast load, impaired LV function, and the need to lie absolutely flat. It is more common in patients with LV dysfunction, valvular heart disease (especially aortic stenosis), and renal dysfunction. It is treated by sitting the patient up, oxygen, IV nitrates, and diuretics.
- Pseudoaneurysm formation is most common with the femoral access route. It causes pain and a swollen pulsatile lump. Diagnosis is by ultrasound scan and it can be treated by manual pressure to cause thrombosis in the false aneurysm. It is sometimes possible to inject procoagulant substances (such as thrombin) into the false aneurysm to cause thrombosis – on advice from an interventional radiologist.
- Renal failure is more likely in patients with pre-existing renal disease or where a large amount of contrast agent has been used. Pre-hydration and the use of N-acetyl cysteine at the time of the procedure reduce the chances of renal dysfunction.
- Retroperitoneal bleeding (see above).
- Systemic embolism following coronary angiography is rare (0.03–0.3% after diagnostic angiography and 0.3–0.4% after PCI). Emboli are usually cerebral but may occur anywhere. They are thought to be fragments of atherosclerotic plaque from the aorta but may also be air or cholesterol emboli (the latter are visible if they affect the retinal circulation). Asymptomatic microemboli are common in MRI or transcranial Doppler studies. Presentations include visual disturbance, aphasia, and focal weakness but confusion may also occur. Urgent CT and neurological consultation should be obtained.

Long-term complications

Stent thrombosis and in-stent restenosis remain the challenge for PCI.

PCI and non-cardiac surgery

Antiplatelet therapy

- Approximately 5% of patients undergoing PCI will need some kind of non-cardiac surgery in the ensuing year.
- Most of the implications relate to use of dual antiplatelet therapy.
- Patients with drug-eluting stents are committed to 12 months of dual antiplatelet therapy with aspirin and clopidogrel (four weeks for a bare metal stent).
- Most centres gather all their interventional data using computer systems that upload to the central cardiac audit databases so the type of stent can be tracked. The patient usually receives a copy including the type of stent used and a clopidogrel information card with the planned duration of therapy.
- Stopping aspirin or clopidogrel during the minimum recommended post-PCI period is associated with a substantial increased risk of stent thrombosis.
- Stent thrombosis can convey 50% mortality.
- With a bare metal stent surgery should be postponed until six weeks post-stenting.
- The antiplatelet effects of clopidogrel can persist for up to a week after cessation.
- There are no randomized trials of dual antiplatelet therapy versus placebo in non-cardiac surgery. Decisions are based on experience, observational studies, and case clusters. Patients undergoing neurosurgery have a high risk of adverse bleeding events whereas in many other types of surgery bleeding may increase by around 30%, but this is not associated with significant mortality or morbidity.
- If bleeding will occur in a region where it cannot be controlled or in a closed space (i.e. intracranial or spinal surgery), the bleeding risk may exceed that of stopping the antiplatelet agents. A growing body of opinion suggests that in all other circumstances where the patient is within the period of mandated antiplatelet agents they should be continued perioperatively, as even in relatively major surgery the risk from bleeding may be less than that of stent thrombosis.
- Continuation of statin therapy throughout the perioperative period may also reduce cardiovascular events.
- In the situation of intervention to facilitate an emergent non-cardiac operation, a stent may not be used. In this case the likelihood of recoil and restenosis leading to a return of symptoms is relatively high (approximately 30%) but this risk may be outweighed by the need for surgery without dual antiplatelet therapy and risk of stent thrombosis.

Anaesthetic support during a PCI

It is rare in adult practice for elective anaesthesia to be used during a PCI. Anaesthetic support is usually required if the patient's airway or breathing is compromised prior to angiography, e.g. if they are in pulmonary oedema or have presented after a cardiac arrest. In addition peri-procedural arrests need urgent attention to airway and breathing and frequently require intubation.

What to expect on arrival in the catheter lab

- X-ray fluoroscopy and angiography are essential to PCI and it is important to wear a lead apron. If you enter a cath lab without radiation protection equipment you are likely to be escorted out by the radiographer, who otherwise has to disable the X-ray equipment with consequent delay and inconvenience.
- Exposure to radiation decreases with distance from the image intensifier according to the inverse square law, so your best protection is to step back from the patient while X-rays are in use, particularly during angiograms.
- If you attend an emergency the patient will already have monitoring of ECG, oxygen saturation, and blood pressure. These will be displayed on the monitor opposite the first operator, usually adjacent to the angiogram image and on a monitor visible to the cardiac physiologist. While it may be convenient to the anaesthetist to establish additional monitoring, interim information can be gained immediately from these screens, although the arterial pressure lumen is used for injection of contrast at which time the pressure trace is not available, and the trace may be distorted during balloon or stent manipulation.
- Patients undergoing angiography usually have peripheral intravenous access only – commonly in their arms – which may be connected via extension tubing to an access site near their feet – ask the nurse. In an emergency the quickest large-bore central access is usually gained by the operator inserting a sterile venous sheath into the femoral vein.
- There are usually joint priorities of resuscitation and rectification of the cause of cardiac arrest; the latter requires further attempts at PCI using fluoroscopy. Insertion of internal jugular lines can therefore be impractical as it requires the angiogram table to be moved away from the image intensifier.
- The table will be moved away if chest compression is required but remote defibrillation with pads connected to the chest will be used. If relocation of the patient is essential to anaesthetic care, discuss this with the operator and/or radiographer.

Further reading

1. King SB, Smith SC, Hirshfeld JW Jr., et al. 2007 focused update of the ACC/AHA/SCAI 2005 guideline update for percutaneous coronary intervention. A report of the American College of Cardiology/American Heart Association Task Force on Practice Guidelines. *Circulation* 2008; 117: 261–295.
2. Mauri L, Hsieh W, Massaro J, Ho K, D'Agostino R, Cutlip D. Stent thrombosis in randomized clinical trials of drug-eluting stents. *New England Journal of Medicine* 2007; 356: 1020–1029.
3. Ong A, McFadden E, Regar E, de Jaegere P, van Domburg R, Serruys P. Late angiographic stent thrombosis (LAST) events with drug-eluting stents. *JACC* 2005; 45: 2088–2092.
4. Serruys P, Morice MC, Kappetein A, et al. Percutaneous coronary intervention versus coronary artery bypass grafting for severe coronary disease. *New England Journal of Medicine* 2009; 360: 961–972.
5. Stettler C, Wandel S, Alleman S, et al. Outcomes associated with drug-eluting and bare-metal stents: A collaborative network meta-analysis. *Lancet* 2007; 370: 937–948.

Interventions in congenital heart disease

Dr S Cullen

Background *180*
Interventions *181*
Further reading *187*

Background

Advances in medicine and surgery have led to a dramatic improvement in outcome for patients born with even very complex congenital heart disease (CHD). Approximately 90% of all infants with CHD will survive into adult life and there will soon be more adults with CHD than children.

Collaboration between surgeons and physicians has led to the development of novel percutaneous transcatheter interventions, which obviate the need for surgery and/or multiple re-sternotomies. Many of these interventions are performed under general anaesthesia to permit guidance by trans-oesophageal monitoring.

Interventions

(Balloon atrial septostomy)

The creation of an atrial communication to permit mixing and improve oxygenation using a balloon catheter in critically ill neonates with transposition of the great arteries was devised by William Rashkind. This innovation transformed the outlook for neonates born with TGA, a previously universally lethal condition. This can now be performed in the neonatal unit using cross-sectional echocardiographic monitoring.

Balloon valvuloplasty

Balloon dilation of a stenotic pulmonary valve can be easily performed using a catheter-mounted balloon placed across the annulus over a guidewire. Balloon size is dictated by the size of the pulmonary annulus (100–120%) measured on cross-sectional echocardiography and angiographic measurements. This is an effective intervention in all patients except those with a dysplastic valve, such as adults with Noonan's syndrome.

Balloon dilation of a stenotic aortic valve has limited application in adults. It can be used in the rare case of a patient presenting with severe disease in pregnancy to defer the need for definitive operation. It can be offered in the growing adolescent if the valve is pliable and not calcified, albeit at the expense of producing important aortic regurgitation. An antegrade approach via trans-septal puncture improves balloon stability and outcome. Definitive surgery will be required subsequently.

Septal defects

Depending on position and size, the majority of secundum atrial septal defects (ASDs) are amenable to transcatheter closure with an occluding device. This technique is only suitable for secundum defects and not for sinus venosus-type or partial atrioventricular septal defects. The defect is sized by balloon using trans-oesophageal or intracardiac echocardiography. Defects in excess of 40 mm with insufficient rims, particularly inferiorly, are not suitable for device closure. Procedural complications are rare but serious problems include device embolization, pulmonary venous obstruction, interference with the mitral valve, and rarely cardiac perforation. Transient arrhythmias are common. Antibiotic prophylaxis and intravenous heparin (50–100 units/kg) are administered. Antiplatelet therapy is administered for six months after the procedure. Concomitant electrophysiological interventions may be performed.

Patent foramen ovale (PFO) has been implicated in the causation of transient ischaemic episodes, cerebrovascular accidents, and migraines. Simple PFO is common in the general population, although it is the less common PFO associated with aneurysmal atrial septum and a positive echocardiography bubble study that is associated with neurological events. Balloon sizing of the PFO can permit definition of tunnel-type defects, allowing improved choice of device type. Evidence is accumulating in favour of closure of PFO in the presence of severe migraines with aura. The technique and complications are as for transcatheter closure of atrial septal defects.

There are limited indications for percutaneous closure of ventricular septal defects (VSDs) in adults. The Amplatzer ASD device has been used in peri-membranous, muscular, and post-infarction VSD. However, difficult access and serious complications limit its application. Complications include complete heart block requiring pacemaker, aortic insufficiency, and device embolization. These procedures should only be undertaken in specialist centres.

Coarctation

Both native and recoarctation of the aorta (CoA) can now be successfully treated by transcatheter balloon dilation and stenting, depending on morphology of both coarctation and major vessels. Magnetic resonance imaging or multislice CT scanning assist in patient selection and balloon/stent size. Native CoA can be treated using a covered stent to reduce the risk of subsequent dissection and rupture. The risk of acute dissection or rupture during the procedure should be appreciated by the anaesthetist. If there is a true interruption of the aorta, surgery is required. Dilation of a recoarctation previously treated by patch aortoplasty carries the highest risk of aortic rupture. In patients in whom aneurysms have developed over time, the aneurysms can be occluded and covered with a stent employed to exclude them from the true lumen of the aorta. Some patients develop intense chest pain (limited dissection) post-procedure and analgesia may be required. Careful monitoring of blood pressure and lifelong surveillance is required.

A small or moderate-sized patent arterial duct without pulmonary hypertension is amenable to percutaneous transcatheter occlusion using coils or Amplatzer device.

Valves

Rheumatic heart disease causing mitral stenosis can potentially be palliated with transcatheter valvuloplasty. Suitability is defined by trans-oesophageal echocardiography. Antegrade approach with femoral venous catheterization and trans-septal puncture employing multitrack catheters is used.

Residual pulmonary regurgitation is common following right heart surgery and correction of tetralogy of Fallot. This may result in right heart volume overload, impaired right ventricular function, decreased exercise tolerance, late arrhythmias, and sudden death. Patients who have undergone surgical placement of a right ventricle to pulmonary arterial connection can be treated in the catheter laboratory with percutaneous pulmonary valve implantation. A bovine jugular venous valve mounted within a platinum iridium stent can be placed in the right ventricular outflow tract using a purpose-made balloon and delivery system. In selected patients this obviates the need for high-risk redo sternotomy. Complications include stent fractures, endocarditis, and device embolization. Percutaneous aortic valve implantation is currently being developed, although it is not yet as advanced as pulmonary valve implantation – 📖 see also Surgical essentials and therapeutic options, p. 366, Chapter 25.

Miscellaneous

In addition there are a miscellaneous group of cardiac abnormalities or post-surgical complications that can be treated by percutaneous techniques. Patient selection is important. These include certain patients with paravalvar prosthetic leaks (both mitral and aortic) or fistulae such as coronary arterial fistulae. These are only undertaken in specialist centres.

Further reading

1. Inglessis I, Landzberg M. Interventional catheterization in adult congenital heart disease. *Circulation* 2007; 115: 1622–1633.
2. Graham T, Driscoll D, Gersony W, Newburger J, Rocchini A, Towbin J. Task force 2: Congenital heart disease. *Journal of the American College of Cardiology* 2005; 45: 1326–1333.
3. Warnes C, Williams R, Bashore T, et al. ACC/AHA 2008 guidelines for the management of adults with congenital heart disease: A report of the American College of Cardiology/American Heart Association Task Force on Practice Guidelines. *Journal of the American College of Cardiology* 2008; 52: e143–e263.

Further reading

Electrophysiological procedures

Dr P Lambiase and Dr M Lowe

Introduction 190
Ablation 192
Further reading 194

Introduction

Electrophysiological procedures can be divided into diagnostic electrophysiology studies (EPSs) or therapeutic procedures, which involve ablation (most commonly using radio-frequency (RF) or freezing with cryotherapy).

Indications

- Bradyarrhythmias:
  - Sinus node dysfunction.
  - AV (His-Purkinje) block.
  - Intraventricular conduction delay.
  - Left or right bundle branch block.
  - Guide to device therapy (permanent pacing).
- Tachyarrhythmias
  - Narrow QRS complex tachycardia, e.g. atrial flutter, atrioventricular re-entrant tachycardia (AVRT), atrioventricular nodal re-entrant tachycardia (AVNRT).
  - Broad QRS complex tachycardia, e.g. ventricular tachycardia (VT).
  - Non-sustained ventricular arrhythmias, e.g. ventricular premature beats (VPBs), non-sustained VT.
  - Prolonged QT syndrome.
  - Unexplained syncope.
  - Survivors of cardiac arrest (near-miss sudden death).
  - Guide to drug therapy.
  - Guide to device therapy (automated implantable cardioverter-defibrillator, AICD).

EPS

Patient preparation

EP procedures are performed in a fully equipped (preferably bi-plane) cardiac catheterization laboratory with experienced personnel, full resuscitation facilities, and a computer-based EP system capable of displaying and storing data.

The procedure

- An EP study involves the positioning of multipolar catheters at pre-specified sites in the heart, usually via the femoral venous approach, although some operators will position a catheter in the coronary sinus from the subclavian or internal jugular vein.
- Catheters are placed under fluoroscopic guidance in the right atrium, right ventricular apex, and near the AV node to record signals from the His and coronary sinus (Figure 13.1). Newer systems can image catheter positions using changes in intracardiac impedance (NavX®). The atrium and ventricle are paced at fixed intervals followed by extrastimuli to assess the conduction system of the heart and initiate an arrhythmia. The mechanism of the arrhythmia is evaluated through intracardiac electrograms and the response to pacing stimuli at timed intervals.

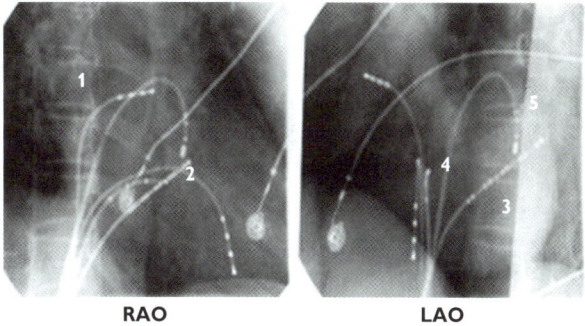

Figure 13.1 Location of intracardiac EP catheters shown in RAO and LAO views.
1. Right atrial catheter. 2. Right ventricular apical catheter. 3. Coronary sinus deca-
polar catheter. 4. His catheter. 5. Ablation catheter on mitral valve annulus at site of
an accessory pathway.

Diagnoses

Supraventricular arrhythmias

- Focal atrial tachycardia.
- Atrial flutter.
- Atrial fibrillation.
- AVNRT.
- Accessory pathway-mediated AVRT.

Ventricular tachycardia

- Focal – usually arising from the right ventricular outflow tract (RVOT VT).
- Re-entrant ischaemic and dilated cardiomyopathy.

Ablation

Most arrhythmias are *re-entrant*, passing through a critical isthmus or pathway that is amenable to ablation. Ablation requires the identification of the critical site and delivery of energy to cauterize the tissue so it becomes electrically inert. The most common ablation procedures include the following.

Atrial flutter

A series of lesions is delivered between the tricuspid valve annulus and inferior vena cava to prevent re-entrant activation within the right atrium passing through the isthmus of tissue.

AVNRT

The most common site of ablation is the slow pathway of the AV node, which lies between the coronary sinus and the His recording site. Complications include 0.5–1% of AV block and pacemaker dependence.

AVRT

The accessory pathway is specifically targeted. This usually lies on the AV ring either on the tricuspid or mitral valve annulus. A mapping catheter is delivered to the mitral valve either via trans-septal puncture or a retrograde approach through the aortic valve. The atrial entry point is identified by ventricular pacing and mapping the earliest returning atrial signals. The most common pathway is in the left free wall. Complications for left-sided pathways include AV block (1%, rising to 5% if the pathway is paranodal), tamponade, and cerebrovascular accident (0.01%).

RVOT ventricular tachycardia

These focal tachycardias are targeted by mapping with an ablation catheter or a specialized basket/mapping array deployed in the RVOT. Pacing at the site is employed to reproduce the surface ECG of the clinical VT at the VT focus. Complications include cardiac tamponade and right bundle branch block (rare).

Atrial fibrillation ablation

- The volume of AF ablation is increasing exponentially and the technique is evolving. Patients usually require a trans-oesophageal echo preoperatively to exclude intra-atrial thrombus.
- Pulmonary vein mapping and ablation catheter are delivered through trans-septal punctures into the left atrium.
- Pulmonary vein anatomy is defined by contrast injection at the vein ostia.
- The geometry of the left atrium is created by moving the ablation catheter in contact with endocardium and this can be aligned with an imported CT or MRI scan to render a precise anatomical localization of catheters.
- Lesions are delivered completely encircling the pulmonary vein ostia with conventional or cooled-flow catheters (Figure 13.2).

- Electrical isolation is confirmed with the mapping catheter placed at the vein ostia. Additional lines may be generated in the roof, between the upper and lower veins, mitral annulus to lower veins, and on the floor of the atrium.
- Patients are anticoagulated with unfractionated heparin to maintain an ACT between 300 and 350 seconds. Post-sheath removal, subcutaneous fractionated heparin is employed until a therapeutic INR of 2–3 is achieved with warfarin.
- Complications include cardiac tamponade (1–3%), CVA (1%), and pulmonary vein stenosis (1%).

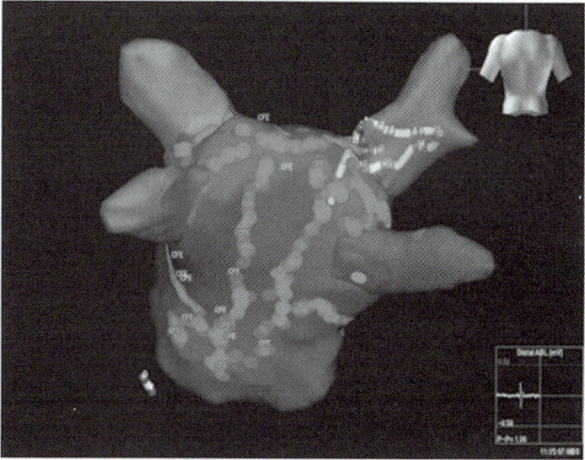

Figure 13.2 PA view of LA created by NavX® system illustrating circular PV catheter in PV os (yellow) and encircling lesions (red) around the left- and right-sided pulmonary veins, with additional lesions delivered at sites of high frequency drivers (complex fractionated electrograms, CFEs). A roof line between the two upper PVs is also present.

Further reading

1. Calkins H, Brugada J, Packer DL, et al. HRS/EHRA/ECAS Expert Consensus Statement on catheter and surgical ablation of atrial fibrillation: Recommendations for personnel, policy, procedures and follow-up. A report of the Heart Rhythm Society (HRS) Task Force on Catheter and Surgical Ablation of Atrial Fibrillation. *Heart Rhythm* 2007; 4: 816–861.

2. Dong J, Dickfeld T, Dalal D, et al. Initial experience in the use of integrated electroanatomic mapping with three-dimensional MR/CT images to guide catheter ablation of atrial fibrillation. *Journal of Cardiovascular Electrophysiology* 2006; 17: 459–466.

3. Haissaguerre M, Hocini M, Sanders P, et al. Catheter ablation of long-lasting persistent atrial fibrillation: Clinical outcome and mechanisms of subsequent arrhythmias. *Journal of Cardiovascular Electrophysiology* 2005; 16: 1138–1147.

4. Oral H, Pappone C, Chugh A, et al. Circumferential pulmonary-vein ablation for chronic atrial fibrillation. *New England Journal of Medicine* 2006; 354: 934–941.

5. Pappone C, Augello G, Sala S, et al. A randomized trial of circumferential pulmonary vein ablation versus antiarrhythmic drug therapy in paroxysmal atrial fibrillation. *The APAF Study Journal of the American College of Cardiology* 2006; 48: 2340–2347.

6. Stabile G, Bertaglia E, Senatore G, De Simone A, Zoppo F, Donnici G. Catheter ablation treatment in patients with drug-refractory atrial fibrillation: A prospective, multi-centre, randomized, controlled study (Catheter Ablation For The Cure Of Atrial Fibrillation Study). *European Heart Journal* 2006; 27: 216–221.

Cardiac surgery

Mr J Yap

Risk assessment *196*
Conduct of surgery *198*
Emergency surgery *199*
Myocardial preservation *200*
Off-pump coronary artery bypass *203*
Minimally invasive cardiac surgery (MICS) *204*
Reoperative surgery *205*
New techniques in surgery *206*
Further reading *206*

Risk assessment

Increasingly, patients who present for cardiac surgery are elderly and have significant comorbidities. The ability to predict outcome for patients is a powerful tool for clinical and resources planning. Cardiac surgeons are increasingly asked to operate on sicker patients who previously may not have been considered suitable for surgery. However, recent experience suggests that the mortality outcome for the common cardiac operations has improved. The quality of postoperative care, especially in intensive care, may have offset the higher patient risk profile. It is important to assess individual patients' comorbidities in order to stratify risk of operative morbidity and mortality, and facilitate more accurate informed consent.

Risk stratification models (📖 see also Chapter 15 p. 210 Multifactorial risk indices)

The risk of surgery is influenced by comorbidities. These include diabetes, chronic obstructive pulmonary disease, and cerebrovascular, thyroid, and renal diseases. The effect of risk factors on surgical outcome has been rigorously defined by risk stratification models.

The Parsonnet model is based on a database developed in the US that was compiled 20 years ago, and therefore tends to overestimate mortality in most comparative studies. This is likely due to surgical and medical advances improving outcome in cardiac surgery. This model has been superseded by the EuroScore model.

EuroScore was developed using data from 128 European cardiac surgical centres. It is the most commonly used scoring algorithm in Europe, and accurately predicts mortality after cardiac surgery. The Bayesian model is the preferred method for risk stratification by the Society of Cardiothoracic Surgeons of Great Britain and Ireland (SCTS). Variations of the model exist, differing in the number of factors used to calculate the final risk score. Bayes models require more complex computer calculations of risk scores but reflect accurately on the target population. Most of these prediction models measure death as an outcome because mortality is an easily measured endpoint. Each model has fairly similar risk factors in its dataset.

Conduct of surgery

Successful cardiac surgery is dependent on a multidisciplinary team of surgeons, anaesthetists, nurses, ancillary staff, and perfusionists working cooperatively:

- Review of preoperative data (including coronary angiogram and echocardiogram) and confirmation of the anticipated procedure.
- Anaesthetist and surgeon discuss planned procedure.
- Plan for anticipated problems, especially with high-risk patients. Cardiopulmonary bypass (CPB) and myocardial protection strategy formulated. TOE requested if necessary.
- Antibiotic prophylaxis.
- General anaesthesia. Venous access and arterial monitoring.
- Patient is prepped with antiseptic solution.
- Incisions – usually median sternotomy for most cardiac operations. Any deviation should be pre-planned.
- Preparation for cardiopulmonary bypass – heparin IV given. ACT checked.
- Cannulation of the ascending aorta for aortic return and right atrium for venous drainage.
- Bypass commenced and patient cooled systemically to appropriate temperature (28–32°C). Ventilator is turned off.
- Aorta is cross-clamped and cardioplegia given (as per myocardial protection strategy chosen).
- Cardioplegia can be given antegrade via aortic root or coronary ostia, or retrograde via coronary sinus.
- Main operative procedure is carried out.
- Preparation for termination of bypass – de-airing if cardiac chambers were opened. Rewarming to 36–37°C. Ventilation recommenced. Ensure that lungs are fully inflated. Inotropic support if required. Check heart rate and rhythm, latest blood gas, and biochemistry.
- 'Off-bypass'. Assessment of cardiac function – visual, haemodynamic, TOE.
- Administer protamine to reverse the action of heparin and facilitate haemostasis. Make sure perfusionist is aware you are giving protamine! The pump suction must be stopped so that blood returned to the reservoir does not form clots (it can still be transfused into patient).
- Haemostasis. Temporary pacing wires inserted as required. Chest drains placed.
- Closure of sternotomy wound, usually with wires.
- Transfer to intensive care unit.
- Appropriate handover to ITU team including any special instructions or potential problems.

Emergency surgery (📖 see also Chapter 33)

The main indication for emergency cardiac surgery is haemodynamic instability caused by surgically treatable cardiac conditions. Major causes are:

- Trauma.
- Stabbing and gunshot wounds.
- Road traffic accident – transection of aorta, torn major vessels, structural damage to the heart.
- Major aortic diseases.
- Acute type A dissection.
- Aortic rupture.
- Endocarditis:
  - Aortic root abscess causing acute ischaemia; conduction failure.
  - Instability caused by severe structural damage, usually to the valves.
  - Overwhelming sepsis and failed medical treatment.
- Critical left main stem disease with ongoing chest pain.
- Acute ventricular septal defect secondary to myocardial infarction.
- Acute deterioration following angioplasty – coronary dissection.

Cardiac tamponade

- Post-cardiac surgery – can occur quickly in the intensive unit. Beware a postoperative patient who has been bleeding significantly and suddenly stops draining blood from the chest drains.
- During cardiology intervention – arrhythmia ablation, angioplasty.
- Trauma – relief of tamponade may save the patient's life.
- Suspect tamponade in any postoperative patient who is 'not quite right'. It will catch you out! If you think about it you will not miss it.

Myocardial preservation

Favourable outcome from cardiac surgery is dependent on effective protection of the heart. In the 1960s and 70s, the importance of myocardial damage from cardiac surgery was realized. In the extreme case of inadequate myocardial protection, a 'stone heart' was experienced. Early methods of myocardial protection included 'electric arrest' and cooling. Pharmacological intervention strategies revolutionized myocardial protection and opened up the possibility of performing complicated intracardiac procedures.

Melrose introduced a potassium citrate-based solution in 1955. Its ineffectiveness and potential for myocardial injury resulted in its abandonment. Without an effective cardioplegic-based technique, other techniques including normothermic ischaemia and coronary perfusion were employed. The lack of uniformly good results encouraged a renewed interest in cardioplegia, especially with a lower concentration of potassium. Initially Bretschneider's solution was introduced. However, significant progress was made when Hearst and Braimbridge introduced the St Thomas' crystalloid solution into clinical practice with excellent results. Later, Buckberg proposed the use of blood cardioplegia because of the buffering and oxygen-carrying potential of blood. Further refinement in the components are continuing in search of the ideal cardioprotective solution. Interestingly, other methods of myocardial protection have remained in less frequent use.

Ischaemic reperfusion injury

Ischaemic reperfusion injury is a result of sudden and uncontrolled restoration of blood flow to the myocardium following a period of ischaemia. This results in structural alterations at cellular level and deranged metabolic processes. Ischaemic reperfusion injury can be experienced following thrombolysis for acute MI, and during angioplasty and cardiac surgery. Ischaemic reperfusion injury may play a significant role in post-cardiac surgery myocardial dysfunction. It can result in myocardial stunning, apoptosis, or infarction depending on the degree of damage. In the laboratory setting, there are clear indications of the possibility of ameliorating the effect of ischaemic reperfusion with therapeutic agents. However, this has not been convincingly replicated in the clinical setting. Calcium overload and oxidative stress work in synergy and cause myocardial injury and death.

Mechanisms

- Calcium overload: Inability to maintain intracellular calcium homeostasis resulting in overload. During ischaemia there is an increase in intracellular calcium due to dysfunction of the calcium pump in the sarcolemma and sarcoplasmic reticulum, which maintains intracellular calcium status. On reperfusion, the restoration of intracellular pH via Na^+/H^+ exchange contributes to further intracellular Ca^{2+} overload via reversed calcium ion exchange. The generation of reactive oxygen species on reperfusion further contributes to the overload.
- Oxidative stress: Multiple mechanisms are implicated in free radical generation following reperfusion. In addition, deranged metabolic

events during the period of ischaemia reduces the endogenous
antioxidants including superoxide dismutase and glutathione system.

Methods of myocardial protection

- **Intermittent cross-clamp fibrillation:** Intermittent aortic cross-clamp with the heart in fibrillation. Systemic temperature cooled to 32 to 34°C with cardiopulmonary bypass. This technique is still used successfully by some surgeons in performing coronary artery bypass grafting. Its success may be related to ischaemic preconditioning.
- **Continuous coronary perfusion:** The coronary ostia are intubated with appropriate cannulae and continuous infusion of oxygenated blood is given during the operative procedure. Not commonly used.
- **Cardioplegia:** Most common form of myocardial protection. Potassium-based solution (supplemented with potentially beneficial components) that arrests the heart in diastole. Offers a relatively bloodless and quiescent operating field. Provides reliable myocardial protection. Can be given either as crystalloid or blood cardioplegia.
  - *Cold crystalloid cardioplegia:* Osmotically balanced with potassium concentration of 10–40 mmol/l and bicarbonate and other components added. Provides good myocardial protection. Superseded by blood cardioplegia.
  - *Cold blood cardioplegia:* Most commonly used technique for myocardial protection. Prepared by mixing autologous blood with potassium and other beneficial components. The cardioplegic solution is cooled to 4–10°C before delivery. Variable ratios of blood to solution (8:1 to 2:1) can be used.
  - *Warm blood cardioplegia:* As above, but the cardioplegic solution is warmed up to 37°C. A few small studies in the early nineties suggested the superiority of warm over cold blood cardioplegia. However, concern was raised in a report of an increased rate of neurological deficit. This technique is still used by some surgeons.

Potential advantages of blood cardioplegia over crystalloid
- Provides oxygenation.
- Good buffering properties.
- Physiological pH.
- Contains endogenous antioxidants.

Techniques of delivery

The ideal technique for cardioplegia delivery is dependent on factors related to the case. The nature of the disease may influence the technique to adopt. Cardioplegia can be given intermittently (every 20–30 minutes) or continuously. The former is more commonly used because it maintains a more bloodless operating field. Effective techniques include:

Antegrade via the aortic root
A cannula is inserted into the ascending aorta. Cardioplegia is delivered via the cannula into the aortic root with the ascending aorta cross-clamped. The cardioplegia perfusion pressure should be equivalent to the systemic diastolic pressure. In some cases, for example aortic valve replacement, cardioplegia is delivered directly into the coronary ostia.

Retrograde via the coronary sinus

A retrograde cannula is introduced into the coronary sinus. Cardioplegia is given with a perfusion pressure of less than 40 mmHg (continuous pressure monitor). Retrograde cardioplegia can be less effective in protecting the right ventricle because of the venous drainage of the heart. It is effective for subendocardial protection.

Antegrade and retrograde

Using both techniques together may be the ideal strategy, especially for patients with poor left ventricular function.

Practical considerations

- Severely hypertrophied hearts are more susceptible to ischaemic and reperfusion injury because of increased energy utilization and difficulty in adequately protecting the subendocardial myocardium.
- Heart failure patients are more susceptible to myocardial dysfunction.
- Antegrade delivery via the aortic root may not be effective in patients with significant aortic regurgitation (cardioplegia leaks into left ventricle) or severe left main stem disease.
- Retrograde cardioplegia carries a risk that Thebesian drainage into the right ventricle may not adequately perfuse the left ventricle and septum.

Off-pump coronary artery bypass
(📖 see also Chapter 24)

Coronary artery bypass grafting (CABG) is conventionally done with cardiopulmonary bypass, which gives the surgeon an optimal environment to perform delicate coronary anastomoses. The attraction of off-pump coronary artery bypass (OPCAB) is based on the principle that it avoids the harmful effects of cardiopulmonary bypass. This in turn may be reflected in a reduction in perioperative morbidity or mortality. The early difficulty in operating on a moving target in a beating heart has been mainly circumvented with the introduction of mechanical stabilizers. There have been numerous trials comparing OPCAB with conventional on-pump. Most of the studies were limited by the fact that on-pump mortality and morbidity are low, and significant differences in outcomes can only be detected in large population studies. Patient-selection bias and variability in surgical techniques and experiences also limited these studies. The current evidence suggests the following:

Potential benefits of OPCAB

- Reduction in post-operative bleeding and blood transfusion requirement.
- Reduction in early mortality.
- Reduction in stroke rate and cognitive dysfunction.
- Reduction in renal failure.
- May have cost benefits.

Potential limitations of OPCAB

- Incomplete revascularization and graft patency – dependent on unit experience.
- Haemodynamic instability on manipulation of the heart.
- Learning curve.
- Competes with excellent 'on-pump' results.

Minimally invasive cardiac surgery (MICS)

- Minimally invasive is a broad term that could mean either minimal access with smaller incisions or not using cardiopulmonary bypass (or both). The great strides made in catheter-based methods for treating cardiovascular diseases, coupled with an increasingly well-informed and demanding patient population, are the main drivers for pursuing a MICS strategy.
- It is imperative that any new procedures adopted must deliver similar or better outcomes than conventional procedures. Recent major advances in innovative techniques and equipment have facilitated the progress of MICS. There is close collaboration between surgeons and industry in this endeavour. It is the industry's and physicians' responsibility to develop these procedures with a focus on safety and efficacy.

Aims of minimally invasive cardiac surgery

- Reduced procedural invasiveness: either smaller incision or no pump or both.
- Decrease complications of operation:
  - Infection.
  - Wound pain.
  - Complications of CPB.
- Improve patient compliance.
- Reduce length of hospital stay and costs.

Examples of operations considered as MICS

- MIDCAB – minimally invasive direct coronary artery bypass.
- OPCAB – off-pump coronary artery bypass.
- EndoACAB – endoscopic LIMA harvesting atraumatic coronary artery bypass.
- TECAB – total endoscopic coronary artery bypass.
- Heartport mitral valve surgery – port access endoscopic mitral surgery with cardiopulmonary bypass.
- Limited sternotomy aortic valve replacement.
- Robotic-assisted cardiac surgery including CABG, mitral valve surgery, and ligation of PDA.
- Endoscopic surgical atrial fibrillation ablation.

Reoperative surgery

The commonest reason for elective redo cardiac surgery is failed grafts from previous CABG that are not amenable to percutaneous intervention and medical therapy. Other causes requiring redo surgery include failed bioprosthetic valves from degeneration or endocarditis, paravalvular leak, new cardiac pathology following previous cardiac surgery, and adult congenital heart surgery. **The success of redo operation in cardiac surgery is dependent on safe re-entry into the chest**.

Factors that require consideration in redo operations are:

- Patent bypass grafts:
  - There is a risk of damaging patent grafts on re-entry via the sternum.
  - This is especially so if a patent left internal mammary arterial (LIMA) graft is severed, which can result in intractable ventricular fibrillation.
  - Embolization from diseased grafts during mobilization of the heart may cause myocardial damage.
- Myocardial protection: This is more difficult during reoperation. For example, a patent LIMA to LAD graft that is not isolated and clamped will make it difficult to achieve an arrested heart even with continuous cardioplegia.
- Aneurysm of the ascending aorta or the presence of an RV to PA conduit may pose a significant risk during sternotomy.
- Dilated right ventricle adherent to the sternum may pose a significant risk during sternal re-entry.
- CT or MRI scan can delineate the main cardiac structures from the sternum.
- Ensure external defibrillator pads are placed as it will not be possible to use internal paddles until the heart is mobilized. There may be a lot of interference from diathermy during this stage, and VF can be difficult to detect. Keeping an eye simultaneously on the arterial trace helps.
- VF is frequent in congenital heart reoperations during right ventricular outflow tract mobilization.
- Check that blood is available and in theatres.
- High-risk cases such as patent grafts or aneurysmal aorta may warrant the exposure of vessels for cardiopulmonary bypass. These are usually the femoral artery and vein. Some surgeons would cannulate the arterial vessel or go on full bypass before re-sternotomy.
- Consider alternative techniques, for example left thoracotomy for CABG to left-sided coronaries, or right thoracotomy or MICS for mitral valve surgery.
- Strategy for dealing with potential postoperative bleeding.

New techniques in surgery

- Robotic surgery.
- Percutaneous valve implantation.
- Endovascular stenting EVAR.
- Gene therapy.
- Small incisions surgery.
- Off-pump coronary artery bypass.

Further reading

1. Bridgewater B, Grayson A, Brooks N, et al. Has the publication of cardiac surgery outcome data been associated with changes in practice in northwest England: An analysis of 25,730 patients undergoing CABG surgery under 30 surgeons over eight years. *Heart* 2007; 93: 744–748.
2. Cohn LH. *Cardiac Surgery in the Adult.* Third edition. Maidenhead, UK, McGraw-Hill Professional, 2008.
3. Nilsson J, Algotsson L, Höglund P, Lührs C, Johan Brandt J. Comparison of 19 pre-operative risk stratification models in open-heart surgery. *European Heart Journal* 2006; 27: 867–874.
4. Stuge O, Liddicoat J. Emerging opportunities for cardiac surgeons within structural heart disease. *The Journal of Thoracic and Cardiovascular Surgery* 2006; 132: 1258–1261.

Preoperative assessment and investigations

Dr M Barnard, Dr W Davies, and Dr B Martin

Preoperative evaluation *208*
Multifactorial risk indices *210*
Non-invasive testing and radionuclide studies *214*
Cardiac catheterization *219*
Further reading *222*

Preoperative evaluation

Cardiac evaluation

- *Cardiac history and presenting symptoms*
  Unstable angina, acute myocardial infarction, congestive heart failure, and cardiogenic shock are high risk.

- *Coronary artery anatomy*
  - Left main disease, triple vessel disease, and proximal left anterior descending lesions are high risk.
  - Look for status of collateral circulation and diffuse distal disease.

- *Ventricular function*
  - Ejection fractions: >50% low risk; <50% moderate risk; <25% high risk.
  - In coronary patients assess valves and structural anomalies.
  - Look at echocardiogram and catheterization data.
  - Look for concomitant: aortic stenosis; mitral regurgitation; aortic insufficiency; ventricular septal defect; or ventricular aneurysm.

- *Electrocardiogram*
  Look for:
  - Q waves, ST changes.
  - Left bundle branch block.
  - PR interval.
  - Rhythm – atrial fibrillation/flutter; supraventricular tachycardia.

- *Chest radiograph*
  - Cardiomegaly.
  - Calcification, e.g. aorta.
  - Acute/chronic heart failure; pleural effusions.

Comorbidities

- *Carotids*
  Assess for presence of high-grade occlusive disease. Symptoms, previous history, and carotid duplex ultrasound examination of high-risk patients. With severe or symptomatic carotid disease, consider CT brain scan as baseline assessment.

- *Peripheral vascular disease*
  Increased risk. May be difficult to place intra-aortic balloon pump.

- *Diabetes*
  Hyperglycaemia associated with attenuation of preconditioning and adverse outcomes – renal impairment, obesity, autonomic neuropathy, peripheral vascular disease, impaired wound healing.

- *Renal disease* (📖 *see also Chapter 8*)
  For dialysis patients, ensure recent dialysis and check serum potassium. Watch for acidosis and hyperkalaemia. Require more frequent blood gas and electrolyte sampling.

- *Pulmonary disease* (📖 *see also Chapter 9*)
  Bronchospasm, air trapping, atelectasis, and segmental collapse are more likely. Chronic lung disease associated with higher risk and longer intensive care stays.

Perioperative cardiac medications

- *Beta-blockers*
  Perioperative continuation or initiation recommended for patients with coronary disease unless contraindicated.
- *Calcium channel blockers*
  Pacing more likely.
- *ACE Inhibitors*
  Perioperative hypotension.
- *Diuretics*
  Maintain postoperatively.
- *Statins*
  Continue perioperatively. Some evidence suggests anti-inflammatory benefits and protection against atrial fibrillation.
- *Aspirin*
  Surgeon and unit dependent. Some stop one week beforehand, others continue – with recognized increased blood loss.
- *Clopidogrel*
  Discontinued 3–7 days before surgery in most cases. Continued in presence of drug-eluting stents. Associated with significant perioperative bleeding risk and high re-sternotomy rate.
- *Heparin*
  Discontinue 4–6 hours before surgery. Continued in a few critically unstable patients.
- *Insulin*
  Routinely administered in most units perioperatively (to achieve adequate, not necessarily 'tight', control).
- *Oral hypoglycaemics*
  Discontinued the day before surgery. Insulin infusion perioperatively. Reinstituted when normal diet resumes.
- *Antibiotics*
  Unit-specific protocols. Typical regime: flucoxacillin and gentamicin prior to skin incision, and 24 hours postoperatively. Clarithromycin for penicillin allergy and teicoplanin for MRSA or unknown status.
- *Anxiolytic*
  Oral diazepam (5–10 mg) or temazepam (10–20 mg) are common premedicants. Oxygen commenced with administration.

Multifactorial risk indices

Risk assessment has evolved over the last three decades. The first risk-scoring system for cardiac surgery was introduced in 1983 by Paiement. Risk scoring is based on adjusting for presence and severity of illness between patients. Risk indices examine multiple preoperative and perioperative variables (often derived from expert consensus) and analyse their correlation with adverse outcomes, usually death. An expected mortality is derived based on a logistic regression model. These indices are used for both comparison of outcomes between centres (they can be used to adjust for case-mix) and for advising patients of their individual operative risk.

Many different variables have been associated with increased risk but a few are common to most systems. These include age, female gender, LV function, body habitus, reoperation, type of surgery, and urgency of surgery (Table 15.1). The only diseases consistently shown to be risk factors are renal impairment and diabetes.

Parsonnet

Parsonnet and colleagues developed a scoring system using 14 risk factors. An additive model was constructed using univariate regression analysis. Five categories of risk were established, which correlated with mortality and morbidity. The Parsonnet score has been frequently used for institutional comparison. However, it is an early model and does not reflect current risk levels.

STS

In North America the Society of Thoracic Surgeons has a long-established national database that currently has data on over 1.5 million CABG patients. Models were developed in the mid-1990s using univariate and multivariate analyses. This risk model has good predictive value.

EuroSCORE

The current gold standard for risk stratification and preoperative scoring in Europe is the European System for Cardiac Operative Risk Evaluation (EuroSCORE). This was constructed from an analysis of 19,030 patients from 128 centres across Europe. Risk factors associated with increased mortality are listed in Table 15.1. The EuroSCORE has been widely validated across countries and centres, making it a very useful clinical tool. Most European national cardiac surgical registries obligate EuroSCORE data collection. The EuroSCORE is accessible by an interactive web-based calculator (www.euroscore.org) and is simple and fast to use. There are two EuroSCORE calculations – the simple additive model and the more advanced logistic score.

Table 15.1 Simple EuroSCORE

Patient-related factors		Score
Age	(per 5 years or part thereof over 60 years)	1
Sex	female	1
Chronic pulmonary disease	long-term use of bronchodilators or steroids for lung disease	1
Extracardiac arteriopathy	any one or more of the following: claudication; carotid occlusion or >50% stenosis; previous or planned intervention on the abdominal aorta; limb arteries or carotids	2
Neurological dysfunction	disease severely affecting ambulation or day-to-day functioning	2
Previous cardiac surgery	requiring opening of the pericardium	3
Serum creatinine	>200 micromol/l preoperatively	2
Active endocarditis	patient still under antibiotic treatment for endocarditis at time of surgery	3
Critical preoperative state	any one or more of the following: ventricular tachycardia or fibrillation or aborted sudden death; preoperative cardiac massage; preoperative ventilation before arrival in the anaesthetic room; preoperative inotropic support; intra-aortic balloon counterpulsation; or preoperative acute renal failure (anuria or oliguria <10 ml/hour)	3
Cardiac-related factors		Score
Unstable angina	rest angina requiring IV nitrates until arrival in the anaesthetic room	2
LV dysfunction	moderate or LVEF 30–50%	1
	poor or LVEF <30%	3
Recent myocardial infarct	(<90 days)	2
Pulmonary hypertension	systolic PA pressure >60 mmHg	2
Operation-related factors		Score
Emergency	carried out on referral before the beginning of the next working day	2
Other than isolated CABG	major cardiac procedure other than or in addition to CABG	2
Surgery on thoracic aorta	for disorder of ascending, arch, or descending aorta	3
Postinfarct septal rupture		4

Cardiac Anesthesia Risk Evaluation

A simplified concept was advanced by Dupuis, who developed an approach similar to the widely used ASA physical status classification. The Cardiac Anesthesia Risk Evaluation score (CARE) has five classes plus emergency status. It combines clinical judgement with three important factors identified by multifactorial risk indices – comorbid conditions, surgical complexity, and urgency.

Cardiac Anesthesia Risk Evaluation Score

1. Patient with stable cardiac disease, no other medical problem, and non-complex surgery.
2. Patient with stable cardiac disease and one or more controlled medical problems with non-complex surgery.
3. Patient with any uncontrolled medical problem or patient in whom a complex surgery is undertaken.
4. Patient with any uncontrolled medical problem and complex surgery.
5. Patient with chronic or advanced cardiac disease for whom cardiac surgery is undertaken as a last hope to save or improve life.
6. Emergency: surgery as soon as diagnosis is made and operating room is available.

Non-invasive testing and radionuclide studies

The electrocardiogram (ECG)

- The ECG is a graphical display of the surface recording of the electrical activity produced by the heart.
- It is a graphical display of a changing potential difference, and how that potential difference changes with respect to time.
- The axes of the ECG graph are 'Time' on the x-axis, measured in seconds, and 'Potential difference' on the y-axis, measured in millivolts.
- An ECG 'lead' refers to a potential difference recorded between two defined points.

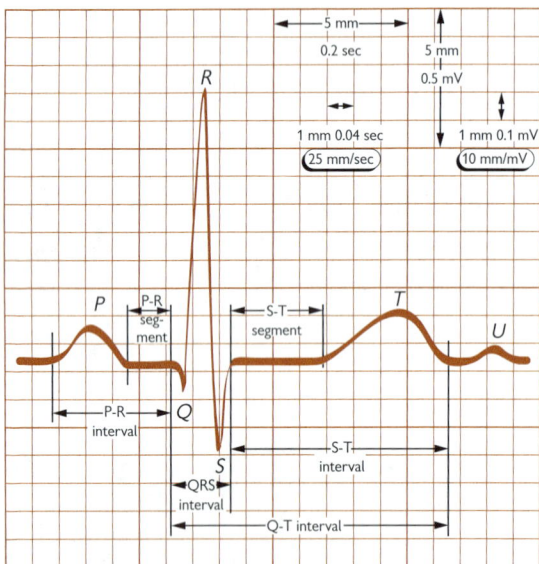

Figure 15.1 The standard ECG.

- An ECG electrode refers to the point of contact between the wires of the ECG cable and the surface of the body.
- Commonly silver/silver chloride electrodes are used, which set up their own small surface potential in order to reduce interference called polarization; this helps to minimize fluctuations of potential due to changes in surface contact.

- An ECG recording measures about 2–4 mV in surface potential difference; if the two electrodes are placed with one on the surface of the heart and one intracardiac, then a standard cardiac action potential would be displayed. The amplitude of this potential difference would be approximately 120 mV, i.e. the difference in potential between the resting cardiac potential and full depolarization.
- Over 95% of the source of the signal is therefore lost in conduction to the surface electrodes.
- The standard calibration for an ECG display is 1 mV per centimetre, and the standard paper speed is 25 mm per second, i.e. one small square represents 40 ms, and one large square 200 ms.
- A straight line on an ECG display does not represent a zero potential, but merely shows that the two measurement points are equipotential.
- ECG leads are traditionally measured from two distinct points (hence measuring the difference in potential between them, and how it changes with respect to each cardiac cycle).
- Since ECG biological signals are small, they require amplification; a differential amplifier is generally used in an ECG to minimize noise by common mode rejection. The signal is then transferred to an oscilloscope for display, or to a printer for interpretation. The distance from the source of the signal affects the size of electrical potentials. Body tissues are generally good at transmitting electrical signals but air is a poor conductor. Moving the standard electrodes from the limbs changes the quality of the ECG signal, and makes the resultant leads non-standard. Placing the recording electrodes on bony prominences minimizes interference from electromyographic (EMG) signals.

Standard limb leads

There are three standard limb leads for the ECG. These are known as *standard bipolar limb leads* I, II, and III. They each measure a potential difference between two electrodes placed on appropriate limbs. Surface electrodes are placed on both arms and the left leg. The standard nomenclature for an ECG dictates that if electrical current is moving towards the positive electrode, then the deflection of the oscilloscope is upwards; if it is away from the positive electrode, then the deflection is downwards.

In standard limb lead I, the left arm is the positive electrode with the right arm being the negative electrode. In standard limb lead II, the left leg is the positive electrode with the right arm being the negative electrode. In standard limb lead III, the left leg is the positive electrode with the left arm being the negative electrode. Standard bipolar limb lead I measures the difference in potential between the right arm and the left arm. Standard bipolar limb lead II measures the difference in potential between the right arm and the left leg. Standard bipolar limb lead III measures the difference in potential between the left arm and the left leg. The difference in potential between the limbs is produced by the sum of all biological electrical potentials in the body.

At a heart rate of 60 bpm, the frequency of the QRS complex is 1 Hz. The physiological range of the ECG is roughly 0.5–4 Hz (heart rate 30–240 bpm). The ECG is a complex wave, which may be broken down into its component sine waves (Fourier analysis). Signals between 0.05 and 40 Hz need to be amplified in order to produce an ECG display. This is known as the bandwidth. In order to enhance the ECG display, e.g. for assessment of the S-T segment, the bandwidth may be widened to 0.05–100 or even 150 Hz, although this may require a greater need for filtering extraneous electrical noise.

The position of electrode placement on a limb is generally not important. However, if the electrodes are moved from the limbs, then the subsequent change in measured potential may become important, and the lead can no longer be regarded as a standard lead for comparative purposes. In the setting of bipolar recordings a third electrode is often placed on the patient; this third electrode is used to reduce electrical noise. It does not take part in the recording of the bipolar signal, but it makes the signal easier to interpret by allowing further attenuation of interference. This is also part of common mode rejection. When using a three-electrode ECG, only one ECG lead may be displayed at any one time.

Non-standard limb leads

Non-standard unipolar leads measure a potential difference between one recording electrode and a fixed reference point, this fixed reference point being the centre of Einthoven's triangle. The fixed reference point is obtained by joining all three limb electrodes to a common point. This essentially creates a potential at 0 mV; i.e. it is an Einthoven triangle, with the heart essentially at the centre of the triangle. It is important to remember that the triangle should involve the right arm electrode, the left arm electrode, and the left leg electrode, as the heart is in the left side of the chest. This creates the equilateral triangle necessary for Einthoven's triangle to apply. Therefore, in order to make a unipolar ECG recording, it is necessary to place five recording electrodes on a patient. A recording electrode is placed on the body in a unipolar position. For convenience set positions for unipolar leads are used for comparative purposes. Remember that these are non-standard, unipolar recordings. The six unipolar chest lead positions are V1–V6. There are three further unipolar limb lead recordings, VR, VL, and VF, where the unipolar electrode is placed on each of the limbs. The unipolar electrode potential is then compared to the zero potential created by Einthoven's triangle (right arm, left arm, and left leg joined to form a common electrode). A further fifth electrode is positioned on the right leg to reduce interference due to electricity from other sources, as in the three-electrode ECG (common mode rejection).

The three unipolar limb leads VR, VL, and VF are not commonly used. One of the reasons for this is that the difference in potential between a limb and the centre of the effective Einthoven triangle is small in comparison to the other lead potentials. For clinical use it is necessary to increase this potential difference by 'augmenting' this potential, producing aVR, aVL, and aVF. This is achieved by removing one of the limb electrodes from Einthoven's triangle, i.e. the limb electrode from the corresponding unipolar limb lead is removed from the sum of the potentials from the three limbs, producing the reference zero potential. For example, in aVR the right arm electrode is compared against a combined potential from the left arm and left leg electrodes joined to a common point, the right arm electrode having been removed from Einthoven's triangle. This 'augmentation' effectively increases the difference in potential between the recording electrodes by about 50%. Similarly in aVL, the left arm electrode potential is compared to a combined potential gained by connecting the right arm and left leg electrodes to a common point. In aVF, the left leg electrode (foot) is compared to a combined potential gained by connecting the right and left arm electrodes to a common point.

Which leads to use?

A five-electrode cable allows the display of at least seven ECG leads at the same time, i.e. I, II, III, aVR, aVL, aVF, and a single unipolar lead, usually a lateral chest lead, may be displayed using a five-electrode ECG.

Monitoring of cardiac rhythm and detection of ischaemia are the main reasons for monitoring the ECG during anaesthesia. Lead II (right arm, left leg) is generally used for detecting arrhythmias, as it monitors along the axis of depolarization in people with a normal cardiac axis. However, if the axis of depolarization is already known from a preoperative ECG, the bipolar lead that monitors along the axis of depolarization will usually be the best for monitoring rhythm, e.g. in left axis deviation lead I may be better for monitoring rhythm, and in right axis deviation lead III may be better for monitoring rhythm.

For monitoring ischaemia, one of the lateral chest leads is probably best employed, but this necessitates a five-lead ECG. If only a three-lead ECG is available, then it is necessary to use a modified non-standard bipolar lead. The modified bipolar lead configuration CM5 is commonly used in this instance. The ECG box is set on the lead II setting. The right arm electrode is moved to the manubrium (M) or right subclavian region, and the left leg electrode is moved to the V5 position (fifth intercostal space, anterior-axillary line). For convenience the third non-recording electrode is commonly placed on the left clavicle (C). This electrode configuration will usually result in a lead (CM5) suitable for monitoring cardiac rhythm and ischaemia in a single lead display. This configuration is not as useful as using a five-electrode cable, but is less cumbersome in the theatre environment, and usually suffices for patients with non-cardiac disease.

Exercise testing

Used as a diagnostic test for evaluation of chest pain. Also determines functional capacity and prognostic information in those known to have ischaemia.

Key clinical findings

- Ischaemic threshold.
- ST depression.
- Hypotension.
- Angina.
- Arrhythmias.

Most predictive value when ST depression >1.5 mm occurs in early stages of exercise.

Strongly positive when:

- Systolic blood pressure falls more than 10 mmHg.
- More than five leads show ST changes.
- ST changes within three minutes.
- ST changes take more than nine minutes to resolve.

Nuclear cardiology

Intravenous radioisotopes (thallium-201, sestamibi, or tetrofosmin) can help assess myocardial perfusion and viability. Radionuclide imaging also provides information on global ventricular function.

During vasodilation less perfusion agent reaches myocardium supplied by vessels with stenotic lesions. Stress (vasodilator) images are compared with rest. Fixed perfusion defects suggest non-viable or infarcted myocardium. Defects that resolve on rest suggest viable myocardium at risk of ischaemia (reversible defects). Sensitivity in unselected patients is approximately 85 to 90%, but false positives are slightly higher than with exercise testing (specificity 75 to 80%).

Positron emission tomography

This specialized technique uses different radioisotopes. They can assess regional blood flow and metabolism in real time. It is costly, involving a cyclotron.

Computed tomography (CT)

- **Conventional CT Scanners**: A ring rotates around the patient and back to its starting position. The table moves a set distance for the next slice.
- **Spiral scanners**: The ring rotates continuously as the patient moves through the scanner. It provides superior image resolution and is faster. 3D images can be constructed.
- **Multislice scanners**: These have several rows of detectors and faster tube rotation. They are expensive and slower to reconstruct images but acquire images faster and produce higher resolution images.

Magnetic resonance imaging (MRI)

Cardiac MRI provides high resolution and 3D imaging of cardiac structures, and quantification of blood flow. It is useful in the preoperative assessment of congenital heart disease and other structural heart disease. Regurgitant blood flow and chamber volumes can be accurately quantified.

Echocardiography (📖 see also Chapter 17)

Transthoracic echocardiography provides information on:
- Regional wall motion.
- Ejection fraction and global left ventricular function.
- Quantitative assessment of valve stenosis and regurgitation.
- Congenital defects.
- Pericardial diseases and effusions.

Stress echocardiography uses exercise or drugs to increase myocardial work. Non-contracting myocardial segments during stress are considered ischaemic if they revert to normal at rest, or infarcted if they are abnormal before, during, and after stress. Dobutamine stress echocardiography is widely held to have similar sensitivity and increased specificity compared to radioisotope studies. It cannot be used in those with poor echocardiography windows or in those at risk during stress (aneurysms, recent MI).

Cardiac catheterization

Angiography may be eventually supplanted or supplemented by high resolution CT, but currently remains the gold standard for diagnosis of coronary artery disease. Catheterization provides information on:

• Coronary anatomy.
• Ventricular function.
• Valve anatomy and function.
• Cardiac output and pulmonary vascular resistance.

Contrast is injected into the coronary ostia in several views. Common projections are right anterior oblique (RAO), left anterior oblique (LAO), and LAO caudal (spider) views. In RAO views the spine is on the right of the image, and it is on the left in LAO views. The circumflex is always the vessel nearest the spine in both views. The LAD travels towards the apex and has septal perforating branches exiting at 90° (Figures 15.2–15.4).

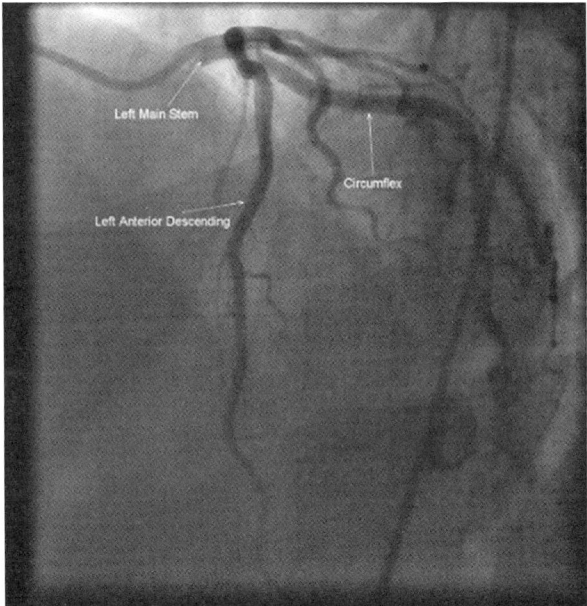

Figure 15.2 LAO left coronary artery.

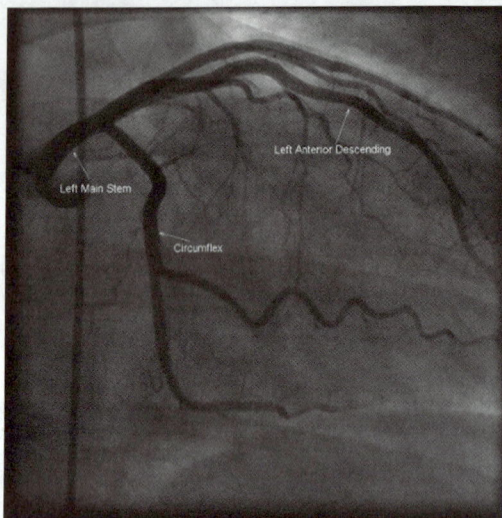

Figure 15.3 RAO left coronary artery.

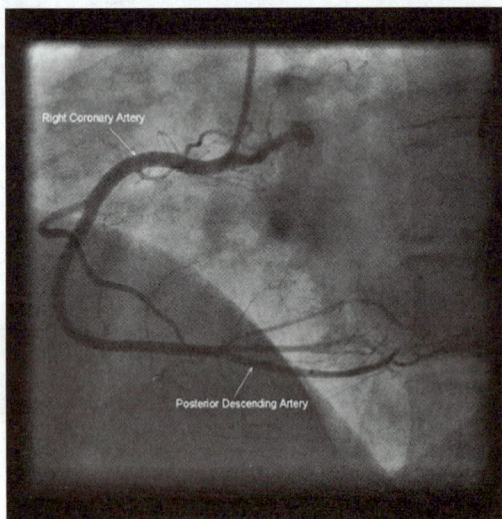

Figure 15.4 Right coronary artery.

Lesions greater than 50% diameter (75% cross-sectional area) are significant. Lesions can be focal or segmental. Blocked vessels may fill retrogradely from other vessels – e.g. the PDA and RCA can fill from the LAD.

Additional information to collect from catheterization reports includes:

- Left ventricular end-diastolic pressure (LVEDP). Values above 15 mmHg indicate ventricular dysfunction or another cause of reduced compliance.
- Cardiac output.
- Left ventricular ejection fraction.
- Regurgitant blood flow (aortic and mitral).
- Regional assessment of ventricular function from the ventriculogram.
- Pulmonary artery pressure and pulmonary vascular resistance if right heart catheterization has been performed.

Further reading

1. Nilsson J, Algotsson L, Hoglund P, Luhrs C, Brandt J. Comparison of 19 pre-operative risk stratification models in open-heart surgery. *European Heart Journal* 2006; 27: 867–874.
2. Ouattara A, Niculescu M, Ghazouani S, et al. Predictive performance and variability of the Cardiac Anesthesia Risk Evaluation Score. *Anesthesiology* 2004; 100: 1405–1410.
3. Suojaranta-Ylinen RT, Kuitunen AH, Kukkonen SI, Vento AE, Ulla-Stina Salminen U-S. Risk evaluation of cardiac surgery in octogenarians. *Journal of Cardiothoracic Vascular Anesthesia* 2006; 20: 526–530.

Monitoring

Professor J Mark and Dr A Barbeito

Perioperative electrocardiography 224
Haemodynamic monitoring and invasive vascular access 228
Cardiac output monitoring 236
Temperature monitoring 238
Neurologic monitoring 239
Further reading 240

Perioperative electrocardiography
(📖 see also Chapter 16 p. 214)

The goals of perioperative electrocardiographic monitoring are continuous measurement of heart rate, identification of arrhythmias, conduction disturbances and pacemaker function, and detection of myocardial ischaemia. It can also suggest electrolyte imbalances.

Table 16.1 ECG colour coding systems and lead location

Lead	US (AHA)	Europe
Right arm	white	red
Right leg	green	black
Left arm	black	yellow
Left leg	red	green
Precordial	brown	white

Recordings may be altered significantly if limb leads are not placed outside the cardiac border!

Lead selection

With a five-lead system, leads II and V4 or V5 should be selected for continuous display. This combination has 90% sensitivity for detection of myocardial ischaemia.

With a three-lead system, a modified V5 lead is obtained by placing the right arm lead in the right subclavicular region and the left arm lead in the standard V5 position (fifth left intercostal space, anterior axillary line). Lead I must be selected on the monitor. This modified V5 lead is superior to any standard limb lead for detection of myocardial ischaemia.

Atrial ECG leads

An atrial lead can be monitored using the temporary epicardial atrial pacing wires placed routinely after cardiac surgery. This lead discloses atrial electrical activity that is augmented relative to ventricular electrical activity and can aid detection of atrial arrhythmias that are otherwise not discernible with standard surface lead recordings.

Diagnosing myocardial ischaemia on the bedside monitor

Modern ECG monitors can now provide tracings that are similar to a 12-lead ECG in quality and diagnostic accuracy, provided that the filters and gain are adjusted appropriately.

Filters

Figure 16.1 shows the three different filter modes generally offered by modern monitors and the corresponding low- and high-frequency filters. These filters are designed to improve the ECG waveform display, but they may also introduce waveform distortion that will lead to misdiagnosis.

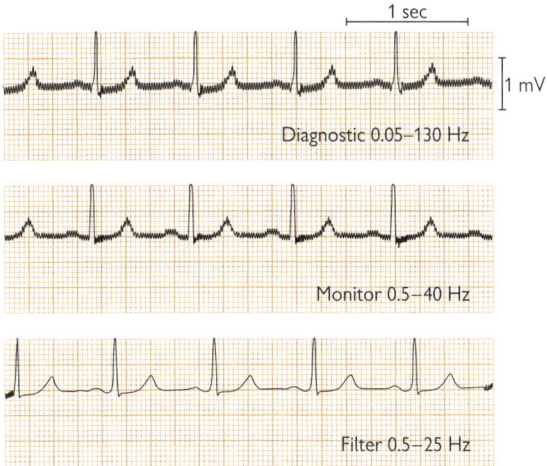

Figure 16.1 ECG filter modes.

Effect of filter selection on ECG electrical interference from the wall power source. Compared to the diagnostic mode (bandpass 0.05 to 130 Hz), the narrower bandpass of the monitor mode (0.5 to 40 Hz) reduces the high frequency artifact, and the filter mode (0.5 Hz to 25 Hz) eliminates this electrical artifact entirely.

The low-frequency filter:
- Diminishes baseline drift caused by patient movement and respiration.
- May exaggerate ST-segment changes (owing to the low frequency of this ECG component), potentially resulting in erroneous diagnosis of myocardial ischaemia.

The high-frequency filter:
- Reduces 50 or 60 Hz wall power source noise.
- Precludes visualization of pacemaker spikes on the ECG trace and interferes with QRS and J-point recognition.

The diagnostic bandwidth filter should be used whenever accurate ST-segment analysis is required.

Gain

The signal gain can also be adjusted on the bedside monitor to increase or decrease the size of the ECG trace. Although useful for better wave visualization, gain changes simultaneously exaggerate or minimize ST-segment shifts. The standard 1 mm ST-segment depression required for the diagnosis of myocardial ischaemia refers to a 0.1 mV depression, which corresponds to 1 mm *only* when the standard gain of 10 mm per mV is selected.

Subendocardial versus transmural ischaemia

Subendocardial ischaemia:
- 'Demand' ischaemia.
- ST-segment depression.
- −1 mm (−0.1 mV), horizontal or down-sloping.
- Measured 60 ms after J-point (junction of QRS and ST segment).
- V5 and V4 leads are most sensitive.
- Non-localizing to coronary distribution.

Transmural ischaemia:
- 'Supply' ischaemia.
- ST-segment elevation.
- +1 mm (+0.1 mV) in two limb leads or +2 mm (0.2 mV) in two precordial leads.
- Measured at the J-point.
- Localizing to coronary distribution.

Haemodynamic monitoring and invasive vascular access

Technical considerations for invasive haemodynamic monitoring

- After the artery or vein has been cannulated, the catheter should be connected to the transducer via saline-filled, low compliance tubing with the minimal length and number of connections. This will optimize the system dynamic response (natural frequency and damping coefficient) and minimize wave distortion.
- The transducer should be connected to a pressurized saline flush system that provides a continuous low flow flush to prevent clot formation at the tip of the catheter.
- The transducer must be zeroed by opening it to air and pressing the zero pressure button on the monitor.
- The transducer should be positioned at a level approximately 5 cm posterior to the left sternal border at the fourth intercostal space, since this position best eliminates the confounding effects of hydrostatic pressure when measuring cardiac filling pressures. This transducer level is preferred over the more commonly used transducer alignment at the mid-axillary line.

Arterial pressure monitoring

Cardiac surgery requires beat-to-beat monitoring of blood pressure because: (a) the concurrent disease (e.g. coronary artery disease, aortic stenosis, etc.) necessitates close haemodynamic observation; (b) the anticipated haemodynamic changes resulting from the operative procedure may be sudden and/or large in magnitude; and (c) pharmacologic and mechanical manipulation of the cardiovascular system is routinely performed.

A non-invasive blood pressure monitor should always be available to corroborate direct blood pressure readings and to serve as backup in case of equipment failure.

Technique for arterial cannulation

- Explain the procedure to the patient and obtain consent.
- Gather all the necessary equipment: 20 gauge catheters; a pressurized saline bag-transducer-tubing system; 1% lidocaine with a small gauge needle for skin infiltration; tape; a sterile occlusive dressing; and prep solution.
- Position the patient's wrist in dorsiflexion using a small roll under it and tape it to maintain stability. Prep the skin.
- The radial artery lies between the tendon of the flexor carpi radialis and the head of the radius. Locate the pulse with two fingers and retract the skin slightly. Infiltrate local anaesthetic at the planned insertion site.
- Insert the catheter approximately 1 cm distal to the pulse, at a 30–45° angle, until flashback is seen. Then reduce the angle of insertion and advance the catheter and needle as a unit another 2–4 mm.

- Carefully slide the catheter off the needle without moving the needle. Once the catheter is fully inserted, apply pressure to the artery just distal to the catheter and remove the needle.
- Connect the catheter to the transducer system, secure the catheter with tape and dressing, and aspirate to remove air bubbles.

Normal arterial pressure waveform morphology (Figure 16.2)

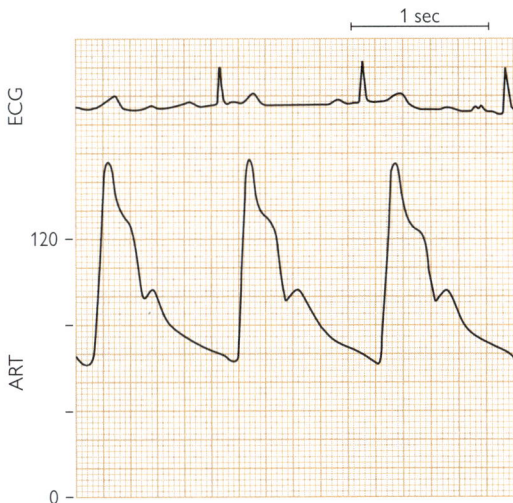

Figure 16.2 Arterial pressure waveform and ECG.

Digital readouts of systolic and diastolic pressures are derived from the highest and lowest values on the arterial pressure trace, which are then displayed as a running average, updated at a regular interval. The mean arterial pressure (MAP) is measured by the monitor as the integrated area under the pressure curve.

Abnormal arterial pressure waveform morphology

Several disease states have characteristic arterial pressure waveforms (and typical underlying causes). Pulsus alternans (congestive heart failure), pulsus bisferiens (aortic insufficiency), pulsus parvus and tardus (weak and slow rising – aortic stenosis), pulsus paradoxus (cardiac tamponade), and the 'spike-and-dome' pattern (hypertrophic cardiomyopathy) may be identified from direct recordings of the systemic arterial pressure. While these abnormal arterial pressure waveforms are not absolutely diagnostic when considered in isolation, they provide useful supplementary diagnostic clues to haemodynamic abnormalities.

Differences between central and peripheral arterial pressure

The stiffness of the arterial tree increases as the distance from the aortic valve increases. This and other mechanical factors cause an increase in systolic pressure, a decrease in diastolic pressure and widening of the pulse pressure as blood flows toward the periphery (distal pulse amplification). Hypothermia, which is used intentionally during cardiopulmonary bypass, triggers thermoregulatory vasoconstriction and causes radial arterial systolic blood pressure to overestimate central arterial pressure. Conversely, during rewarming, vasodilation reverses this gradient and causes radial artery systolic pressure to be lower than central arterial pressure. This gradient reversal is usually of limited magnitude and resolves spontaneously within an hour. However, central arterial pressures (direct aortic) should be used for separation from bypass whenever this artefactual peripheral arterial hypotension is severe.

Using the arterial pressure trace to estimate preload

Cardiopulmonary interactions that result from changes in intrathoracic pressure and lung volume during mechanical ventilation result in a cyclic variation in blood pressure, termed systolic pressure variation (SPV). Increased SPV ($\geq$10 mmHg) has been shown to be a sensitive indicator of hypovolaemia and responsiveness to fluid administration.

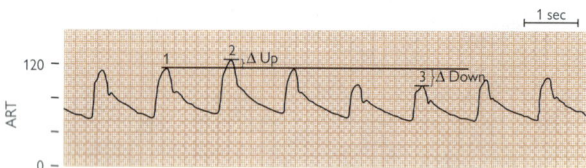

Figure 16.3 Systolic pressure variation in arterial waveform.

Systolic pressure variation (SPV) during positive pressure mechanical ventilation. End-expiratory systolic blood pressure (1) serves as a baseline from which an early inspiratory increase (2, ΔUp) can be measured, followed by a delayed decrease (3, ΔDown). The large ΔDown and total SPV of nearly 30 mmHg suggests the diagnosis of hypovolemia, despite the fact that tachycardia and hypotension are not present. ART, arterial blood pressure.

Central venous pressure monitoring

A central vein is usually cannulated during cardiac surgery in order to monitor cardiac filling pressures and to administer vasoactive drugs, fluids, and blood products. It can also serve as a site to insert a temporary transvenous pacemaker, a pulmonary artery catheter, or a coronary sinus catheter for cardioplegia administration during minimally invasive surgery.

Technique for central vein cannulation

• Explain the procedure to the patient and obtain consent.
• Gather the necessary equipment: central venous catheter kit and sterile gloves and gown.
• Position the patient supine with the head turned slightly to the left for right internal jugular vein cannulation.

- Prepare the catheter, guidewire, local anaesthetic, syringes, and needles *before* you prep and drape the patient to minimize the time he/she is under the drapes.
- Prep and drape the planned puncture site and infiltrate with local anaesthetic. Place the patient in the Trendelenburg position.
- Currently most UK operators use ultrasound guidance to locate the vein.
- Palpate the triangle formed by the two heads of the sternocleidomastoid muscle and the clavicle. Insert a 22 ga 'seeker' needle at the apex of the triangle at a 45° angle, aiming at the ipsilateral nipple until blood return is encountered.
- Using the seeker needle as a guide, insert the large-bore hollow needle less than 2 cm until blood return is obtained again. Alternatively, an 18 ga catheter over a needle can be used to cannulate the vein; the needle can then be removed and the catheter connected to a short piece of tubing to measure venous pressure and confirm intravenous placement.
- Insert the guidewire to 20 cm through the needle or catheter, watching for arrhythmias. Remove the catheter or needle while maintaining control of the wire at all times. Create a small nick with a scalpel at the puncture site to allow passage of the dilator through the skin.
- Insert the dilator over the wire far enough to reach the vein but not the full length, to avoid vein rupture. Remove the dilator and apply pressure at the puncture site.
- Pass the catheter over the wire and advance it into the vein to a depth of 15 cm. The wire will protrude through the proximal hub of the catheter.
- Remove the wire, aspirate and flush the catheter ports, and suture the catheter to the skin.
- Check a CXR for correct line placement and to rule out pneumothorax.

Pulmonary artery catheterization

The current pulmonary artery catheter (PAC) for use in adult patients is 110 cm in length, contains three or four lumens, and has an embedded thermistor and a 1.5 ml balloon at the tip. The catheter is inserted through a one-way valve on a large-bore introducer placed into a central vein.

Technique for PAC insertion
- Make sure all vascular lumens of the catheter are flushed.
- Check the balloon for full and symmetric inflation.
- Using sterile technique, advance the catheter through the introducer sheath with the balloon deflated until the tip enters the right atrium (RA, approximately 20 cm). Note the RA pressure (CVP) recorded from this site.
- Inflate the balloon and advance the catheter several centimetres at a time, using the blood flow to carry the balloon-tipped catheter through the right heart chambers. As the PAC crosses the tricuspid valve, note the pressure in the right ventricle (RV, approximately 35 cm).
- Advance the catheter further through the pulmonic valve into the main pulmonary artery (approximately 45 cm) and note the PA systolic and diastolic pressures.

- Slowly advance the catheter until it occludes a branch of the PA (approximately 50 cm) and note the PA wedge pressure (PAWP) or wedge pressure.
- Deflate the balloon and lock it. Note return of a PA pressure tracing. Subsequent balloon inflation attempts should be done slowly, while observing the PA pressure trace. A catheter that 'wedges' before the entire 1.5 ml of air is injected into the balloon has migrated too far distally. This catheter position may lead to PA rupture, which carries a 50–70% mortality rate. The PAC has a national tendency to move forward with time.

Remember that the balloon is filled with air and it will tend to 'float'; a head-down position will aid passage of the catheter through the tricuspid valve into the RV, and a head-up and right lateral decubitus position will aid passage into the main PA and reduce the incidence of arrhythmias.

If the distinction between RV and PA pressures is not clear, focus on the diastolic component of the waveforms. If pressure continues to drop after the dicrotic notch, the catheter is in the PA. A rise in pressure during diastole is created by diastolic filling and indicates that the catheter is in the RV.

- TOE may assist positioning.

Filling pressures as indicators of preload: CVP, PADP, and PAWP

Why do we measure filling pressures?
Since the force of contraction is proportional to the initial length of the cardiac muscle fibre (Frank-Starling Law), the first measure to optimize stroke volume should be to provide optimal fibre length with adequate filling volume or preload. Filling pressures are mainly used as indirect measures for preload or end-diastolic chamber volume, since the latter cannot be monitored easily in clinical practice. Left ventricular end-diastolic pressure (LVEDP) provides the closest pressure estimate for left ventricular end-diastolic volume (LVEDV).

Pressure is not volume
- When utilizing a filling pressure as a surrogate for estimating cardiac volume, one must take into consideration three points:
- The diastolic pressure-volume relationship in cardiac muscle is not linear, but rather curvilinear, with a progressively steeper slope at higher volumes.
- Ventricular compliance may change independent of end-diastolic volume (e.g. as a consequence of ischaemia). The same effective preload may be represented by two different filling pressures if ventricular compliance changes (Figure 16.4).
- Filling pressure measurements are referenced to atmospheric pressure, but physiologically it is transmural pressure (the difference between intracardiac and intrathoracic, extracardiac pressure) that determines ventricular preload. Increased intrathoracic or intrapericardial pressures (e.g. high PEEP levels, cardiac tamponade, or large pleural effusion) may reduce cardiac filling but at the same time paradoxically increase measured filling pressures (Figure 16.5).

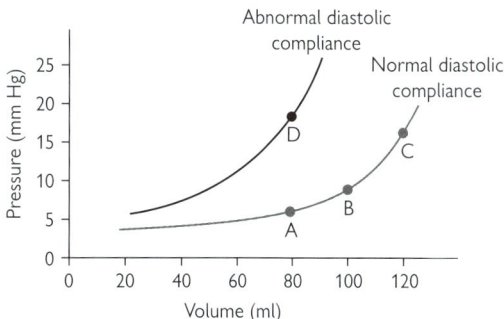

Figure 16.4 Ventricular compliance: end diastolic pressure volume relationship.

Pressure-volume relationship in a ventricle with normal or abnormal compliance. When ventricular compliance is normal, a 20 ml increase in right ventricular end-diastolic volume (RVEDV) produces a 2 mmHg rise in central venous pressure (CVP) (point A to point B) when RVEDV is 80 ml, but an 8 mmHg rise in CVP (point B to point C) when RVEDV is 100 ml. (B) When ventricular compliance changes, as with ischemia or ventricular hypertrophy, higher filling pressures are required to generate the same RVEDV (point A to point D).

	A	B	C
Transduced PAWP	20	20	20
Transmural PAWP	25	10	25
LV Compliance	Normal	Normal	Stiff
LV Volume	Increased	Normal	Normal
		(or reduced)	(or reduced)

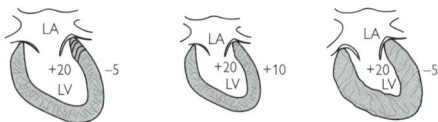

Figure 16.5 Measured filling pressures and transmural pressures.

Limitation of using pulmonary artery wedge pressure (PAWP) as an estimate of left ventricular preload. The figure shows three different situations in which the transduced PAWP is the same, but the actual transmural pressure is different, and hence the left ventricular volume is different. LA, left atrium; LV, left ventricle.

In order to minimize the effect of intrathoracic pressure on central vascular pressure values, all measurements should be done at end-expiration. Intrathoracic pressure approaches zero at end-expiration in both spontaneous and mechanically ventilated patients, hence eliminating this confounding factor from the equation.

Remember that the same filling pressure may indicate very different loading conditions depending on the patient's ventricular compliance and intrapericardial and intrathoracic pressures.

Estimating LVEDP

Since LVEDP is not measured directly in daily practice, other surrogates need to be used. Figure 16.6 shows the pressure measurement surrogates for LVEDP and the common confounding physiologic factors. As one moves further upstream from direct measurement of LVEDP (measurement points A, B, C, and D), many additional factors alter the ability of these measurements to predict LV preload accurately.

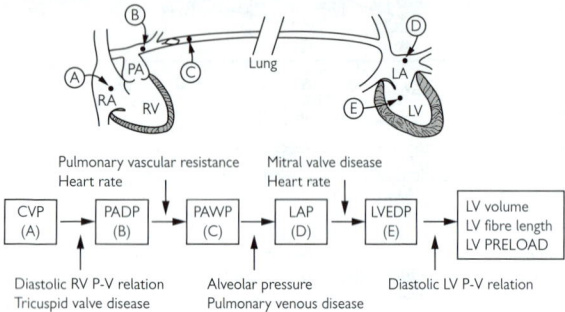

Figure 16.6 LVEDP measurement surrogates and confounding influences.

Pressure measurement surrogates for left ventricular preload and the common major confounding physiologic factors. RA, right atrium; RV, right ventricle; PA, pulmonary artery; LA, left atrium; LV, left ventricle; CVP, central venous pressure; PADP, pulmonary artery diastolic pressure; PAWP, pulmonary artery wedge pressure; LAP, left atrial pressure; LVEDP, left ventricular end-diastolic pressure.

So what does the CVP tell me?

The normal CVP waveform contains three positive deflections (a, c, and v waves) that correspond to atrial contraction, tricuspid valve closure, and venous filling respectively. The mean CVP value correlates well with RVEDP in most cases, although the peak of the a wave reflects RVEDP most accurately. Assuming no valvular disease, pulmonary hypertension, or right ventricular dysfunction, RVEDP and LVEDP move in the same direction, and consequently CVP can be considered to be an indirect measure of LV preload. However, the RV is more compliant than the LV even in healthy patients, and hence any given increase in ventricular volume will generate a certain increase in LVEDP but a much less pronounced, sometimes undetectable, change in CVP.

Cardiac output monitoring

Normal cardiac output (CO) is 4.0 to 6.5 litres per minute in the resting adult. Preload, afterload, myocardial contractility, and heart rate regulate CO, and as such CO provides an important assessment of the status of the circulation as a whole. Several methods have been devised to measure CO, and all have advantages and disadvantages.

Thermodilution cardiac output

- Room temperature saline solution is injected via the CVP port of the PAC. The difference in blood temperature is measured via a thermistor at the tip of the PAC, and CO calculated from the area under the thermodilution curve.
- Slight measurement variation is common, so three consecutive measurements with <10% variation among them should be averaged to obtain a reliable CO.
- Tricuspid regurgitation, intracardiac shunts, and varying rates of fluid infusion invalidate the underlying assumptions of this technique and may produce misleading results.
- Continuous CO can be measured with special PACs that incorporate a blood-warming filament in the RV portion and a temperature detector at the tip. A 3–6 minute average of the CO is displayed and refreshed every 30 seconds. Consequently, this method will not show sudden CO changes quickly.

Lithium dilution cardiac output

- Lithium chloride is injected into a peripheral vein and blood drawn from an arterial catheter at a constant rate. A lithium-sensitive electrode attached to the arterial line measures a lithium dilution curve and calculates a CO.
- Accuracy is high with this method. It also obviates the need for a central line or PAC.
- Chronic lithium therapy and several neuromuscular blocking agents may interfere with the lithium electrode measurements.

Oesophageal Doppler cardiac output

- An oesophageal Doppler probe is inserted into the mid-oesophagus, with its transducer facing the posteriorly-located descending thoracic aorta. The velocity of blood flow is measured using Doppler interrogation, and a descending aortic stroke volume is calculated.
- The technique assumes a constant aortic diameter and a constant distribution of blood flow between the upper body and descending aorta (approximately 70% of total CO).
- Measurements are reliable and easy to perform when an adequate acoustic window is obtained, but probe instability often requires bedside adjustment.
- Because this method relies on several assumptions, it generally underestimates CO measured by other methods. It is also limited to use in intubated patients and is contraindicated in patients with severe oesophageal pathology.

Pulse contour analysis

- Pulse contour methods derive the CO from analysis of the arterial pressure waveform. Most (not all) need to be calibrated against a known CO prior to monitoring.
- These methods provide beat-to-beat monitoring of CO and show acceptable agreement with thermodilution measurements.
- Some devices require recalibration every four to eight hours and whenever marked changes in vascular resistance occur.

Temperature monitoring

Temperature should be monitored for any surgical procedure where the risks of hypothermia and malignant hyperthermia are substantial. The use of extracorporeal circulation and deliberate hypothermia makes temperature monitoring especially important during cardiac surgery.

Hypothermia is used to reduce the metabolic rate and protect organ function during cardiopulmonary bypass (CPB). Rewarming is essential before separation from CPB, because persistent hypothermia has many adverse effects in the postoperative period. Absolute temperature, as well as temperature gradients between the core and periphery, should be monitored closely during the entire CPB procedure, but especially during rewarming.

• Excessive temperature gradients (>10°C) between aortic inflow blood and core temperature will alter solubility of gases dissolved in blood. Bubbles may form and cause thromboembolic complications.

• Warming of inflow blood above 37°C will increase brain temperature and the cerebral metabolic rate of oxygen ($CMRO_2$) leading to neurologic complications postoperatively.

• Large temperature gradients between core and periphery are indicative of inadequate rewarming time and may lead to hypothermia after CPB as re-equilibration occurs.

Body temperature should be measured with a nasopharyngeal probe. An oesophageal temperature probe is in close contact with the iced solution used for direct heart cooling and may be inaccurate during CPB. When a PAC is in place, the PA blood temperature should also be measured. Rectal or bladder temperatures are considered more intermediate temperatures. Bladder temperatures are highly dependent on urinary flow. Skin temperature is inaccurate and should not be used during cardiac surgery.

Neurologic monitoring

Neurologic monitoring techniques can be divided into CNS function monitors, such as the EEG and evoked potentials (SSEP and MEP), and perfusion/oxygenation monitors, such as transcranial Doppler and near-infra-red reflectance spectroscopy (NIRS). Aortic surgery produces major alterations in brain and spinal cord perfusion, making neurologic monitoring of particular importance during these procedures. Unfortunately, although these monitoring techniques may produce useful information intraoperatively, their predictive value remains questionable. Use of multiple monitoring modalities simultaneously may improve diagnostic accuracy, permitting targeted intervention and reducing neurologic injury.

Further reading

1. Auler J, Galas F, Hajjar L, Santos L, Carvalh T, Michard F. Online monitoring of pulse pressure variation to guide fluid therapy after cardiac surgery. *Anesthesia and Analgesia* 2008; 106: 1201–1206.
2. Funk D, Moretti E, Gan T. Minimally invasive cardiac output monitoring in the perioperative setting. *Anesthesia and Analgesia* 2009; 8: 887–897.
3. Mayer J, Boldt J, Wolf M, Lang J, Suttner S. Cardiac output derived from arterial pressure waveform analysis in patients undergoing cardiac surgery: Validity of a second generation device. *Anesthesia and Analgesia* 2008; 106: 867–872.
4. Murkin J, Adams S, Novick R, et al. Monitoring brain oxygen saturation during coronary bypass surgery: A randomized, prospective study. *Anesthesia and Analgesia* 2007; 104: 51–58.
5. Rex S, Brose S, Metzelder S, et al. Prediction of fluid responsiveness in patients during cardiac surgery. *British Journal of Anaesthesia* 2004 93: 782–788.

Trans-oesophageal echocardiography

Dr S Wright

Ultrasound physics 242
Imaging modes 244
Uses and indications for trans-oesophageal
    echocardiography 248
Monitoring applications 250
Standard examination and views 252
Complications of TOE 256
Further reading 259

Ultrasound physics

Ultrasound

Echocardiography uses ultrasound to generate images.
- Sound is a mechanical vibration (i.e. compression and rarefaction) and travels in waves.
- Ultrasound frequencies are higher than those perceptible to the human ear (i.e. greater than 20 kHz) and for echocardiography purposes lie in the frequency range of 2 to 10 MHz.
- Ultrasound obeys the laws of reflection; a sound wave reflected by an interface between two materials of differing density or *acoustic impedance* (e.g. blood and endocardium) can be received back by a transducer within the echo probe. Because the velocity of sound transmission through human tissue is roughly constant (540 m/s) the time taken for an emitted pulse of sound to be reflected and return to the transducer is related to the distance between the reflecting interface and the transducer. This information is then processed to generate a 2D image of the reflecting interfaces.
- Refraction at interfaces and scatter of the ultrasound signal by small particles can also occur and can lead to the generation of artefacts.

Transducers

Within transducers ultrasound is generated by piezoelectric crystals (quartz or ceramic), which expand when an electrical current is applied. The application of alternating current to a piezoelectric crystal causes rapid alternating expansion and contraction, which sets up a pressure wave or vibration (sound). Similarly, a sound wave meeting a piezoelectric crystal makes the crystal vibrate, leading to generation of an electrical signal. A piezoelectric crystal can therefore both generate and receive ultrasound signals.

Most echocardiography probes are made up of several piezoelectric crystals (a *phased array*), which in turn each send out a short pulse of ultrasound and then switch to receive reflected signals from tissue interfaces. The ultrasound beam is steered electronically and 'swept' across the imaging plane like a windscreen wiper to produce an arc of ultrasound; a typical scan width of 90° may contain 180 lines of ultrasound. How often the image is refreshed (or *frame rate*) depends on the depth of image field – the further the ultrasound signal travels, the longer a crystal must remain in receive mode before the next pulse of ultrasound can be transmitted.

The frequency of the wave generated by a transducer is determined by the nature of the emitting crystals. A wave's velocity, frequency, and wavelength are defined by the relationship:

$$v = f \times \lambda$$

where v = velocity (1540 m/s in human tissue), f = frequency, and λ = wavelength.

Spatial resolution along the length (axis) of the ultrasound beam (the smallest distance that can be discriminated between adjacent structures) is determined by the ultrasound wavelength. This axial resolution is typically 0.5–1 mm, and is higher than lateral resolution (but is typically 2–3 mm in the image far field).

High frequency probe transducers are able to resolve small distances but the signal is rapidly attenuated as it passes through tissue, and structures far from the echo probe are poorly imaged. Conversely, low frequency probes achieve a greater depth of imaging field, but at the expense of resolution.

The Doppler principle (Figure 17.1)

Use of the Doppler principle allows measurement of velocity, both of blood and tissue:

The shift in frequency of a reflected wave is determined by the velocity of the reflecting object.

- Ultrasound reflected by red cells moving away from the echo probe will have a lower frequency than the original wave.
- Red cells moving towards the probe will cause an increase in reflected frequency.
- Echo machines are able to interpret the frequency shift of the reflected ultrasound wave to calculate the velocity of the reflecting surface.
- The greatest frequency shift is observed when the Doppler signal is parallel to the direction of movement of the reflecting surface.

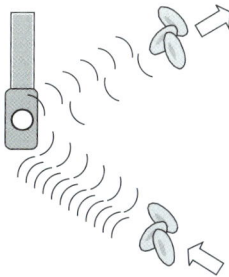

Figure 17.1 The Doppler principle. The frequency of the reflected wave is dependent on the velocity of the reflecting interface. Sound reflected by red cells moving away from the probe (top) will have a lower frequency; that reflected from cells moving towards the probe (bottom) will have a higher frequency.

Imaging modes

Box 17.1 Imaging modes

- 2D.
- M-mode.
- Doppler:
  - Pulsed-wave Doppler
    - spectral display
    - colour flow mapping
  - Continuous wave Doppler.
  - Tissue Doppler.
- 3D.

2D imaging

This is the greyscale tomographic representation (2D slice) of anatomy. The image arc can be set between 0 and 90°. The wider the arc, the lower the image frame rate.

M-mode (Figure 17.2)

M-mode (Motion mode) imaging is the graphical plot of motion against time of all points along a cursor line within a 2D image. This slice through the heart obtained from a single beam of ultrasound has high temporal resolution and allows accurate measurements of displacement of structures over time.

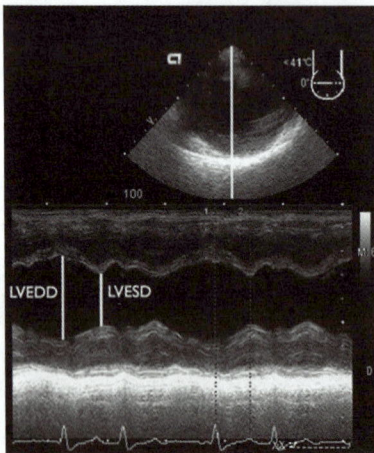

Figure 17.2 M-mode image showing motion of all points along a cursor line positioned on a 2D image, plotted against time. LV end-diastolic and end-systolic diameters can be measured and used to calculate fractional shortening (LVEDD – LVESD/LVEDD).

Doppler imaging

Pulsed-wave Doppler

This involves emission and reception of a Doppler ultrasound signal by a single crystal that switches between 'send' and 'receive' modes. Velocity is measured at a predetermined point (*sample volume*) in the 2D imaging plane, which is set by the operator (the crystal switches to receive only at the time it would take sound to reach the defined point in the image and return). This pinpoint localization of measurement is offset by the disadvantage that the maximum velocity that can accurately be measured is limited to low velocities (the *Nyquist limit*).

The velocity of the reflecting surface may be plotted graphically against time as an outlined *spectral display* (Figure 17.3).

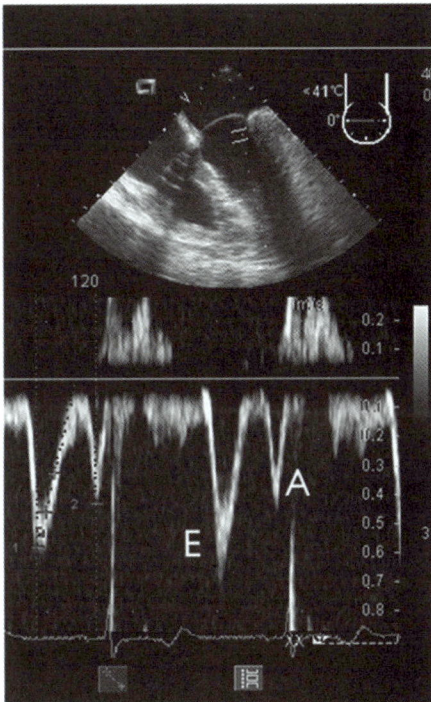

Figure 17.3 Pulsed-wave Doppler spectral display of trans-mitral flow. Blood flow velocity is measured after the sample volume cursor (=) has been positioned at the mitral leaflet tips. Two distinct waves representing diastolic flow are displayed, the early E wave of passive LV filling and the later A wave, which is generated by atrial contraction.

Alternatively, the velocity data can be superimposed onto a 2D echo image as *colour flow mapping*, whereby different colours represent different velocities (Figure 17.4). By convention, blue colours denote flow away from the echo probe and red colours code for flow towards the probe (BART: Blue Away, Red Towards). As it is a form of pulsed wave Doppler imaging, colour flow mapping is also limited by the Nyquist limit.

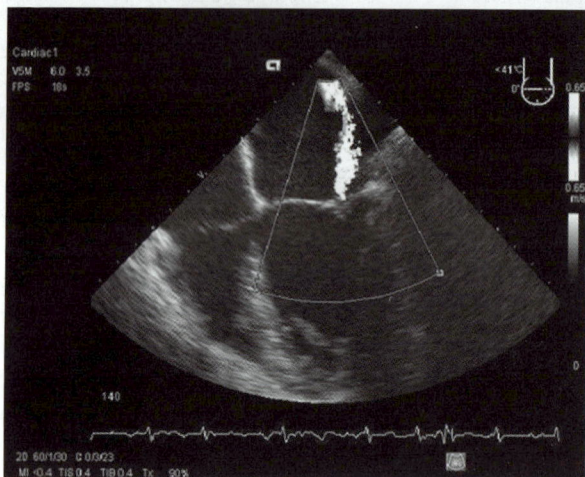

Figure 17.4 Colour flow mapping of mitral regurgitant jet in a four-chamber view.

Continuous wave Doppler (Figure 17.5)
The disadvantage of the Nyquist limit in measuring velocity of flow can be overcome by using continuous wave Doppler imaging, whereby one crystal continuously emits ultrasound along a line within the 2D image, while an adjacent crystal receives the reflected signal for frequency analysis. While this removes the maximum velocity limit that can be measured (and is therefore useful for assessing high velocities such as through stenotic valves), this is at the expense of precise localization because flow velocity is measured at all points along the cursor line.

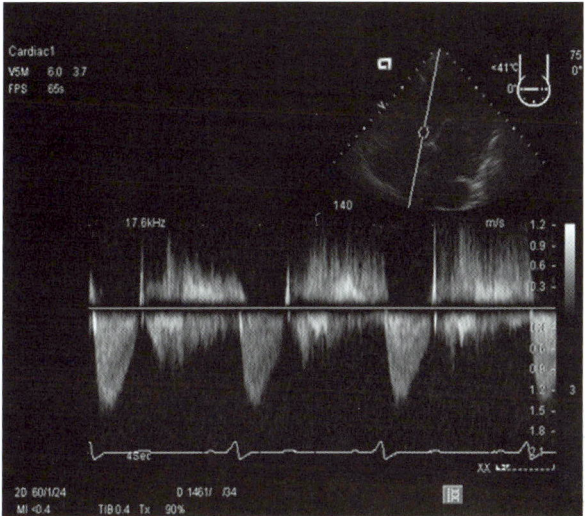

Figure 17.5 Continuous wave Doppler spectral display of blood flow velocity through the aortic valve in a Deep TG LAX plane. Velocity of flow at all points along the cursor line is plotted against time. Producing an "infilled" spectral display, cf pulse wave.

Tissue Doppler imaging (TDI)

The principles of Doppler imaging may also be applied to myocardial tissue. When in TDI mode, the echo machine has different filter and gain amplification settings compared to the standard Doppler mode, since the velocity of myocardial motion is lower and the amplitude of the reflected signal is greater than that of blood cells.

TDI can be used either in colour or pulsed wave modes. In colour TDI the myocardial velocity is expressed as colour mapping superimposed on the 2D image (using the BART convention). Spectral pulsed wave TDI displays myocardial velocity as a plot against time. This measurement is most commonly used to measure mitral annular descent velocity, which provides quantification of ventricular systolic and diastolic function.

3D imaging

3D images of cardiac structures can be generated by analysis of the series of views produced by automatic rotation of a multiplane transducer within the oesophagus. Reconstruction of the 3D image was time-consuming but recently real-time 3D representation of intracardiac structures from TOE is being developed. However, it is likely that in the intraoperative setting 3D imaging will be of most value for demonstration of complex valve anatomy during valve repair procedures.

Uses and indications for trans-oesophageal echocardiography

The American Society of Cardiovascular Anesthesiologists has published a list of indications for intraoperative TOE based on expert opinion:

Box 17.2 Indications for intraoperative TOE

Category I

Indications in which TOE is frequently useful in improving clinical outcome (strongest evidence or expert opinion):

Preoperative
- Persistent haemodynamic instability not responding to treatment.
- Unstable patients with suspected thoracic aortic pathology.

Intraoperative
- Persistent haemodynamic instability not responding to treatment.
- Valve and HOCM repair.
- Congenital heart surgery requiring CPB.
- Endocarditis surgery.
- Pericardial window surgery.
- Aortic dissection surgery for aortic valve evaluation.

Postoperative
- Haemodynamic instability of unknown aetiology.

Category II

Indications in which TOE may be useful in improving clinical outcome (weaker evidence or expert opinion):

Preoperative
- Assessment of acute aortic pathology.

Intraoperative
- Patients with increased risk of myocardial ischaemia, infarction, or haemodynamic instability.
- Valve replacement.
- Repair of cardiac aneurysms.
- Removal of cardiac tumours.
- Detection of foreign bodies.
- Detection of air emboli.
- Cardiac thrombectomy.
- Pulmonary embolectomy.
- Cardiac trauma.
- Thoracic aortic dissections.
- Assessment of aortic atheroma and other sources of aortic emboli.
- Pericardial surgery.
- Assessment of anastamotic sites during heart and lung transplantation.
- Placement of ventricular assist devices.

Category III

Indications in which TOE is infrequently useful in improving clinical outcome (little evidence or expert support):
- Evaluation of myocardial perfusion, coronary artery anatomy, or graft patency.
- Repair of cardiomyopathies other than HOCM.
- Uncomplicated endocarditis in non-cardiac surgery.
- Monitoring for emboli during orthopaedic procedures.
- Assessment of repair of thoracic injuries.
- Uncomplicated pericarditis.
- Evaluation of pleuropulmonary disease.
- Placement of balloon pumps, internal cardiac defibrillators, or pulmonary artery catheters.
- Monitoring of cardioplegia administration.

These indications for intraoperative TOE are based primarily on its application as a diagnostic tool. However, TOE during cardiac surgery is a haemodynamic monitor of value, and it is frequently employed in *all* patients undergoing cardiac surgery.

Monitoring applications

TOE provides an accurate, instantaneous indication of haemodynamic status and response to therapy. Function and volume status can be rapidly assessed. Both 2D appearance and Doppler-derived data from TOE imaging are used to guide inotrope therapy and fluid replacement.

In 2D images the area of the LV cavity is assumed to reflect LV volume and can be used to assess filling status of the patient. Continuous tracking of LV area during the cardiac cycle is available on many machines and ejection fraction (or *fractional area change*) can be calculated on a beat-to-beat basis. The development of 3D echo has meant that LV volume can now be directly calculated.

Echocardiography is a highly sensitive monitor of myocardial ischaemia. Analysis of regional ventricular wall motion allows early detection of ischaemia-induced regional wall motion abnormalities, which may prompt surgical revision or changes to haemodynamic management.

The pressure gradient across an orifice is related to the velocity of blood flow by the modified Bernoulli equation:

gradient = $4 \times$ velocity^2

Doppler spectral display of velocity over time gives rise to waveforms that change in shape and magnitude with changes in haemodynamic status (Figure 17.6). Analysis of these waveforms allows calculation of gradients, pressures, stroke distance, and stroke volume (and cardiac output).

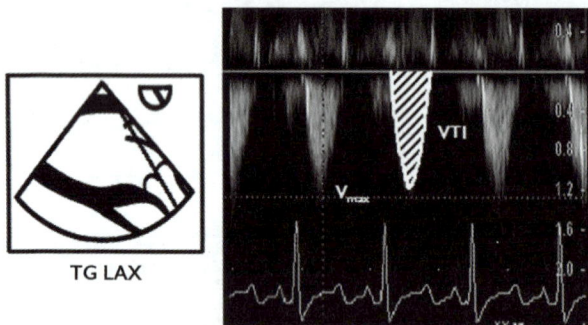

TG LAX

Figure 17.6 Continuous wave Doppler trace of flow through from a transgastric long axis view. Velocity is measured at all points along the cursor line, which passes through the aortic valve.

Analysis of the shapes of trans-mitral flow and pulmonary venous flow waveforms gives information on left ventricular diastolic function and left atrial pressure.

Standard examination and views

The ultrasound transducer positioned in the tip of a multiplane TOE probe produces an arc of ultrasound that can be rotated smoothly from the horizontal plane (0°) through the vertical plane (90°) and beyond to 180° (which generates a mirror image of 0°) (Figure 17.7). In addition, by manipulating control wheels on the probe handle, the probe tip can be ante- and retroflexed in order to tilt the plane of interrogation (Figure 17.8). In this way the imaging plane can be aligned with various intrathoracic structures in order to clarify the anatomy.

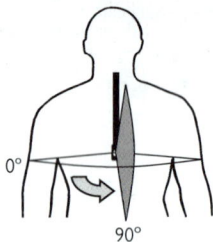

Fig. 17.7 Rotation of the ultrasound probe

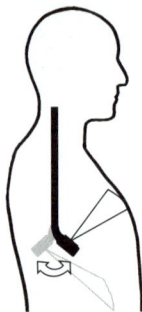

Fig. 17.8 Probe ante- and retroflexion.

The probe position and degree of imaging plane rotation that best display individual structures are constant. This has led to the definition of 20 conventional TOE imaging planes (Figure 17.9). A systematic and comprehensive examination should be performed in all patients (unexpected TOE findings that lead to alteration of the surgical procedure are found in a small proportion). Most people use 10–12 of the conventional imaging planes in their standard examination sequence, and will add additional views according to their findings. It is essential to have a clear understanding of cardiac anatomy.

The sequence in which the imaging planes are achieved and displayed is determined by personal preference and by the patient's pathology. Proposed sequences are typically based on either:

• Depth of the probe tip in the patient: imaging planes are achieved in the upper oesophagus before the probe is advanced to obtain mid-oesophageal planes, and finally into the stomach.

- Individual structures: imaging planes that define a certain structure
  (e.g. aortic valve) are obtained before focusing on the next structure.
  This forms the basis of the sequence described below:

Examination sequence

1. Left ventricle
- Transgastric mid-short axis:
  - 2D: global systolic function (fractional area change), regional wall
    motion, volume status (end diastolic area), wall thickness.
  - M mode: fractional shortening, wall thickness.
- Transgastric basal short axis:
  - 2D: global and regional function.
- Mid-oesophageal four chamber:
  - 2D: global systolic function (including Simpson's method), regional
    wall motion, volume status, wall thickness.
- Mid-oesophageal two chamber:
  - 2D: global systolic function, regional function.

2. Mitral valve
- Mid-oesophageal four chamber:
  - 2D: leaflets (excursion, thickening, calcification, vegetations,
    prolapse, override), area of leaflet contact, height of plane of
    coaptation. Annulus (diameter, calcification). Chordae (integrity,
    calcification, redundancy). Papillary muscles (function, integrity).
  - Colour flow mapping for MR: jet size and direction, vena
    contracta, PISA.
  - Doppler: gradient, pressure half-time, VTI, LV diastolic function.
- Mid-oesophageal mitral commissural:
  - As four chamber.
- Mid-oesophageal aortic long axis:
  - As four chamber.
- Transgastric basal short axis:
  - Colour flow mapping for regurgitant orifice.

3. Left atrium
- Mid-oesophageal four chamber:
  - 2D: size, thrombus, left atrial appendage, spontaneous echo
    contrast.
  - Doppler: pulmonary venous flow.
- Mid-oesophageal bicaval:
  - 2D: as above.

4. Aortic valve
- Mid-oesophageal aortic short axis:
  - 2D: leaflets (excursion, thickening, calcification, planimetry of
    orifice area, vegetations). Coronary arteries (ostial position,
    course).
  - Colour flow mapping: LV outflow tract for AR.

(continued)

- Mid-oesophageal aortic long axis:
  - 2D: measure diameters of AV annulus, sinuses of Valsalva, sino-tubular junction, ascending aorta.
  - Colour flow mapping: LV outflow tract for AR.
- Transgastric long axis:
  - Colour flow mapping: LV outflow tract for AR.
  - Doppler for velocity, gradient, velocity time integral, SV and CO, valve area using continuity equation, pressure half-time of AR jet.
- Deep transgastric long axis:
  - Colour flow mapping for AR.
  - Doppler for velocity, gradient, velocity time integral, SV and CO, valve area using continuity equation, pressure half-time of AR jet.

5. Right ventricle
- Mid-oesophageal four chamber:
  - 2D: systolic function, free wall thickness, chamber size.
- Transgastric mid-short axis:
  - 2D: systolic function.
- Mid-oesophageal RV inflow-outflow:
  - 2D: systolic function, RVOT obstruction, chamber size.

6. Tricuspid valve
- Mid-oesophageal four chamber:
  - 2D: annular size, leaflet morphology and motion, subvalvar apparatus.
  - Colour flow mapping for TR.
  - Doppler of TR jet to estimate RV systolic pressure.
- Mid-oesophageal RV inflow-outflow:
  - 2D: leaflet morphology and motion.
  - Colour flow mapping for TR.
  - Doppler of TR jet to estimate RV systolic pressure.

7. Right atrium
- Mid-oesophageal four chamber:
  - 2D: size, Eustachian valve, coronary sinus, thrombus, Chiari network, cannulae, catheters, leads.
- Mid-oesophageal RV inflow-outflow:
  - 2D: as four chamber.
- Mid-oesophageal bicaval:
  - 2D: as four chamber.

8. Pulmonary valve
- Mid-oesophageal RV inflow-outflow:
  - 2D: leaflet morphology and motion.
  - Colour flow mapping for PR.
- Mid-oesophageal ascending aortic short axis:
  - 2D: leaflet morphology and motion, post-stenotic PA dilation.

9. Interventricular septum
- Mid-oesophageal four chamber:
  - 2D: wall thickness and motion.
  - Colour flow mapping for defects/shunts.

- Transgastric LV short axis:
  - 2D and colour flow mapping as four chamber.
- Mid-oesophageal aortic valve short axis:
  - 2D and colour flow mapping as four chamber.

10. Interatrial septum
- Mid-oesophageal four chamber:
  - 2D: position, mobility, defects. Pulmonary vein and coronary sinus anatomy.
  - Colour flow mapping and air/saline contrast for shunts.
- Mid-oesophageal bicaval:
  - 2D and colour flow mapping as four chamber.

11. Great vessels
- Mid-oesophageal ascending aortic short axis:
  - 2D: PA, aorta, SVC. Size and position. Dissection.
  - Doppler in PA for SV.
- Mid-oesophageal aortic valve long axis:
  - 2D: aortic root and ascending aorta. Size, atheroma, dissection.
- Upper oesophageal aortic arch long axis:
  - 2D: size, atheroma, dissection, coarctation.
  - Doppler in distal arch if AR present.
- Upper oesophageal aortic arch short axis.
- Descending aortic long axis:
  - 2D: size, atheroma, dissection, coarctation.
- Descending aortic short axis:
  - 2D: as long axis.

Complications of TOE

General complications
- Direct mechanical trauma:
  - chipped teeth, pharyngeal abrasion, oesophageal perforation or haemorrhage, aneurysm rupture, mucosal thermal injury.
- Displacement or traction on contiguous structures:
  - recurrent laryngeal nerve injury, hypotension from great vessel compression.
- Stimulation of visceral reflexes:
  - dysrhythmias, vomiting.
- Bacteraemia.

Complications specific to the perioperative setting
- Distraction from anaesthesia and other monitoring.
- Accidental extubation:
  - inadvertent removal of intravascular catheters and cannulae.

UPPER OESOPHAGEAL VIEWS

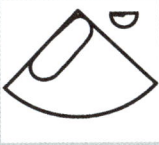

UE aortic arch LAX

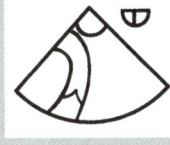

UE aortic arch SAX

MID OESOPHAGEAL VIEWS

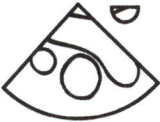

ME asc aortic SAX

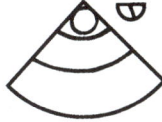

ME asc aortic LAX

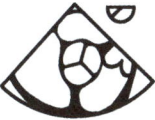

ME AV SAX

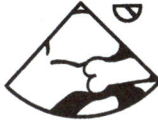

ME AV LAX

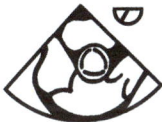

ME RV inflow-outflow

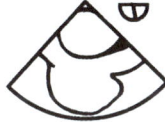

ME bicaval

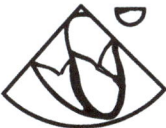

ME four chamber

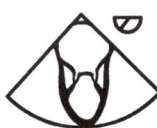

ME mitral commissural

Figure 17.9 Conventional TOE imaging planes, as described by the Society of Cardiovascular Anesthesiologists. UE = upper oesophageal; ME = mid-oesophageal; TG = transgastric; LAX = long axis; SAX = short axis; asc = ascending; RV = right ventricle; LV = left ventricle; AV = aortic valve; mid = mid-papillary.

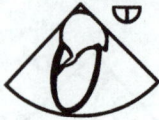

ME two chamber

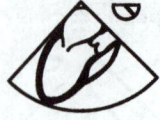

ME LAX

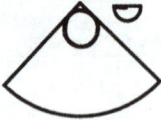

Desc aortic SAX

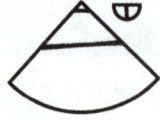

Desc aortic LAX

TRANSGASTRIC VIEWS

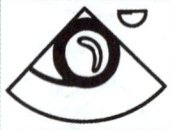

TG basal SAX

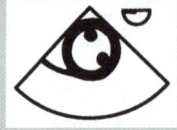

TG mid SAX

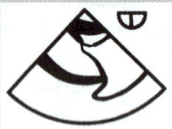

TG 2 chamber

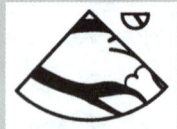

TG LAX

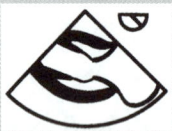

TG RV inflow

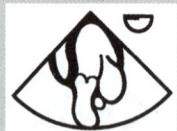

Deep TG LAX

Figure 17.9 (continued)

Further reading

1. Glas K. Training in perioperative echocardiography. *Current Opinion in Anaesthesiology* 2006; 19: 640–644.
2. Cahalan MK, Stewart W, Pearlman A, et al. American Society of Echocardiography and Society of Cardiovascular Anesthesiologists Task Force guidelines for training in perioperative echocardiography. *Anesthesia and Analgesia* 2002; 94: 1384–1388.
3. Mathew JP, Glas K, Troianos CA, et al. American Society of Echocardiography/Society of Cardiovascular Anesthesiologists recommendations and guidelines for continuous quality improvement in perioperative echocardiography. *American Society of Echocardiography* 2006; 19: 1303–1313.
4. Douglas PS, Khandheria B, Stainback RF, et al. ACCF/ASE/ACEP/ ASNC/SCAI/SCCT/SCMR 2007 appropriateness criteria for transthoracic and transesophageal echocardiography. *Journal of the American College of Cardiology* 2007; 50: 187–204.
5. Shanewise JS, Cheung AT, Aronson S, et al. ASE/SCA guidelines for performing a comprehensive intraoperative multiplane transesophageal echocardiography examination: Recommendations of the American Society of Echocardiography Council for Intraoperative Echocardiography and the Society of Cardiovascular Anesthesiologists Task Force for Certification in Perioperative Transesophageal Echocardiography. *Anesthesia and Analgesia* 1999; 89: 870.

Cardiopulmonary bypass

Dr M Barnard and Dr B Martin

Cardiopulmonary bypass circuits 262
Pre-bypass checklists 263
Conduct of bypass 264
Further reading 271

Cardiopulmonary bypass circuits

Circuit

A cardiopulmonary bypass (CPB) system drains blood from the venous system, oxygenates it, and pumps it under pressure into the arterial system. Blood drains from the venous cannula by gravity into a reservoir with pumped blood from suckers and 'vents' in the surgical field adding to the reservoir. The venous blood is oxygenated, its temperature adjusted, and it is pumped into the arterial system. It passes through a filter into the aorta or femoral artery via an arterial cannula (narrower than venous to maintain pressurization).

The venous cannula can be either a single right atrial cannula or separate SVC and IVC cannulas. Bicaval cannulation allows more complete venous diversion to the reservoir and surgical access to the atria and septum (e.g. mitral valve surgery).

CPB pumps can be roller pumps or centrifugal. Centrifugal pumps reduce blood component trauma and potentially reduce the inflammatory response. Leuco-depleting filters may do the same. Heparin-coated circuits may reduce activation of coagulation factors (⊞ see also Chapter 7).

Priming solution

The prime is a mixture of crystalloid and/or colloid fluids, together with electrolytes, buffer, mannitol, and heparin. Individual choices of composition vary widely. Packed red blood cells are added if the preoperative haemoglobin and body size dictate that initial haemodilution will take the haemoglobin to below 5 g/dl.

Pre-bypass checklists

Perfusionist's checklist

- All air and bubbles removed from priming solution in circuit.
- Tubing connected to flow in the right direction! Retrograde flow causes arterial air injection.
- Oxygen supply.
- Alarms and automatic pump shutdown (with inadequate venous return) active.
- Arterial cannula shows appropriate pulsatile pressure when in the aorta (check for aortic dissection).

Anaesthesia checklist

- Understand proposed procedure:
  Cannulation sites? Cardioplegia? Temperature goal? Circulatory arrest? Special organs at risk (e.g. spinal cord)?
- Anticoagulation:
  Heparin given? ACT (activated clotting time) >480 seconds? (Measure ACT three minutes after administration of heparin.)
- Anaesthesia: Blood drug concentrations are diluted by the priming volume at commencement of CPB. Additional doses of anaesthetic drugs or muscle relaxants?
- Cannulation:
  Correct arterial cannula position? Aortic pressure pulsatile and correlates with radial pressure? Bubbles in cannula? Carotid pulses equal (cannula can obstruct carotid)?
- Infusions:
  'Give one hundred.' Fluid boluses from the pump can be given quickly and easily via the aortic cannula in the pre-CPB period to treat hypotension. Ensure central line is not occluded by SVC cannula or surgical snare. Many give drugs direct to CPB circuit for this reason.
- Monitoring:
  Check and zero transducers. Nasopharyngeal temperature probe before heparin given. Zero the urine output. If a PA catheter is present, withdraw into sheath several centimetres to avoid PA rupture. Check TOE probe is not flexed and switched to 'freeze' (probe is warm when on). Check pupils as baseline.

Conduct of bypass

Initial checklist
- Colour difference between arterial and venous cannula blood?
- CVP <5?
- Heart distension?
- Stop ventilation – if cardiac ejection has stopped.

Maintenance checklist
- **Anticoagulation**:
  ACT >480 every 30 minutes?
- Additional heparin 5–10,000 IU increments according to ACT.
- **Blood gases, electrolytes, glucose, haemoglobin**: (📖 see also acid-base management Chapter 19 p. 280).
  - Checked every 30 minutes.
  - Watch mixed venous saturations – sensitive indicator of perfusion adequacy.
  - CO_2 regulated by altering gas flow to oxygenator. Capnograph line can be attached to oxygenator exhaust.
  - Potassium kept above 4.5. Levels affected by cardioplegia, so be more cautious.
  - Insulin infusion can be started during CPB for all, even non-diabetic patients. 1 unit/hr will maintain normoglycaemia in the majority.
- **Anaesthesia**:
  Depth required to prevent awareness, prevent movement including breathing, and partially suppress autonomic response to stimulation. Nitrous oxide is not used due to risk of increasing size of air bubbles in circulation. Hypothermia decreases anaesthetic requirements by 10% per °C, so anaesthetic requirements are maximal during normothermia (beginning and end of CPB). Volatile agents may be given by attaching to oxygenator inlet of CPB circut. Muscle relaxants are rarely needed following induction.
- **Ventilation**:
  Stop when CPB is 'full flow' and heart not ejecting. Turn off anaesthetic machine volatile agent vaporizers. Arterial gases sampled from the CPB pump will not detect arterial desaturation due to pulmonary shunt from partial CPB or other causes.
- **ECG**:
  - Watch for VF. If an aortic clamp is not placed promptly and cardioplegia administered, the heart is at risk of distension (direct venous return into ventricles). This compromises subendocardial perfusion.
  - When using cardioplegia, watch the ECG continuously for spontaneous activity. It is an important sign of need for re-administering cardioplegia. If the heart is not protected adequately, the most elegant surgery will be in vain.
  - If sinus rhythm recurs during cross-clamping for any reason, VF often follows when the clamp is released (reperfusion injury).
  - Most arrhythmias are due to surgical manipulation. Do not hassle the surgeon to desist. Simply inform them of the haemodynamics,

and only request them to rest the heart if it is unduly prolonged (more likely with junior surgeons).

- **Urine**:
Urine production is a useful guide to adequate organ perfusion. In the presence of hypothermia, healthy kidneys sometimes become oliguric during CPB. If there are no other signs of malperfusion, an expectant attitude can be adopted. A diuresis usually follows.

- **Temperature**:
  - Monitor in one or two locations. Nasopharyngeal reflects brain temperature and can be influenced by warm aortic blood. Bladder reflects core temperature well but can be inaccurate during low urine flow. Shell temperature lags behind core temperature. It can be measured by rectal or skeletal muscle probe. Large gradients (8 to 10°C) often develop during cooling and rewarming. Oesophageal temperature can be affected by ice ('slush') in the mediastinum.
  - Temperature decreases faster (particularly core) during cooling than it increases during rewarming. Vasodilators can hasten rewarming, particularly in the 'shell' compartment. Never use a gradient between water in the heat exchanger and blood of more than 8°C during rewarming, to minimize risk of neurological sequelae.

- **De-airing**:
Air enters the heart and goes back into the pulmonary veins during open heart surgery. Raising venous pressure and inflating the lungs ('squeeze the lungs please') fills the LV and facilitates de-airing. TOE provides useful information on the quantity and distribution of intra-cardiac air (although it is very sensitive).

Circulatory control

- Blood pressure = cardiac output × SVR.
- During CPB cardiac output is generally fixed by the pump. Therefore blood pressure will be dependent on SVR. Don't assume this!
- Always check with the perfusionist whether pump flow has been changed or diverted. It could be diverted and not entering the patient directly, for example to a haemofilter or sampling line. Also, the flow must compensate for any blood returning via an aortic root vent, as this blood is diverted to the pump and does not perfuse the body.
- SVR is dependent on haematocrit, therefore haemodilution on commencing CPB will always lower SVR and blood pressure. Generally this does not need to be treated as it is transient (<2 minutes).
- Check that hypotension is not due to:
  - Low pump flow rate.
  - Cannula disaster.
  - Transducer error/drift.
- Check that hypertension is not due to:
  - Excessive pump flow rate.
  - Innominate artery cannulation by aortic cannula.
  - Transducer error/drift.
  - 'High line pressure.'
  - Normal 'line pressure' is up to three times patient pressure.

- Occlusion of arterial cannula.
- Clotted arterial filter.
- High SVR.
- Transducer error.

LV distension

- This is a potential disaster. **Never** let the LV distend during cardiac surgery. Otherwise subendocardial and myocardial ischaemia will pose a significant problem.
- Inadequate venous drainage (blood enters LV via lungs).
- Aortic regurgitation.
- 'Collateral flow' – bronchial arteries, septal defects, pulmonary-systemic shunts, coronary Thebesian veins, pericardial collaterals, left SVC to LA connection.
- Treat cause and/or insert LV or PA vent.

Blood pressure control

- Lower/upper limit of MAP during CPB is controversial and there are no absolute guidelines.
- In general MAP >50 mmHg.
- During hypothermic bypass:
  - Mild to moderate (30–32°C) MAP maintained at 50 to 70 mmHg. If colder, lower pressures may be tolerated – MAP 30–40 mmHg.
  - Rewarming:
    - Hypotension usually occurs when cross-clamp removed (metabolite washout). This is not treated unless it persists for several minutes.
    - Hypotension often also follows pleural blood retrieval. This is thought to be due to activation of factors while the blood is resting outside of the vascular system. These are then introduced into the arterial system from the pump. It is problematic in that typically the surgeon will retrieve the blood just prior to discontinuing bypass!
  - Warm reperfusion:
    - MAP slightly lower than that desired post-CPB, so will be reasonable coming off. MAP usually increases post-CPB due to pulsatile waveform and height of systolic pressure.

Adjusting blood pressure

- Vary pump flow rate – not commonly used. Low flows compromise perfusion. High flows increase blood trauma. Can be used briefly for periods of very low or high blood pressure.
- Increasing SVR – the primary control of BP in most cases. Phenylephrine or metaraminol boluses. Norepinephrine (noradrenaline) or vasopressin can be used when SVR becomes less responsive to these. Vasopressin therapy is currently popular for 'vasoplegia' secondary to cardiopulmonary bypass.
- Decreasing SVR – anaesthesia. Within reason! It is easy to use vasodilators and vasoconstrictors. Dialling up very high or very low volatile agents produces a slow response and does not treat the cause if adequate anaesthesia is assured. Opioids are quite useful – remifentanil produces particularly stable conditions. Vasodilators – GTN boluses or infusions, phentolamine, sodium nitroprusside.

Complications of cardiopulmonary bypass

Arterial cannula – aortic dissection detection
- Check waveform is pulsatile and correlates with radial pressure. High arterial 'Line' pressure.
- Low/absent radial line pressure.
- Organ hypoperfusion.
- Visual identification.
- TOE.
- Solution: remove aortic cannula. Repair or replace aorta.

Carotid/subclavian occlusion
- Facial blanching.
- Pupillary dilation.
- Conjunctival oedema.
- Low blood pressure in radial artery.
- Solution: surgical repositioning of cannula.

Reversed cannulation
- This is a catastrophe!
- Detection:
  - Hypotension.
  - Severe facial oedema.
  - High CVP.
  - Surgical direct inspection.
- Solution: gas embolism protocol. (see massive air embolism below)

Venous return obstruction
- Air lock.
- Mechanical – obstruction to venous cannula.
- Turn flows down so CPB reservoir does not empty.
- Detection: empty venous reservoir, increased CVP (false low reading if CVP tip distal to tight caval tapes, organ ischaemia due to reduced perfusion).
- Solution: reduce CPB flow or 'come off' CPB.
- Air lock: raise and tap venous tubing, thus moving the air downstream.

Massive air embolism
- Causes:
  - If the CPB reservoir empties, then air will be pumped into the patient. Alarms can warn of or even (automatically) prevent this – but no system or alarm setup is foolproof.
  - Heart contracts and ejects before de-airing when heart has been opened. While undesirable this is unlikely to be 'massive'.
  - Pump turns the 'wrong way'. The pump can turn in either direction. The circuit can also be connected incorrectly. Unlikely though it sounds, this can happen by mistake, or if different pump protocols are used by individuals in the same institution.
  - Leak or kink in the tubing before the pump head. This can entrain air.
  - Clotted oxygenator.
  - Malfunctioning pump ('runaway').
  - Paradoxical embolism across (previously unsuspected) septal defect. Particularly with no aortic cross-clamp.

- Solution:
  - **Stop** CPB.
  - Head down.
  - Remove aortic cannula and flush.
  - Connect arterial line to SVC cannula or SVC. Inject blood at 1–2 l/min into SVC to reverse cerebral blood flow. Drain blood and air from aortic cannulation site.
  - Compress carotids intermittently to allow retrograde purging from vertebral system.
  - If you suspect whole body embolism, then this can be repeated with the IVC. This is more complicated.
  - Restore normal CPB when all air appears to have been removed.
  - Systemic vasoconstriction 'pushes bubbles through' vessels and bifurcations.
  - Consider CNS protective measures postoperatively (temperature, CO_2, sedation).

Oxygen failure
- Detection: oxygen analyser on pump gas flow, colour of arterial cannula blood, blood gases.
- Solution: restore supply. Use external cylinder if necessary. Cool patient. Manual ventilation of lungs if able to come off or reduce CPB.

Pump/oxygenator failure
- Solution: what is the temperature? If possible wean emergently from CPB. If perfusion will be absent for more than two minutes, induce hypothermia to maximal extent possible. Pack head and heart with ice. Open cardiac massage if feasible/appropriate.
- Pump failure – hand crank pump until replacement or new tubing available. Unplug if necessary and switch the tubing to the next pump head along (there are usually three or four in a row).
- Oxygenator – replace. This will take even the most skilled perfusionist several minutes.

Clotted CPB circuit
- Detection: visual observation, high arterial line pressure.
- Solution: stop CPB. Cardiac massage. Reheparinize. Replace oxygenator and CPB circuit. Follow massive air embolism if necessary. Ring medical defence organization.

Fluids

Haemodilution
- Viscosity increases with hypothermia. Microcirculatory flow is impaired. Haemodilution counteracts this and improves organ perfusion at low temperatures.
- Haemodilution decreases blood pressure, predominantly when CPB commences (SVR is affected by viscosity).
- Plasma proteins are diluted by the prime lowering oncotic pressure. Fluid requirements increase and tissue oedema is more likely.
- If Hb is reduced by more than 50%, pump flow must double to compensate. This is not practical or desirable, so hypothermia is necessary to reduce total body oxygen consumption.

- There is no absolute or universal 'target Hb' during CPB. Values must be tailored to individual patients. In general terms most tolerate levels of 7–9 g/dl.

Fluid management

- Autotransfusion – autologous blood may be removed prior to or during commencement of CPB. This is then retransfused back during or after CPB. This is effective (and provides undiluted clotting factors) but requires adequate Hb concentration.
- Blood prime is used in anaemic patients, where commencing CPB might lower Hb <5.
- Haemodilution is usually most prominent at beginning of CPB. Renal filtration can be supplemented (where venous reservoir levels permit) with extracorporeal ultrafiltration added to the CPB circuit.
- Cardioplegia can increase serum potassium.

Drugs

Volatile anaesthetic agents

- Inhalation anaesthetics such as isoflurane can be administered during CPB by means of a vaporizer placed in the gas flow to the oxygenator. Anaesthetic uptake is affected by gas flow, pump blood flow, temperature, oxygenator, and distribution of blood flow. Nitrous oxide is not used (bubble enlargement).
- Oxygenator damage has been reported with volatile anaesthetic agent spills.

Pharmacokinetics

- Dilution – enlarged circulating volume during CPB dilutes drugs and proteins and increases volume of distribution. Total drug concentrations may increase but non-protein-bound drugs may remain constant because of decreased protein-bound fraction. The increased volume of distribution is relatively minor compared to total volume of distribution for many drugs.
- Elimination – clearance can be impaired due to alterations in hepatic and renal blood flow and enzyme function.
- Absorption – drugs may be absorbed onto the oxygenator and CPB circuit. Fentanyl and GTN are both affected. Lower plasma levels will result.
- Lungs – drugs may be sequestered in the lungs and not circulated or metabolized during CPB. A bolus will then be added to the circulation on discontinuation of CPB.
- Tissues – poor skeletal muscle and fat perfusion during CPB dictate that drugs may become sequestered in tissues. They will be released during and following rewarming as normal perfusion resumes.
- Pharmacology – the pharmacology of most drugs during CPB has not been sufficiently studied. Different drugs vary, and the effects are different during the various CPB phases and temperature changes.

Temperature

Slowed cooling
- Temperature sensor error/malposition.
- Inadequate carotid perfusion.

Slow rewarming
- Sensor error/malposition.
- Inadequate pump flow rate.
- Excessive vasoconstriction.
- Heat exchanger failure/misuse.
- Large patients.

Further reading

1. De Vroege R, van Oeveren W, van Klarenbosch J, et al. The impact of heparin-coated cardiopulmonary bypass circuits on pulmonary function and the release of inflammatory mediators. *Anesthesia and Analgesia* 2004; 98: 1586–1594.

2. Khan N, De Souza A, Mister R, et al. A randomized comparison of off-pump and on-pump multivessel coronary-artery bypass surgery. *NEJM* 2004; 350: 21–28.

3. Levy J, Tanaka K. Surgical myocardial protection – inflammatory response to cardiopulmonary bypass. *Annals of Thoracic Surgery* 2003; 75: S715–S720.

4. Lo B, Fijnheer R, Castigliego D, et al. Activation of hemostasis after coronary artery bypass grafting with or without cardiopulmonary bypass. *Anesthesia and Analgesia* 2004; 99: 634–640.

5. Puskas J, Williams W, Mahoney E, et al. Off-pump vs conventional coronary artery bypass grafting: Early and 1-year graft patency, cost, and quality-of-life outcomes. *JAMA* 2004; 291: 1841–1849.

6. Shann K, Likosky D, Murkin J, et al. An evidence-based review of the practice of cardiopulmonary bypass in adults: A focus on neurologic injury, glycemic control, hemodilution, and the inflammatory response. *The Journal of Thoracic and Cardiovascular Surgery* 2006; 132: 283–290.

Deep hypothermic circulatory arrest

Dr J Gothard and Dr A Kelleher

Deep hypothermic circulatory arrest (DHCA) *274*
Cerebral metabolism and hypothermia *276*
Management of DHCA *278*
Outcome *284*
Further reading *285*

Deep hypothermic circulatory arrest (DHCA)

Hypothermia is used extensively in cardiac surgery to protect organs such as the heart and brain during cardiopulmonary bypass (CPB). Deep, or profound, hypothermia (15–20°C) allows complete cessation of the circulation to the body for a variable length of time. The combination of deep hypothermia and circulatory arrest is used to facilitate surgery when it is difficult or even impossible to use conventional CPB.

Indications for DHCA

- Aortic arch surgery.
- Surgery of the descending aorta.
- Re-sternotomy after previous cardiac surgery.
- Neurosurgery (e.g. cerebral aneurysm surgery).
- Complex neonatal cardiac surgery.

A major indication for DHCA in adults is aortic surgery, particularly the resection of aneurysms involving the arch and descending aorta, when it may be necessary to operate with an open aorta. The use of DHCA in paediatric practice has recently declined with improvement in surgical techniques and CPB technology, and the knowledge that neonates are not as tolerant of circulatory arrest as previously thought (📖 see also Chapter 29).

Cerebral metabolism and hypothermia

At normothermia, resting cerebral metabolism per unit mass is approximately 7.5 times the average metabolism in non-nervous tissue. The brain is incapable of significant anaerobic metabolism because of its high metabolic rate and lack of glycogen stores. There are no significant stores of oxygen in brain tissue so neuronal activity relies on the second-by-second delivery of oxygen and glucose from the circulation. Cessation of the blood supply to the brain causes an immediate reduction in the production of energy-rich molecules such as adenosine triphosphate (ATP). The depletion of ATP stores leads to failure of membrane ionic transfer, membrane depolarization, and intracellular accumulation of calcium, lactate, and water. These result in neuronal damage. When the blood supply is re-established to the brain, ATP stores are restored, but secondary neuronal damage may occur due to reperfusion injury.

Cerebral reperfusion injury

The mechanisms leading to neuronal death following ischaemic injury are complex, with neurons continuing to die over weeks and months, and reperfusion injury contributing significantly to the total neuronal loss.

The inflammatory responses to cardiopulmonary bypass and DHCA are central to reperfusion injury and include leucocyte, platelet, complement, and endothelial cell activation, as well as breakdown of the blood-brain barrier. Cerebral vascular resistance increases and autoregulation is impaired. There is some evidence that the severity of the reperfusion injury may be attenuated by steroids (given 4–6 hours preoperatively), and the inclusion of leucocyte filters within the cardiopulmonary bypass circuit.

Hypothermia

Deep hypothermia reduces metabolic rate and oxygen consumption of neuronal and other tissues, thus reducing energy depletion and lengthening the tolerated period of ischaemia. The reduction in metabolic rate is roughly exponential with decreasing temperature so that there is a relatively greater decrease at higher temperatures. Neuronal metabolism is never completely suppressed, even at temperatures as low as 15°C, and animal experiments have shown that after a period of approximately 30 minutes of DHCA the level of high-energy phosphates in cerebral tissue becomes undetectable. Deep hypothermia also attenuates the release of toxic neurotransmitters and reactive oxygen species during ischaemia and reperfusion periods. Traditionally acceptable periods of circulatory arrest at different temperatures are summarized in Table 19.1.

Table 19.1 Hypothermia and circulatory arrest

Temperature (°C)	CMR (% baseline)	Duration of 'safe' circulatory arrest (minutes)
32	70	7.5
28	48	10.5
25	37	14
20	24	21
18	17	25
15	14	31

CMR: cerebral metabolic rate

It is important to remember that in order to achieve uniform and effective hypothermia, the cooling period should be at least 20 minutes long and continue for at least a further 10 minutes after the desired temperature has been reached.

Management of DHCA

This is one of the most controversial areas in cardiac anaesthesia and not only encompasses the problem of cerebral protection but also that of spinal cord and other organ protection, particularly when surgery involves the descending aorta. Various surgical groups have produced good results for thoracic aortic surgery, with acceptable mortality and morbidity, using widely varying management protocols. Box 19.1 summarizes the general effects of hypothermic bypass.

Box 19.1 General effects of hypothermic bypass

Blood and circulation
- Vasoconstriction.
- Increased viscosity of blood and stiffer, less deformable red cells.
- Coagulopathy and reduction in platelet function and number (due to sequestration).
- Left shift of the Hb dissociation curve – reduced oxygen delivery.
- Predisposition to heparin rebound.

Metabolism
- Tendency to metabolic acidosis.
- Impaired glucose metabolism.
- Electrolyte imbalance, including a decrease in serum K^+.
- Decreased drug metabolism.

Cerebral
- Vasoconstriction.
- Reduction in cerebral oxygen consumption.
- Renal.
- Reduction in glomerular filtration rate.
- Impairment of sodium, water, and glucose reabsorption.

GI tract
- Gastric dilation, ileus.
- Submucosal gastric erosion and haemorrhage.

Cardiac
- Bradycardia, contractility initially well preserved.
- Dysrhythmias.

Anaesthetic considerations

There is some evidence that volatile anaesthetic agents may confer a degree of preconditioning to neuronal as well as myocardial tissue, therefore a balanced technique including a relaxant, an intravenous opioid, and a low-dose inhalational agent such as isoflurane would be satisfactory. In practice, however, the effects of temperature and acid-base changes have a far greater impact on cerebral blood flow and metabolism than the choice of anaesthetic agent. Nitrous oxide is avoided due to cerebral vasodilation and expansion of air emboli. It is usual to administer an incremental dose of muscle relaxant just prior to circulatory arrest (the diaphragm can move even during arrest!). The use of thiopental for cerebral protection is discussed below.

Monitoring

Monitoring requirements are as for any other major cardiac operation. Particular emphasis is placed on the measurement of temperature, pressure gradients (radial versus femoral artery), cerebral activity, and the effect of cooling. Trans-oesophageal echocardiography (TOE) may be used to monitor ventricular function, ventricular distension, and the presence of atheromatous plaques and air. It may also be used to monitor flow in the arch and arch vessels, although adequate views are not always possible. In some units somatosensory-evoked potentials (SSEPs) are monitored distally during surgery on the descending aorta. Further details of specific monitoring are summarized in Box 19.2.

Box 19.2 Specific monitoring requirements for DHCA

Temperature monitoring
- Brain:
  - Nasopharyngeal.
  - Tympanic membrane.
- Core:
  - Oesophagus.
  - Rectum/bladder.
- Peripheral:
  - Skin.

Cardiovascular monitoring
- Radial artery: left, right, or both depending on surgery.
- Femoral artery: may need to be utilized for PCB.
- Pulmonary artery catheter: more useful postop; sheath may be useful for transfusion.
- TOE:
  - Ventricular function.
  - Flow in aorta/grafts.
  - Air and atheromatous plaques.

Cerebral function monitoring
- EEG/cerebral oximetry: not used universally.
- Jugular bulb catheter: cerebral venous oxygen saturation.

Spinal cord monitoring
- Somatosensory-evoked potentials (SSEPs).

Cooling and rewarming

- Patients are slowly cooled via the cardiopulmonary bypass circuit to 15°C prior to circulatory arrest. A low haematocrit has a theoretical advantage because of the increased viscosity of blood during hypothermia. Some units, however, maintain the haematocrit at approximately 30%, which may limit intracellular acidosis. Theatre temperature is kept as low as possible.
- Rewarming is only recommended following a period of cold reperfusion at 15°C for approximately 10 minutes. The rewarming process is continued slowly until the core temperature approaches 36°C. Hyperthermia is avoided as it worsens neurological injury. The temperature gradient between the rewarming perfusate and the patient's core temperature is restricted to a maximum of 10°C (8°C in some units) in order to limit metabolic/blood flow mismatch.

Acid-base management

- Alpha-stat acid-base management, in which total stores of carbon dioxide are maintained at a constant level, is regarded as beneficial in terms of neurocognitive outcome in adult patients undergoing cardiac surgery at moderate hypothermia (greater than 30°C).
- pH-stat acid-base management, in which carbon dioxide is added to the circulating blood, is used by some prior to DHCA. The added carbon dioxide makes the blood relatively more acidotic compared with alpha-stat management. This leads to cerebral vasodilation and relative over-perfusion of the brain, with potentially more effective and even cerebral cooling. It achieves this at the cost of increasing the embolic load to the brain, which may be associated with adverse neurological outcomes.
- Some centres use pH-stat management during the initial cooling phase and then revert to alpha-stat management once the target temperature has been reached. This is thought to mitigate the intracellular metabolic acidosis associated with pH-stat management. This is termed the 'cross-over' management technique. Alpha-stat pH management is then usually used for reperfusion and rewarming.
- The practice described above is not universal. Some units use alpha-stat management throughout the cooling and rewarming phases, possibly allowing a relatively high $PaCO_2$ as a compromise between adequate cerebral cooling and limiting embolic load.

Hyperoxia

There is some evidence from animal studies that the use of hyperoxia during bypass may limit the extent of ischaemic injury following DHCA. The primary mechanism of injury is ischaemia, and the benefits due to the increase in dissolved oxygen at hypothermic temperatures appears to outweigh any injury associated with oxygen free radicals. Hypothermic hyperoxic bypass is also associated with fewer and smaller gaseous microemboli, as oxygen is much more soluble than nitrogen, particularly at low temperatures.

Glucose homeostasis

Glucose homeostasis is deranged and hyperglycaemia is common during hypothermia. Endogenous insulin production is decreased and glycogenolysis and gluconeogenesis are increased by elevated circulating catecholamines. Hyperglycaemia is associated with the release of excitatory neurotransmitters within the brain, and is known to increase intracellular acidosis, delaying the recovery of normal metabolic homeostasis. There is increasingly strong evidence that hyperglycaemia can contribute to major morbidity and mortality in patients undergoing cardiac surgery. Although we lack data relating specifically to hyperglycaemia associated with DHCA, it seems appropriate to control the blood sugar within the normal range (5–8 mmol/l).

Coagulation

Effective coagulation is deranged during hypothermia. Deep hypothermia causes a reduction in the flexibility of the red blood cells and a rise in haematocrit due to loss of plasma from the circulation. Leucopoenia and thrombocytopenia occur due to sequestration of white cells and platelets in the liver and spleen. In addition, platelet aggregation and adhesion are impaired, as is the function of coagulation factors. Although these effects are reversible with restoration of normothermia, it is prudent to have platelets and clotting factors available.

It is essential to maintain adequate heparinization during deep hypothermia and it is wise to give a bolus of heparin during cooling prior to DHCA.

Cerebral protection

Methods used to protect the brain during DHCA include:
- Adequate cooling.
- Packing ice around the head.
- Cerebral perfusion techniques.
- Steroid therapy.
- High-dose barbiturates.
- Other drug therapy (calcium channel blockers, NMDA receptor antagonists).

Adequate, even cooling of the brain is achieved by cooling slowly and perfusing the patient at the target temperature for at least 10 minutes prior to circulatory arrest. Some centres aim for jugular bulb venous oxygen saturations of 95% or EEG 'electrical silence' prior to arrest. Packed ice or a cooling helmet is placed around the head to aid cooling and to prevent rewarming during arrest.

Thiopental has been given in doses up to 40 mg/kg to induce and maintain EEG burst suppression during moderate hypothermia, but evidence supporting its use for DHCA is conflicting. Thiopental can result in prolonged sedation and myocardial depression. There is some evidence that high-dose steroids given several hours prior to CPB provide a degree of neuroprotection. Methylprednisolone may be given at a dose of 30 mg/kg prior to induction of anaesthesia when DHCA is planned, although it is likely to be more effective if it can be given up to six hours earlier. If DHCA exceeds 30 minutes it is recommended that methylprednisolone is continued at a lower dose for 48 hours (125 mg 6-hourly for 24 hours and then 125 mg 12-hourly for 24 hours).

Calcium influx and excitotoxicity are both mechanisms implicated in ischaemic neuronal damage. Calcium channel blockers and drugs such as NMDA receptor antagonists may potentially be neuroprotective but are not currently used routinely in DHCA.

Even a combination of the techniques described above may not provide optimal cerebral protection. This has led to the use of surgical perfusion techniques discussed below.

Cerebral perfusion techniques

Retrograde cerebral perfusion was introduced to attempt to provide oxygenated blood and metabolic substrates to the brain during DHCA. Doubts have arisen as animal studies have shown that retrograde perfusion may not provide enough brain capillary perfusion to confer any significant metabolic benefit. Therefore antegrade cerebral perfusion, which is more physiological but also technically difficult, was developed.

Retrograde cerebral perfusion

During retrograde cerebral perfusion the superior vena cava is perfused with cold, oxygenated blood at pressures of 25–40 mmHg at a flow rate of 250–400 ml/minute. Return to the pump is usually via suction in the operating field.

An advantage of retrograde cerebral perfusion is that it helps to preserve cerebral hypothermia; however, initial enthusiasm has been tempered by adverse neurological outcomes in some series and the realization that competent internal jugular vein valves and collapsed cortical veins may limit adequate brain perfusion. The technique is now mainly reserved as a method of washing out particulate emboli and air from the cerebral circulation following aortic surgery.

Antegrade selective cerebral perfusion

Antegrade selective cerebral perfusion may be used during aortic arch surgery to provide isolated cerebral blood flow. The right axillary artery is generally the cannulation site of choice as it is usually relatively free from atheromatous disease, is not generally affected by dissection, and avoids the embolic hazards of retrograde perfusion through a diseased atheromatous aorta associated with femoral perfusion.

The right axillary artery is cannulated (either directly or more usually through a side graft) and the left common carotid and proximal brachiocephalic arteries are clamped. Flow is then directed up the right carotid artery to the brain at a rate of 8–10 ml/kg/min, maintaining the right radial pressure at 30–60 mmHg whilst the aortic arch is reconstructed. It is clear that effective cerebral perfusion is dependent upon an intact circle of Willis. The cerebral vessels may then be perfused directly once a vascular graft has been placed incorporating their origins.

Antegrade cerebral perfusion carries the risk of atheromatous or air embolization or cerebral injury due to excessive perfusion pressures. The patient should be carefully assessed preoperatively to exclude significant carotid atheromatous disease. In experienced hands, however, this method of cerebral protection allows brain perfusion during DHCA and may be associated with an improved neurological outcome.

Spinal cord protection (📖 see also Chapter 26)

DHCA can be used to facilitate surgery on the descending aorta but it is usually preferable to maintain perfusion to the lower half of the body using left atrium to femoral artery bypass (left heart bypass). Some centres rely on the use of DHCA and fast, effective surgery alone to minimize the risk of paraplegia following this type of surgery. Others use a combination of techniques to minimize spinal cord injury. These may include:

- Modification of surgical technique.
- Distal circulatory support – e.g. left atrium to femoral artery bypass.
- Monitoring somatosensory-evoked potentials.
- CSF drainage/cooling.

Outcome

The incidence of focal deficit (stroke) after DHCA and aortic surgery is reported in various clinical series at 5–10%. Age, atherosclerosis, and manipulation of the aorta are risk factors. However, diffuse neurological deficits due to global cerebral ischaemia are more common, with a frequency of 10–20%. These disorders cover a wide spectrum including confusion, agitation, seizures, and even coma. Their incidence is related to age, technical difficulties with bypass, and prolonged circulatory arrest. The incidence of more subtle cognitive dysfunction, a common finding following conventional CPB, is also high.

Further reading

1. Cooper W, Duarte I, Thourani V, et al. Hypothermic circulatory arrest causes multisystem vascular endothelial dysfunction and apoptosis. *Annals of Thoracic Surgery* 2000; 69: 696–702.
2. Czerny M, Fleck T, Zimpfer D, et al. Risk factors of mortality and permanent neurologic injury in patients undergoing ascending aortic and arch repair. *The Journal of Thoracic and Cardiovascular Surgery* 2003; 126: 1296–1301.
3. Haverich A, Hagl C. Organ protection during hypothermic circulatory arrest. *The Journal of Thoracic and Cardiovascular Surgery* 2003; 125: 460–462.
4. Immerv F, Barmettler H, Berdat P, et al. Effects of deep hypothermic circulatory arrest on outcome after resection of ascending aortic aneurysm. *Annals of Thoracic Surgery* 2002; 74: 422–425.
5. Percy A, Widman S, Rizzo J, Tranquilli M, Elefteriades J. Deep hypothermic circulatory arrest in patients with high cognitive needs: Full preservation of cognitive abilities. *Annals of Thoracic Surgery* 2009; 87: 117–123.

Intra-aortic balloon counter-pulsation

Dr A Rosenberg

Principles *288*
Indications and contraindications *289*
Placement *290*
Management *292*
Further reading *296*

Principles

An intra-aortic balloon pump (IABP) is a catheter-mounted, helium-filled, polyethylene balloon that is typically inserted via a femoral artery into the descending aorta just below the left subclavian artery. Placement of an IABP is among the most established and expeditious means to mechanically support inadequate cardiac output or coronary perfusion resulting from acute or chronic conditions when preload, contractility, and afterload have been optimally managed. When fluids, pharmacologic treatments, and exclusion of other causes of low cardiac output (distributive and obstructive causes, i.e. sepsis, tamponade, tension pneumothorax etc.) have been achieved, IABPs accomplish the following:

- Balloon inflation at the beginning of diastole augments aortic root diastolic pressure, thus increasing coronary blood flow.
- Balloon deflation at the beginning of systole reduces afterload and may increase stroke volume by as much as 40%, decreasing cardiac work and oxygen consumption.

Recent advances in IABP technology include fibre-optic sensors used to automatically select the optimal trigger source, set inflation to dicrotic notch, and respond to tachyarrhythmias, as well as smaller catheters with the same balloon sizes.

Indications and contraindications

Indications

- Reducing afterload for cardiogenic shock unresponsive to inotropic support, severe mitral regurgitation, or ventricular septal defect.
- Post-cardiotomy low cardiac output including failure to wean from cardiac bypass.
- Unstable angina unresponsive to medical management.
- Support during high-risk procedures/events:
  - Unstable patients prior to CPB or VAD placement.
  - Especially high-risk PTCA, coronary stent placement, or rotoblator procedures.
  - Failed coronary angioplasty with ongoing ischaemia.
  - Ventricular arrhythmias refractory to medical treatments.

Contraindications

- Aortic regurgitation (diastolic augmentation will worsen AR).
- Aortic aneurysm or dissection.
- Severe aorto-iliac and peripheral vascular disease.

Placement

IABPs are usually placed in either a cardiac catherization lab or the operating theatre, where fluoroscopic support is readily available to help guidewire and catheter placement. In extreme cases, they can also be placed in the ICU for patients too unstable to transport. Most IABPs are placed percutaneously in the femoral artery using the Seldinger technique. Occasionally, they can also be placed surgically directly into the descending aorta in patients with extreme peripheral vascular disease or occluded femoral/iliac arteries.

- The tip of the balloon should be 2 cm distal to the origin of the left subclavian artery.
- After the patient is prepped and sterilely draped, laying the IABP catheter on the patient will help estimate the distance the catheter needs to be inserted (from groin to third rib).
- Aspirate any residual air from the IABP using a 20 ml or 60 ml syringe.
- Be sure the wire that is placed into the dilator in the femoral artery moves freely before inserting and advancing the IABP catheter.
- After connecting arterial manometry tubing to IABP, aspirate back arterial blood to remove air, flush with saline, and evaluate the arterial waveform.
- Urgent CXR is used to identify the small radio-opaque metal tip of the IABP to evaluate positioning. TOE can also be used for this.

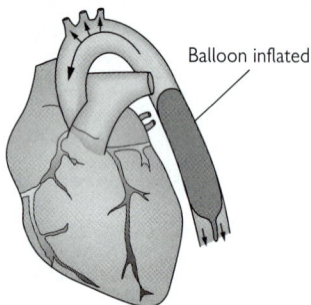

Balloon inflated

Figure 20.1 Positioning and function of IABP (Courtesy of Datascope).

Management

Timing and rate of inflation and deflation can be based on ECG, arterial pressure waveforms, and cardiac pacing devices. Optimal circulatory support can be achieved by any of the above that result in the best augmented blood pressures (Figure 20.2).

- Inflation should be at aortic valve closure (dicrotic notch) and should result in diastolic augmented BP higher than unassisted systolic BP.
- Deflation timed to allow assisted aortic end diastolic pressure to be 10–15 mmHg less than unassisted diastolic pressure, demonstrating reduced afterload.
- Assisted systole should be less than unassisted systole due to lower augmented end-diastolic pressure.
- Arterial pressure triggers may be best when significant arrhythmias are present, in pacing-dependent patients, where there is interference from diathermy, or if very low ECG signals are present.
- ECG timing may be optimal in patients with narrow pulse pressures.
- Reducing IABP support rates from 1:1 to 1:2 or 1:3 may improve cardiac output in patients with tachycardias often above 130 bpm.
- Aggressive prevention and management of tachyarrhythmias is vital, as all triggering modes are frequently inefficient with tachycardias.
- Modern IABP consoles offer automatic timing options that may be able to respond to changing heart rates, pulse pressure, and even atrial arrhythmias in real-time.
- Balloon volume loss alarms, decreased augmentation, and blood in the catheter suggest balloon puncture/tear, which may result in gas embolism. The catheter needs to be replaced.
- Anticoagulation with heparin is often used with IABPs to keep the aPTT around 50 to 70 seconds in order to avoid arterial thromboembolism. Especially important for rates ≤1:3.
- Routine pulse assessment in left arm and legs as well as inspecting insertion site and flank for haematoma is required.

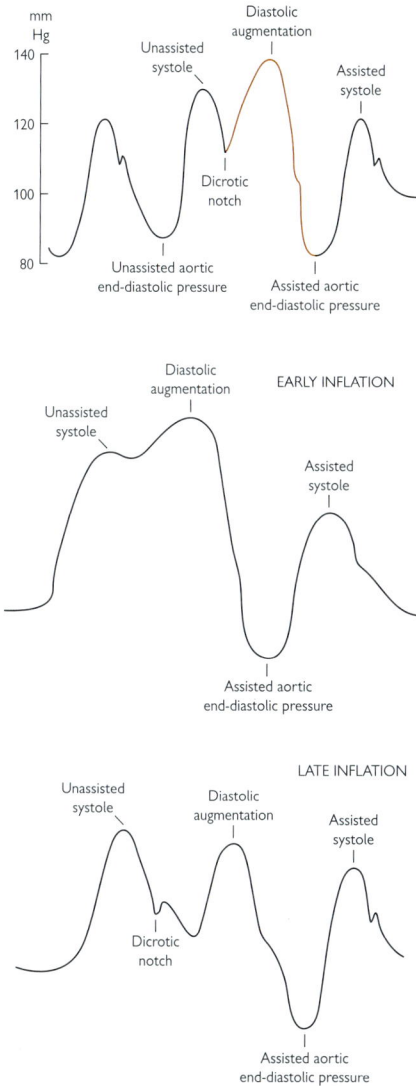

Figure 20.2 IABP timing and common inflation/deflation errors.

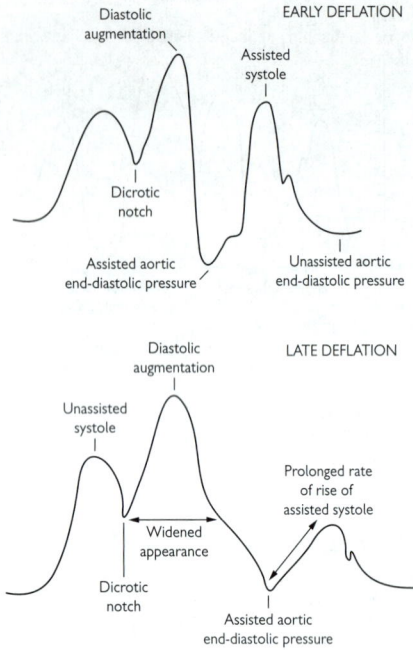

Figure 20.2 (continued)

Weaning and removal

Clinical improvement with reduced pharmacologic support or a lack of benefit from IABP with a complication arising (typically leg ischaemia or haematoma) are the usual reasons for weaning/removing an IABP.

- Reduce inflation ratio from 1:1 or 1:2 to 1:3 or 1:4 (depending on type of IABP) for three to six hours.
- Evaluate adequacy of organ perfusion (cardiac outputs, mixed venous oxygen saturations, pharmacologic support, lactate, urine output, cerebral mentation).
- Hold heparin for two to four hours prior to IABP removal and correct coagulopathy, and/or thrombocytopenia if platelets <50,000–100,000.
- With standby button pushed and IABP inflation off, aspirate remaining gas from balloon via stopcock.
- Identify and gently place non-dominant fingers on femoral artery, with only minimal gauze pads needed. Pull catheter in a rapid, steady manner and press down on femoral artery immediately after a small arterial pulse of blood is ejected from the insertion hole to allow any small thrombus material to exit the artery.
- Hold pressure that keeps blood from exiting insertion hole for at least 45 minutes without relaxing pressure to 'see if bleeding occurs'. Many institutions will then keep the patient supine for an additional six hours, monitoring insertion site for haematoma with/without pressure dressing over insertion site and leg for ischaemia.

Complications

- Vascular:
  - Femoral, iliac, or aortic perforation/rupture.
  - Embolization of thrombus, atherosclerotic plaques.
  - Leg, left arm, and renal/visceral ischaemia if balloon is malpositioned or moved.
- Infection.
- Haemorrhage.
- Haemolysis.
- Thrombocytopaenia.
- Gas embolus.
- AV fistula in groin – presence of pulsating mass, bruit, ultrasound diagnosis.

Further reading

1. Stone G, Magnus Ohman E, Miller M, et al. Contemporary utilization and outcomes of intra-aortic balloon counterpulsation in acute myocardial infarction. *Journal of the American College of Cardiology* 2003; 41: 1940–1945.
2. Trost J, Hillis L. Intra-aortic balloon counterpulsation. *The American Journal of Cardiology* 2006; 97: 1391–1398.
3. Elahi M, Chetty G, Kirke R, Azeem T, Hartshorne R, Spyt T. Complications related to intra-aortic balloon pump in cardiac surgery: A decade later. *European Journal of Vascular and Endovascular Surgery* 2006; 29: 591–594.
4. Papaioannou T, Stefanadis C. Basic principles of the intraaortic balloon pump and mechanisms affecting its performance. *ASAIO* 2005; 51: 296–300.
5. Dyub A, Whitlock R, Abouzahr L, Cinà C. Preoperative intra-aortic balloon pump in patients undergoing coronary bypass surgery: A systematic review and meta-analysis. *Journal of Cardiac Surgery* 2008; 23: 79–86.

Ventricular assist devices

Dr A Rosenberg

Principles *298*
Indications *299*
Types of VADs *300*
Anaesthetic management during VAD placement *302*
Complications *304*
Further reading *305*

Principles

Though ventricular assist devices (VADs) have been available for over 20 years, they have become more prevalent due to increased numbers of patients with end-stage heart failure, limited access to transplantation, and improved device technologies. These may allow patients to ambulate, participate in cardiac rehabilitation, await transplant at home (bridge to transplant), or may constitute a permanent treatment (destination therapy). The REMATCH trial of 129 randomized patients demonstrated a 48% reduced one-year mortality with permanent LVAD treatment versus best medical management.

Indications

(📖 see also Chapter 32)
- *Bridge to recovery*: myocarditis (viral, alcohol, and post-partum have best chance of recovery); acute myocardial infarction; post-transplant reperfusion or rejection syndromes; post-cardiotomy low cardiac output.
- *Bridge to transplant*: progressive heart failure despite maximal medical management.
- *Destination (permanent) therapy*: contraindication to transplantation; age; chronic infections (hepatitis C).

Types of VADs

There are several classifications (Table 21.1) including:
- Ventricle(s) supported: LVAD, RVAD, BiVAD.
- Mechanism: pusher plate-pulsatile, axial rotary-non pulsatile.
- Location: extracorporeal, paracorporeal, intracorporeal.
- Drive train: pneumatic, electric, magnetic.

Table 21.1 Types and characteristics of mechanical assist devices for failing cardiac function (see also Figures 21.1–21.3)

Device name	Flow type, l*	Ventricle support	Support duration	Notables
Extracorporeal/Percutaneous				
IABP	P	L	S	
Cardiac Bypass Machines	NP, 5 l	L, R, B	S	
ECMO	P, 4–5 l	L, R, B	I	Resp. failure support possible
Tandem Heart	NP, 3–4 l	L	S	
Abiomed Impella	NP, 3–5 l	L	S	
Abiomed BVS 5000	P, 4–6 l	L, R, B	I	Extensive worldwide use
Paracorporeal				
Thoratec VAD system	P, 5 l	L, R, B	I, L	Smaller sizes available
Berlin Heart	P, 1.5–8 l			Small size for neonates
Abiomed AB 5000	P, 5 l	L, R, B	I, L	Transition from BVS to AB
Intracorporeal				
Thoratec Heartmate I	P, 5 l	L	I, L	Approved for destination
Worldheart Novacor LVAS	P, 5 l	L	L	
Thoratec Heartmate II	NP, 3–4 l	L	I	Investigational
Thoratec IVAD	P, 3–5 l	L, R, B	I	Only intracorporeal BiVAD
Micromed DeBakey Vad	NP, 3–4 l	L	I	Small size, use in paediatrics
SynCardia CardioWest	P, 7 l	B	I, L	Temporary artificial heart
Abiomed Abiocor	P, 7 l	B	L	Approved for destination

P: pulsatile; NP: non-pulsatile; l*: usual flow rate in litres; L: LVAD; R: RVAD; B: BiVAD; S: short-term (hours to days); I: intermediate (months to a year); L: long-term (months to several years).

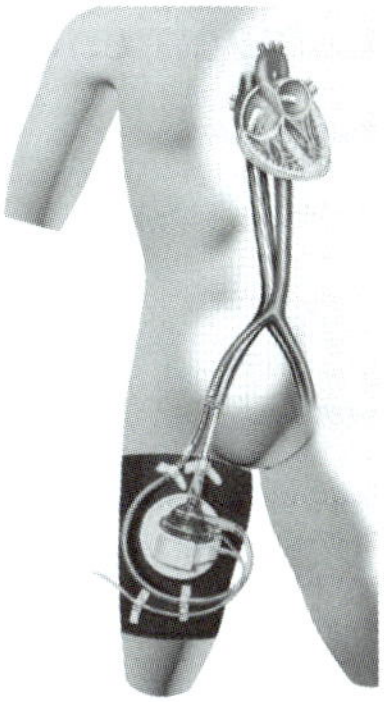

Figure 21.1 Percutaneous-type VADs – Cardiac Assist Tandem Heart (Courtesy of Cardiac Assist Inc.).

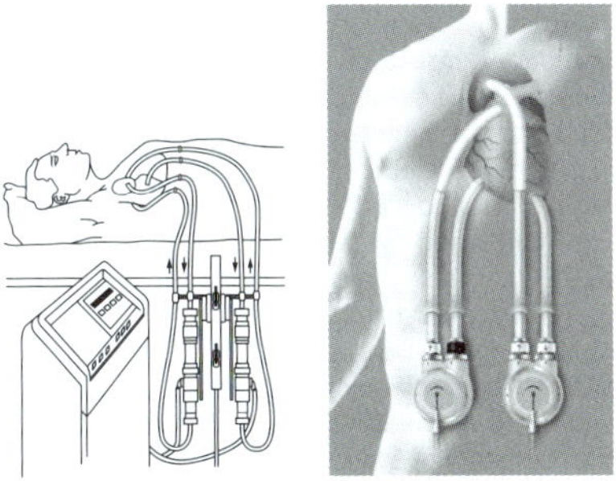

Figure 21.2 Extracorporeal/Paracorporeal VADs (Courtesy Abiomed and Thoratec Corporations).

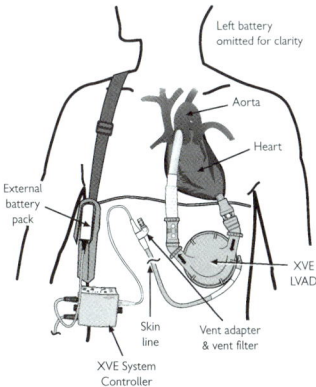

Figure 21.3 Intracorporeal VAD (Courtesy Thoratec Corporation).

Anaesthetic management during VAD placement

Preoperative management

- Comorbidities are the rule:
  - **Neuro**: old or new CVA from vascular disease.
  - **Pulmonary**: acute or chronic pulmonary hypertension; COPD.
  - **Renal**: electrolyte abnormalities; renal impairment; acidosis; altered drug excretion.
  - **Hepatic**: congestion; coagulopathy; altered drug metabolism.
  - **Endocrine**: diabetes; amiodarone-related thyroid dysfunction.
  - **Haematology**: heparin/warfarin administration (mural thrombus prevention); coagulopathies; heparin resistance (anti-thrombin III deficiency).
- New vascular catheters should be placed under meticulous sterile conditions prior to VAD placement to avoid bloodstream infections – existing lines may not be new or sterile.
- Temporary IABP may be used to avoid hypotension and worsening cardiac output during anaesthetic induction.
- Aggressive correction of coagulopathy with avoidance of intraoperative blood products and the associated cytokines/thromboxanes may reduce incidence of RV failure.
- Minimal sedatives prior to induction to avoid hypoventilation, rising pulmonary resistance, and right heart strain.
- Intraoperative TOE useful to maximize preload and inotropic support and evaluate new haemodynamic changes, presence of PFO (see below), VSD, intramural thrombus, valvular lesions, de-airing, and complications of VAD positioning.
- VADs are implanted via median sternotomy with/without CPB, but do not require cardiac cooling/standstill.
- LVAD inflow is from LV apex; outflow cannula is anastomosed to ascending aorta.
- RVAD inflow is from RV apex or atrium; outflow cannula to pulmonary artery.
- Aortic regurgitation requires repair (bridge to recovery/transplant) or closure (bridge to transplant) to avoid recycling of blood into device. Aortic stenosis is usually treated to allow any native function to augment cardiac output.
- Tricuspid regurgitation is often repaired/replaced to avoid or to treat right heart volume overload or low RV output.
- Mitral stenosis requires repair/replacement to improve VAD inflow.
- Following placement, weaning from CPB occurs with VAD in fixed mode to avoid excess ventricular collapse, inflow obstruction, and septal wall distortion.

Postoperative management

- VADs usually placed in a fixed mode for first 24 hours to avoid excess ventricular emptying and collapse. After haemodynamic stability maintained, an auto mode is used to maximize VAD output.
- Typical haemodynamic parameters for first 24 hours: MAP 70 mmHg, VAD output 3–7 l/min. Axial flow devices may use pulsatility index instead of output, which typically varies from approximately 4 l/min at 9000 rpm to 9 l/min at 15,000 rpm.
- Patients with acute LV failure (acute MI, LV hypertrophy) have smaller ventricles with a reduced reserve for LVAD filling. These are more sensitive to volume loading.
- Patients with chronic LV failure have dilated ventricles and a larger reservoir for LVAD filling. They are less sensitive to volume loading.
- After haemostasis is achieved and there is no significant postoperative bleeding, most VADs require antiplatelet therapies, anticoagulation with heparin, and eventually warfarin to maintain an INR of 2.5.

Complications

- Hypotension:
  - Low VAD flows: inadequate left and right ventricular filling; obstructed inflow/outflow; right heart failure.
  - Aortic insufficiency (aortic dissection from cannula).
  - Low vascular resistance or sepsis.
  - Haemorrhage: tamponade; abdominal; groin/retroperitoneal from previous catheterization.
  - Adrenal insufficiency.
- PFO may be 'unmasked' by left atrial decompression on VAD activation, with consequent right-to-left shunting and hypoxaemia.
- Right heart failure:
  - Maximize RV preload (CVP 8 to 15 mmHg), diuretics, and inotropic support.
  - Nitric oxide, inhaled epoprostenol (prostacyclin), and mild respiratory alkalosis to reduce pulmonary vascular resistance.
  - Rule out excess LVAD flow pulling septum toward LV.
- Bleeding:
  - At operative site, abdominal with devices requiring pre-peritoneal pockets, and retroperitoneal sites. Some institutions leave sternum open for 12–24 hours.
  - Use of antiplatelet and anticoagulants increases risk of perioperative bleeding but are required to reduce risk of thromboembolism.
  - Possible increased risk of GI bleeding reported among axial flow devices (arterio-venous malformations, vascular dysplasia).
- Infection:
  - Drive line, device, intravascular catheter, nosocomial sources (ventilator-associated pneumonia, urinary tract). Long durations of prophylactic antibiotics are routinely used in some centres to cover Gram-positive organisms (e.g. vancomycin).
- Arrhythmias:
  - LVADs protect patients from lethal arrhythmias, but these can still significantly reduce cardiac output. Strategies include reducing inotropes, pharmacologic prevention, and cardioversion.
- CNS:
  - Stroke from thromboembolism, air, or haemorrhagic event from anticoagulation.

Further reading

1. Aaronson K, Patel H, Pagani F, et al. Patient selection for left ventricular assist device therapy. *Annals of Thoracic Surgery* 2003; 75: S29–S35.
2. Hon J, Yacoub M. Bridge to recovery with the use of left ventricular assist device and clenbuterol. *Annals of Thoracic Surgery* 2003; 75: S36–S41.
3. Lietz K, Long J, Kfoury A, et al. Outcomes of left ventricular assist device implantation as destination therapy in the post-REMATCH era. Implications for patient selection. *Circulation* 2007; 116: 497–505.
4. Warner Stevenson L, Rose E. Left ventricular assist devices: Bridges to transplantation, recovery, and destination for whom? *Circulation* 2003; 108: 3059–3063.

Postoperative care

Dr G Hopgood and Dr C Hamilton Davies

General principles *308*
Inotropes and cardiovascular medications *312*
Mechanical ventilation *316*
Abnormal gases *318*
The oliguric patient *320*
The hypotensive patient *322*
Atrial fibrillation *326*
Sedation and analgesia *328*

General principles

General principles are similar to non-cardiac intensive care, in terms of maintaining global and regional oxygen delivery. Postoperative care is often protocol-driven or follows unit-specific care pathways. This allows a significant degree of autonomy in nursing care. In addition, when the postop course differs from routine it allows identification of problems and early referral to medical staff. When you first start working on a cardiac intensive care unit, seek out your local protocols as a priority.

Transfer to ICU

Patients will usually be delivered by the attending anaesthetist, a theatre nurse, and a member of the surgical team. Each has important information to impart. The first priority is to establish full monitoring, and ensure relevant infusions are not disrupted. The following occur simultaneously:

- Confirm ventilator settings, disconnect from transport ventilator or bag, and reconnect to ITU ventilator. Usually volume control (📖 see also Mechanical ventilation, p. 316), VT 7–10 ml/kg, 12 breaths per minute, PEEP of 5 cm water. An initial inspired oxygen fraction of 60–100% is reasonable, expecting to revise down with the first blood gas result. Be guided by intraop requirements. Confirm chest motion. Ventilator disconnections can be missed in the turmoil of arrival and alarms are often temporarily disabled.
- Observe transfer monitor and correlate with a palpable peripheral pulse. Confirm pacemaker settings and electro-mechanical association. Aortic balloon pumps should be plugged into power supply and timing and synchrony confirmed.
- Attach patient to monitors including ECG, pulse oximeter, invasive blood pressures, and capnography.
- Ensure uninterrupted infusion of any vasoactive agents commenced in theatre. Continue or commence any analgesic or sedative infusions required.
- Establish core and peripheral temperature.
- Note the initial volume of blood in drains. Alert surgeons if significant.

Gather data

A handover is essential for ITU nurse and intensivist.
- Demographics and patient details:
  - Age.
  - Gender.
  - Diagnosis and planned operation; urgency.
  - Comorbidities and risk factors.
  - Medications and allergies.
- Surgical information:
  - Operation performed; difficulty and complications (especially haemostasis).
  - Location of drains and pacing leads.
  - Expectations or requests for postop management.
- Anaesthetic information.
- Anaesthetic difficulties at induction or pre-CPB.
- Ease of separation from CPB.

- Rhythm disturbance.
- Drug infusions and doses.
- Fluid/blood product requirements and associated filling pressures.
- Perioperative TOE findings.
- Blood gas, electrolytes, ACT, and other lab results.
- Lines and tubes (any insertion difficulties).
- Expectations and recommendations and goals for ongoing care.

This data will establish:
- Target MAP, CVP, and CO.
- Target blood gas parameters.
- Rewarming plan.
- Expectation of probable duration of mechanical ventilation/sedation.
- Likelihood of routine or complex postop course.

Typical early targets are:
- MAP 60–80 mmHg. Hypertension increases bleeding, may disrupt anastomoses/suture lines, and increases LV work. Hypotension can impair organ perfusion and decrease coronary perfusion.
- CVP 7–12 mmHg. High 'right'-sided pressures diminish coronary blood flow (by raising coronary sinus pressure), and may be a marker (albeit indirect and not relied on alone) of filling and function.
- Sinus rhythm at a rate of 60–100 bpm. Tachycardia increases myocardial work; bradycardia may decrease cardiac output and raise cardiac chamber pressures. A-V synchrony is desirable.
- Warm/well perfused peripheries. Clinical indicators of CO may be unreliable, but warm, dry peripheries and normotension are reassuring signs.
- SPO_2 ≥95% (📖 see also Abnormal gases, p. 318).

Investigations
- Blood gases – adjust ventilation to achieve a PO_2 ≥12 kPa, PCO_2 4.7–6 kPa.
- Electrolytes – give KCl 10–30 mmol over 30–60 minutes to achieve serum potassium 4.5–5 mmol/l; give 10–20 mmol magnesium sulphate over 30 minutes if Mg ≤1 mmol/l.
- Lactate is a marker of adequacy of systemic perfusion (in absence of hepatic dysfunction). A useful rule of thumb is that a postoperative level up to three is common, and can be watched as long as it is not increasing. More than four usually indicates a problem, and over ten indicates a near-lethal situation.
- Hb – usually transfuse to keep Hb ≥7.5 g/dl, but be guided by unit practice and data specific to the patient. An initial low Hb may rise as excess intraoperative fluid/cardioplegia is redistributed/diuresed. Alternatively it may fall with ongoing bleeding or infusion of fluids.
- Platelets, coagulation profile.
- CXR – timing varies with unit policy. Either on arrival or following removal of chest drains. Check endotracheal tube, central venous line, drains, lung expansion, pleural collections, and mediastinal shadow.

Ongoing management

- Intensive monitoring is continued for 12–36 hours. The airway will remain intubated and the patient ventilated until they have reached normothermia and have adequate gas exchange, with stable haemodynamics and minimal exogenous support (📖 see also Mechanical ventilation; Extubation criteria, p. 317).
- The circulation will require frequent reassessment and titration of fluids/inotropes/vasopressors. Blood gas analysis, pH, base deficit, and lactate all contribute to the assessment of circulatory status. It can be a time of dynamic instability. Ventricular dysfunction might be the result of aortic cross-clamping or an inflammatory process. Simultaneously there will be a progressive vasodilation (and hypotension) associated with rewarming and to a lesser extent ongoing systemic inflammatory response.
- Total body fluid overload is the norm, reflecting intraoperative fluid (CPB prime and cardioplegia). Nevertheless, capillary leakiness favours intravascular hypovolaemia, and there is typically an ongoing fluid requirement for the first 12–24 hours. Subsequently, capillary integrity is restored with reabsorption of fluid intravascularly. It is common to administer small doses of furosemide on subsequent postoperative days to address the fluid load. If excessive blood loss occurs the surgeon must be advised whilst resuscitation progresses and remediable causes are addressed.
- Temperature may rise passively or active measures may be instituted (forced air warming). Shivering increases oxygen demand. There are various treatment options (adequate sedation, pethidine 25 mg, clonidine 75 μg, tramadol 25–50 mg) that may be used in conjunction with exogenous warming. Hyperthermia is also undesirable as it increases metabolic rate and may worsen neurological outcomes.
- Most cardiac surgery follows a routine. There are usually minor complications that can be detected early and managed with simple interventions. Developing catastrophe includes ventricular failure, graft occlusion, stroke, cardiac tamponade, and major bleeding. Always consider – do I need help? Do not forget to advise the surgeon if you have concerns.

Inotropes and cardiovascular medications

(📖 see also Chapter 3.)

The commonest scenarios requiring pharmacological manipulation are:
• Arterial hypertension.
• Hypotension due to low systemic vascular resistance.
• Hypotension due to ventricular dysfunction.
• Tachycardia.
• Bradycardia.
• Pulmonary hypertension.

Pharmacologic agent selection can be difficult – there are many different types, with overlapping mechanisms of action. Four cardiovascular variables are important when considering manipulation:
• Heart rate.
• Inotropic state.
• Systemic vascular resistance.
• Pulmonary vascular resistance.

Vasopressors

These are agents that increase systemic vascular resistance (SVR) and are used in the setting of hypotension associated with vasodilation.

Norepinephrine (noradrenaline)

This is a potent α-adrenoreceptor agonist with moderate efficacy at β1-adrenoreceptors. It is largely devoid of ß2 effects. Infusions are typically 2–8 mg in 50 ml 5% dextrose, at doses of 0.01–0.3 µg/kg/min. It is an appropriate agent for hypotension due to low SVR. It has some β-agonism to prevent a significant reflex reduction in heart rate. Vasoconstriction can cause a reduction in cardiac output.

Phenylephrine

Synthetic non-catecholamine direct α-agonist. May be infused to increase SVR at rates of 0.5–10 µg/kg/min or as a bolus (50–100 µg). Baroreceptor reflex bradycardia may occur. It is frequently used as repeat boluses for vasodilation associated hypotension during CPB.

Metaraminol

Similar to phenylephrine, but with direct and indirect activity. Bolus at 0.5–1 mg.

Inotropes

Epinephrine (adrenaline)

Potent α-, β1-, and β2-adrenoreceptor agonist. At low dose β2 effects predominate with vasodilation of skeletal muscle beds. This is rarely therapeutic or desired. At about 4 µg/min β1 effects develop with a rise in HR and an increase in inotropic state. Cardiac output rises and systolic blood pressure rises. At higher doses α-agonism results in an increase in SVR and further increase in blood pressure. Drawbacks are: increase in myocardial work and oxygen demand; arrhythmias; lactic acidosis (muscle glycogenolysis); hyperglycaemia (hepatic glycogenolysis, lypolysis); and decreased renal blood flow (high dose). It is often used to support ventricular dysfunction in the first 12 hours post-bypass. Dose: 0.01–0.2 µg/kg/min.

Dopamine

Similar to adrenaline with relatively greater preponderance of α effects over $\beta2$ at higher doses. A significant mechanism of action is uptake into adrenergic nerve terminals and liberation of endogenous noradrenaline. Doses of 1–3 µg/kg/min produce a modest rise in cardiac output, a rise in renal blood flow, and increased salt and water excretion. 'Renal dose dopamine' confers no renal protection and is no longer used. Higher doses raise SVR. It is an acceptable agent in hypotension due to ventricular dysfunction. May cause arrhythmias.

Dobutamine

Synthetic $\beta1$-selective inodilator. It increases heart rate, inotropic state, and cardiac output (2.5–20 µg/kg/min). Acceptable for hypotension due to myocardial impairment. Tachycardia and high myocardial O_2 demand limit the upper dose. It has a lower efficacy (maximum effect) than other catecholamines.

Enoximone

Non-catecholamine phosphodiesterase inhibitor (PDE III selective). These increase cardiac output by decreasing the breakdown of myocardial cAMP. Simultaneous vasodilation and reduced SVR is prominent – used alone blood pressure often falls. The effects on individual SVR can be defined by administering during CPB when CO is 'fixed' and SVR can be titrated with noradrenaline. It is an excellent agent in LV dysfunction – often first choice in the context of very poor LV function. It is particularly useful in RV or biventricular failure with associated pulmonary hypertension. Other proposed advantages include a proposed lusitropic effect (improving diastolic function). It has an advantage over adrenaline in not causing peripheral acidosis or tachycardia. The main drawback is the usual requirement for concomitant noradrenaline infusion. Dose: 1–10 µg/kg/min. Milrinone is used similarly.

Vasodilators

Glyceryl trinitrate (GTN)

Produces predominant venodilation, and reductions in ventricular preload, myocardial work, and cardiac output. Higher doses produce a fall in SVR that limits the fall in CO, though it reduces blood pressure. Coronary vasodilation is minimal, selective dilation of internal mammary grafts seems unlikely, and pulmonary vasodilation is typical. Can be used for pulmonary hypertension, limited by falls in systemic BP. It is an easy choice for hypertension due to high SVR despite predominant venodilation. Often run as a background infusion of 1–3 mg/hr post-CABG. This is not so much for preserving coronary blood flow as for improving ventricular compliance, 'offloading' the heart, and assisting with vasodilation during rewarming or (with boluses) during sudden blood pressure surges. Tachyphylaxis can develop with prolonged infusion due to depletion of thiol donor stores.

Sodium nitroprusside (SNP)

Liberates nitric oxide via an interaction with oxyhaemoglobin. Dilates arterioles and venous capacitance vessels. Used for treatment of hypertension due to high SVR, and rarely to decrease LV work and increase CO in LV failure. Dosing is complicated by cyanide toxicity, and less commonly thiocyanate toxicity and methaemoglobinaemia. Dose rates should not exceed 10 µg/kg/min for more than 10 minutes, and ongoing infusions should be kept below 2 µg/kg/min. Protection from light is traditional.

Labetalol

Mixed α- and β-antagonist with a ratio of activity of 1:7. It produces dose-dependent reduction in SVR, with a fall in inotropic state and heart rate – the net effect is a reduction in BP. It is convenient for the treatment of hypertension. It is suitable for titrated bolus doses of 5 mg. A duration of action averaging 50 minutes is often quoted, although clinically it is often much shorter. It is usually well tolerated in small doses. Postoperatively it is an excellent agent when the nurses are worried about ongoing hypertension. If the heart rate is adequate give 5–20 mg in 5 mg aliquots approximately 5 to 10 minutes apart.

Agents for tachycardia

β-blockers

Esmolol 10 mg boluses or infusion at 25–200 µg/kg/min produce fall in heart rate and cardiac output with a conveniently short duration of action. Metoprolol 1 mg increments to a maximum 150 µg/kg produce similar effects. It should be used with significant caution in the first 12 hours post-CPB, due to possible sustained effects.

Other

Amiodarone and digoxin should be reserved for dysrhythmias. Intravenous calcium channel blockers should be administered with significant caution and cardiological advice obtained. A new ultra-short-acting form of intravenous calcium antagonist (clevidipine) will soon become available.

Agents for bradycardia

A functioning epicardial pacing system works well, although abnormal ventricular function can result from pacing-induced dysynchrony (normal conduction pathways are not followed). This is particularly manifest with pre-existing poor LV function. Atrial or sequential pacing should be considered in this situation (📖 see also Chapter 13).

Isoprenaline

A positive inotrope and potent chronotrope. Dose: 0.02–0.2 µg/kg/min. Can be given via peripheral intravenous line. The rise in CO is often offset by a β2-mediated peripheral vasodilation and a net fall in BP. This, coupled with a rise in myocardial oxygen demand, may exacerbate myocardial ischaemia. It is used for bradycardia with pulmonary hypertension, and when epicardial pacing facilities are not available.

Atropine

Muscarinic cholinergic antagonist. Dose: 0.6 mg (may be repeated). Small doses may cause paradoxical bradycardia. Anticholinergic side effects are rarely problematic.

Mechanical ventilation (📖 see also Chapter 9)

Most units aim to extubate patients within two to six hours. On arrival patients may be hypothermic, with partial neuromuscular blockade, and with residual opioid effect. Longer periods reflect perioperative complications or individual patient factors. Ventilatory support techniques vary between units based on differences in case mix and nature of surgery, anaesthetic technique, and local preferences. Patients may not have adequate respiratory drive, spontaneous ventilatory capacity, or cognitive function to breathe adequately. There is frequently smoking-related airway disease and obesity.

The first step is to establish alveolar ventilation with an oxygen-enriched gas mix to achieve adequate oxygenation of arterial blood. The following are approximate guidelines:

- Ensure adequate sedation and analgesia – to prevent the patient 'fighting' with the ventilator.
- A partial sitting-up position is advantageous for lung volumes.
- Volume control mode delivers a fixed tidal volume and rate and allows direct control of arterial CO_2. Synchronization of mandatory breaths and addition of pressure support (SIMV + PS) is used as it allows spontaneous respiratory effort to be partially coordinated with ventilatory support. Additional pressure support of 12–15 cm H_2O is typical. A maximum ventilatory pressure is set at 40–45 cm H_2O, which cycles the ventilator into expiration.
- Pressure control ventilation is an alternative, but alveolar ventilation alters with changes in pulmonary compliance. It provides protection against barotrauma, is used in children due to airway leaks, and is frequently used when gas exchange is poor or compliance is low.
- Tidal volume of 7–10 ml/kg. Respiratory frequency 10–14.
- PEEP of 5 cm decreases atelectasis and V:Q mismatch. Higher values may be used when oxygenation is compromised (📖 see also Abnormal gases, p. 318). However, there are adverse cardiovascular effects (decreased venous return, increased PA and RV pressures, RV distension) and increased risk of barotrauma. Surgeons frequently request increased PEEP in the presence of postoperative bleeding, but this is not supported by strong evidence and will only be effective if the increased pressure is transmitted to the mediastinal structures and is greater than the pressure in the relevant bleeding vessel.
- An initial FiO_2 of 0.5–0.7 can be weaned with blood gas guidance. The anaesthetist will often deliver the patient on 100% O_2 to provide an additional margin of safety during transfer.
- An I:E ratio of 1:1 or 1:2 usually allows adequate expiration and acceptable peak inspiratory pressures. Patients with a history of chronic airflow limitation may benefit from a longer expiratory time to minimize gas trapping (auto-PEEP).

Weaning

As the patient warms adequately, if no intervening problems develop, sedation can be decreased or discontinued. It is common practice to transition to a pressure support ventilation mode – typically an inspiratory support of 10–12 cm H_2O plus PEEP.

Extubation criteria

These vary between units and are often protocol driven:

- Adequate respiratory effort without significant apnoea.
- Adequate gas exchange with minimal ventilatory assistance and an oxygen requirement easily achievable by facemask O_2. As a guide, minimal assistance is a pressure support of ≤15 cm H_2O, PaO_2 ≥10.5 kPa at an FiO_2 of ≤0.4, and the $PaCO_2$ ≤6.5 kPa.
- Respiratory rate should be ≤20/min at rest.
- With PS 5–10 cm H_2O and PEEP 5 cm H_2O the patient should be generating tidal volumes ≥7 ml/kg, and be capable of generating a negative inspiratory pressure of ≥–20 cm H_2O.
- Stable haemodynamics with no or stable inotrope/vasopressor requirements.
- Minimal blood loss.
- Normal pH.

In addition, when sedation is discontinued the patient must:

- Be oriented and obey commands.
- Demonstrate adequate analgesia.
- Possess an adequate cough reflex.

Abnormal gases

High airway pressure

Multiple potential causes, some common, some serious. These include under-sedation, coughing, bronchospasm (asthma, COPD, allergy, transfusion reaction), endobronchial intubation, and pneumo/haemothorax.

Hypoxaemia (PO2 ≤10.5 kPa) (📖 see also Chapter 9)

- Pulmonary dysfunction is common after CPB and will not completely resolve for two or more weeks. Its aetiology is multifactorial and includes atelectasis, diaphragmatic dysfunction, pain, poor cough, systemic inflammatory response, infection, and LV dysfunction. It is more likely in smokers and the obese.
- In extubated patients, basal atelectasis and later infection are the likely aetiology.
- Pulmonary oedema, pneumo/haemothorax, and pleural effusion can all be responsible.
- FiO$_2$ should be increased whilst a diagnosis is sought and definitive treatment defined.
- Confirm airway patency and bilateral equal ventilation.
- Check position, patency, and appropriate functioning of underwater sealed drains.
- Suction endotracheal tube.
- Review ventilator settings in ventilated patients.
- Review X-rays and request urgent repeat films.
- In extubated patients increased humidified oxygen, mobilization, and physiotherapy should be requested.
- Facemask CPAP or BiPAP if the problem is severe.
- Before fine-tuning the ventilator it is necessary to ensure that the patient is appropriately analgesed and sedated.
- PEEP of 5 cm H$_2$O is usual and may be increased to 7 or occasionally 10 cm H$_2$O if atelectasis/collapse is the predominant problem.
- Slow inspiration (prolonged inspiratory time) may allow better gas distribution to low compliance lung units. As with increased PEEP and larger tidal volumes, the concomitant impairment to venous return must be borne in mind.
- Occasionally bronchospasm requires bronchodilators.
- Rarely, hypoxaemia is due to V:Q mismatch associated with pulmonary hypotension. Systemic hypotension and hypovolaemia will usually coexist, be severe, and be the primary presentation.
- Pulmonary embolus is rare and investigated using CT pulmonary angiography.

Hypercarbia (PaCO2 ≥6.5 kPa)

An elevated $PaCO_2$ reflects either increased production or impaired elimination of CO_2 (inadequate alveolar ventilation). The former is less common but causes include fever, shivering, agitation, and administration of sodium bicarbonate. Inadequate ventilation requires an increase in respiratory frequency or tidal volume, and a review of opioid or sedative administration.

Acidosis (pH ≤7.35)

A distinction should be made between metabolic, respiratory, and mixed acidosis. Respiratory acidosis (pCO_2 ≥6.5 kPa) should be treated as for hypercarbia. There are many causes of metabolic acidosis. Some common scenarios are:

- Inadequate tissue perfusion: Decreased pH, negative base excess, elevated lactate, and anion gap. These patients often respond to filling but may require inotropic agents.
- Renal failure: As above, but may have normal lactate. In addition, the urine output will tend to be low and serum creatinine, urea, and estimated creatinine clearance will be abnormal.
- Hyperchloraemia (> 110 mmol/l): High Cl^- relative to Na^+ will decrease the strong ion difference and increase the dissociation of H_2O into its ionic components, thus increasing plasma H^+ and decreasing pH. Vigorous hydration of the normovolaemic but vasodilated patient with chloride-rich fluids (saline, most colloids) will exacerbate this acidosis. If normal renal function is present, renal compensation will occur over time, and bicarbonate may be useful.
- Epinephrine (adrenaline) increases basal metabolic rate. It favours glycogenolysis in skeletal muscle and liver. Lipolysis and an elevated blood sugar are normal responses. Lactate frequently rises. It can be difficult to differentiate between an undertreated low output state in a patient on adrenaline and a low output state with metabolic side effects of the treatment agent.

The oliguric patient

(📖 see also Chapter 8.)

Definition

Urine flow rate less than 0.5 ml/kg/hr for more than two consecutive hours. This is the minimum flow rate of maximally concentrated urine that can clear the body of non-volatile acid and metabolic wastes.

Significance

Low urine output may be a marker of incipient circulatory dysfunction, or of impending or established renal dysfunction. Circulatory compromise may range from hypovolaemia to serious life-threatening pericardial tamponade. Perioperative renal failure (requiring replacement) has an associated mortality of 50%.

Causes

- Blocked urinary catheter.
- Inadequate renal perfusion (low BP, low CO, hypovolaemia, cardiac tamponade).
- Stress response (ADH, renin/angiotensin/aldosterone).
- Renal vascular occlusion (aortic dissection, embolism, IABP).
- Renal ischaemia (intra- or postop hypoperfusion – prolonged hypovolaemia or hypotension).
- Chronic renal dysfunction/failure.
- Nephrotoxicity (perioperative contrast, gentamicin, non-steroidals).

Management

- Review the preop history with particular emphasis on:
  - Urea, creatinine, and an estimate of creatinine clearance.
  - Blood pressure – poorly controlled hypertensive patients have a right-shifted curve for autoregulation of renal perfusion.
- Review intraoperative management seeking the following:
  - Fluid balance including cardioplegia. Note: Most patients have a significant positive fluid balance postoperatively but could still be intravascularly depleted.
  - Haemodynamics and urine output – prolonged hypotension.
  - Adequacy of haemostasis; risk factors for tamponade.
  - Haemofiltration during CBP.
  - Furosemide administration.
- Examine the patient:
  - Warm and vasodilated or cold and clammy.
  - Ensure the catheter is patent.
- Look at the monitors and identify:
  - Hypovolaemia (↓ BP, ↓ CVP, ↓ CO, systolic BP variability).
  - Low cardiac output (if monitored).
  - Hypotension/relative hypotension.
  - Myocardial ischaemia.

- Asses the laboratory data:
  - Haemoglobin.
  - Acid-base balance and serum lactate.
  - Urea, creatinine, and potassium.
- Now, institute a therapeutic plan:
  - Fill hypovolaemic patients with crystalloid, colloid, or blood as indicated by lab data. There is no single parameter that defines hypovolaemia or quantifies adequate resuscitation, but it is usually reasonable to fill to a CVP of 14–15 or aim to increase by 2.5, or a pulmonary artery occlusion pressure of 12 before declaring fluid-unresponsive oliguria. A CVP or PAOP that does not rise or rises only slowly with filling often implies hypovolaemia. Note that some patients require much higher filling pressures and some may be hypervolaemic at lower filling pressures. The key is to use small aliquots of fluid
  (250 ml in an adult), monitor the response, and adjust the plan to the specific patient at hand.
  - Treat hypotension. Use a combination of fluids, vasopressors, and inotropes to achieve normotension, an adequate CO, and an acceptable SVR. Target a blood pressure that considers the patient's preoperative BP, age-appropriate BP, and risks of hypertension/ bleeding.
  - Furosemide. May be useful to facilitate a negative fluid balance. Note: The target is adequate renal and systemic perfusion whilst protecting the heart against over-distension. It is not just nice numbers on the ITU chart for the morning round! However, high-dose furosemide has been used to convert oliguric renal impairment to polyuric renal impairment. The latter is easier to manage.
- Assess the response. An inadequate response may reflect a correct diagnosis but under-treatment, or an incorrect diagnosis. Review the need for:
  - Increased monitoring, particularly of CO (oesophageal Doppler, Pulse contour, pulmonary artery catheter, etc.).
  - Echocardiography to assess ventricular filling and function, and to exclude tamponade.
  - Sharing the problem – advise senior colleagues and the surgical team.
  - Renal replacement therapy ([] see also Chapter 8). This is not usually required in the early postop period. Indications include refractory volume overload, pH <7.1, K^+ persistently >6.5 mmol/l, Na^+> 160 mmol/l, Cr >300 mmol/l and rising.

The hypotensive patient

Hypotension develops when one of the following is defective:
- The pump: Impaired ventricular function of any cause.
- The volume: Reduced circulating blood volume.
- The space: An increased intravascular space.

The treatment of life-threatening hypotension should be commenced immediately before the definitive aetiology has been identified.

Diagnosis and definitive treatment

Ensure oxygen is being supplied, examine the patient's chest, and confirm ventilation is occurring. Review the arterial oxygen saturation and note the PO_2 and CO_2 on a blood gas. Review the type and duration of operation performed and pre-existing LV function.

Assess:
- Heart rate.
- Ventricular function (echo is best; arterial waveform and cardiac output measurements are surrogates). TOE allows global and regional biventricular function to be assessed, and will exclude tamponade. A cause of poor ventricular function should be identified. It is most commonly due to pre-existing poor function. The appropriate course of action is usually to increase or start an inotrope such as enoximone or adrenaline (📖 see also Inotropes and cardiovascular medications, p. 312). If tamponade (hypotension, tachycardia, low urine output, metabolic acidosis, elevated venous pressures) is suspected, urgent investigation (TOE) and treatment is required. Graft failure and valve dysfunction should be considered. In this case there are usually suggestive ECG changes. Many instances of profound but unexpected hypotension are iatrogenic, due to changes or disconnection of vasoactive infusions.
- Rhythm disturbance.
- Pacing capture.
- Circulating volume. Gather historical data – intra- and postoperative fluids, intra- and postop blood loss, and cardioplegia volume. CVP and PAOP may provide useful trends. It may be useful to administer 250 ml aliquots of colloid and assess the response as a combined diagnostic and therapeutic intervention. Systolic pressure variation during IPPV is a commonly used test, with wide variation implying hypovolaemia. Note that small variations are normal. TOE can help guide filling. Medical causes of bleeding should be excluded or treated as indicated.
- Vasodilation. A peripherally warm patient with a minimal core-periphery temperature gradient, bounding pulses, and brisk capillary refill is usually vasodilated. Acid-base status is usually normal. Venous pressures may be low due to pooling of blood in capacitance vessels. This is a common post-bypass phenomenon, reflecting the systemic inflammatory response, which may be exacerbated by vasodilating medications (GTN, propofol, SNP). Progressive vasodilation is the normal response to rewarming. Sepsis may be a factor, particularly in the context of emergency surgery for endocarditis. Rare causes such as allergy/anaphylaxis or transfusion reactions should not be overlooked.

Offending drugs should be decreased or withdrawn if possible, and noradrenaline commenced.

Emergency treatment

Follow an ABC approach:
- Summon help. The surgeon should be notified.
- Ensure the airway is patent.
- Provide 100% oxygen and confirm that the patient is breathing adequately or that bilateral equal ventilation is occurring. Exclude tension pneumothorax/massive haemothorax.
- Resuscitate. Give 500 ml of colloid or crystalloid. Ensure any inotrope/ vasopressor infusions are connected properly and infusing. Increase those infusions appropriately. Consider a small bolus of vasoactive agent: metaraminol 0.5–1 mg, phenylephrine 50–100 μg, adrenaline 5 μg. DC cardiovert significant tachyarrhythmias.

In severe hypotension if there is no response:
- Commence CPR.
- Prepare for emergent re-sternotomy.

Massive haemorrhage, graft failure, and pericardial tamponade are amenable to prompt surgical intervention.

Hypotension (severe)

Simultaneously treat, diagnose, and call for help:
- Confirm airway patency, adequate ventilation, and adequate oxygenation.
- Place patient supine or slightly head-down.
- Assess HR, rhythm, BP, CVP, CO, SPO$_2$, bleeding/drain losses, and Hb.
- CPR if no output, and activate process for emergency chest reopening.
- Give colloid in 250 ml increments and packed red cells for Hb ≤8 g/dl. Treat haemorrhage as above.
- Vasodilated patients: Give 0.5 mg increments of metaraminol or 50–100 μg increments of phenylephrine whilst norepinephrine infusion is established.
- Low output state: Commence epinephrine infusion. It may be necessary to bolus epinephrine. Start with 5 μg (take 1 ml of 1:10,000 adrenaline, dilute to 20 ml, and give 1 ml). If there is no response, repeat and increase the dose.
- Pulseless tachyarrhythmias: Cardiovert with synchronized DC shock.
- Bradycardia: Give 0.6 mg atropine and/or pace. Do not forget transcutaneous pacing is widely available on most defibrillators.
- Do not forget to: Get help, advise the surgical team, consider alerting for potential reopening, consider pericardial tamponade, do CPR if there is no cardiac output.

Bleeding (📖 see also Chapter 6 p. 102)

This is not something to keep to yourself! Advise the surgical team and senior ICU staff for all but the most trivial bleeding. As a general rule, there should be no more than 3 ml/kg/hr in the first hour, 2 ml/kg/hr for the next three hours, and less than 1 ml/kg/hr for hours 5–12.

- Resuscitate with crystalloid, colloid, and packed red cells as necessary. The target Hb should be around 8.0 g/dl. Remember, the Hb will fall with non-red cell resuscitation.
- Send full blood count and coagulation screen in addition to bedside coagulation estimates if available (ACT, TEG). CXR to assess mediastinal width.
- Reverse residual/rebound heparin with protamine 50 mg.
- Ensure adequate ongoing red cell availability, and request frozen plasma, platelets, and cryoprecipitate as indicated by laboratory findings. Generally, give 2 units FFP for INR ≥1.6 or APTT ≥48 s (with heparin reversed), one adult platelet pool for platelet count ≤100 × 10^9/l, and 5 units cryoprecipitate for fibrinogen ≤1 g/dl.
- Consider tranexamic acid 15–25 mg/kg.
- Remember that bleeding may be contained. Tamponade may coexist and exacerbate hypotension associated with bleeding.

Atrial fibrillation

(📖 see also Chapter 4.)

Incidence and significance

One of the commonest post-cardiac surgery complications: 20–40% of open heart procedures. Peak incidence is 24–72 hours postoperatively. It increases morbidity, mortality, postop length of stay, and cost. There are multiple implications:

- Loss of atrial transport.
- Decreased cardiac output and systemic perfusion.
- Ventricular oxygen demand increases with higher ventricular rates.
- Aortic diastolic pressure (coronary arterial pressure) falls and right atrial pressure (coronary venous pressure) rises, leading to decrease in coronary perfusion.
- Thromboembolism.

Causes and risk factors

Multifactorial: direct atrial damage due to cannulation and manipulation of atria and pulmonary veins; hypothermia; cardioplegia; electrolyte disturbances; or systemic inflammatory response.

Most important risk factors are:

- Preop AF or PAF.
- Age ≥60 years.
- Systemic arterial hypertension.
- Withdrawal of preop β-blockers.
- Valve surgery.

Also: old inferior MI, poor LV, LA hypertrophy, perioperative ischaemia, catecholamine infusions, IABP, blood loss, large volume cardioplegia, and sepsis/infection.

Prevention

There is no consistently effective regimen. The following all probably have some utility:

- High normal potassium (4.5–5 mmol/l).
- Magnesium supplementation.
- Pre- or intraop amiodarone loading.
- Perioperative β-blockade.
- Off-pump surgery.
- Atrial epicardial pacing and perhaps other pacing techniques.

Management

Aim of intervention: restore AV synchrony and control ventricular rate. It is usually not worth persistent attempts to maintain sinus rhythm in those with preop AF – rate control is the priority. Haemodynamic instability favours electrical cardioversion (see below). Stable patients are often best managed with a chemical/drug-based approach, but cardioversion should always be kept in mind. Most units have a standard or semi protocolized approach.

Electrical cardioversion

Correctable factors (see below) should be attended to before cardioversion as this will increase the likelihood of success. **Familiarize yourself with the defibrillator before you need it**. Patient must be adequately sedated/anaesthetized, and the airway appropriately secured. This can be tricky when haemodynamics are poor. Have the resuscitation trolley to hand. Use the sync button and ensure synchrony with the ECG R wave. Use between 50 and 200 J (bipolar) and administer no more than three shocks without reviewing the situation.

Chemical cardioversion and rate control

Stabilize haemodynamics: judicious fluids, inotropes, and vasopressors. Seek remediable causes: inadequate sedation, hypoxia, acidosis hypothermia or hyperthermia, or sepsis. Review the functioning of any attached pacing device and adjust or switch off as appropriate. Consider a change of inotrope, particularly for patients on dopamine/epinephrine/isoprenaline infusions.

Give:

- KCl 10–40 mmol in 100 ml saline over 30–60 minutes via a central line to achieve a serum concentration of 4.5–5 mmol/l.
- $MgSO_4$ 10–20 mmol over 30 minutes to achieve a serum concentration ≥1.0 mmol/l.
- Amiodarone load if LV function adequate. 5 mg/kg or 300 mg in 5% glucose over 1 hour. If rhythm restored, SR will be sustained in one third and recur in two thirds. Consider an ongoing infusion even if SR achieved – 900 mg in 5% glucose (often 500 ml) over 24 hours. Converts easily to PO therapy, which may be continued for 4–6 weeks.

OR:

- Digoxin 125–250 μg over 30 minutes. Can be repeated to a maximum of 1500 μg.
- β-blocker – particularly if taking preop. Caution in combination with amiodarone (especially if there are no ventricular pacing wires).
- Discuss with the patient's cardiologist before using calcium channel blockade, flecainide, procainamide, or other agents.
- Consider cardioversion.

Rate controlled but AF persists:

- Consider cardioversion if AF persists and less than 24–48 hours.
- Anticoagulation is usually warranted for AF that continues beyond 48 hours – discuss with surgical team, and consider any contraindications.
- Cardoversion planned after 24–48 hours can usually proceed if thrombus in cardiac chambers can be excluded by TOE (see also Chapter 34).

Sedation and analgesia

Sedation provides comfort and patient tolerance during mechanical ventilation. By controlling agitation and distress, the sympathetic response to the endotracheal tube and other stimuli can be attenuated. This intention must be balanced against:

- A desire for rapid/clean emergence when weaning from ventilation.
- A need to minimize exposure to respiratory and cardiovascular depression.

In addition it may be necessary to sedate some patients who develop delirium after tracheal extubation, often at night. Risk factors include: age over 80 years, comorbidity, cerebrovascular disease, infection, drug and alcohol withdrawal, and psychoactive medication. In this setting the following factors are relevant (in addition to seeking a remediable cause of the cognitive disturbance):

- Cardiovascular fragility.
- Respiratory depressant effects of most sedative drugs.
- Need to protect patient against self-harm.
- Safety of staff and other patients.
- Desire to restore a normal day/night sleep/wake cycle.

Immediate postoperative regimens

The ideal agent does not exist. It is important to note that sedation is in addition to analgesia, not an alternative.

- Propofol infusion: A 1% or 2% solution at a rate of 0–300 mg/hr. Advantages include a relatively short, context-sensitive half-life and excellent safety profile. Dose may be limited by reduction in vascular resistance and blood pressure.
- Midazolam: 0–5 mg/hr. Perhaps more haemodynamically stable, but limited by delayed emergence when infusion stops.
- Dexmedetomidine: This highly selective α2-agonist provides both analgesia and sedation with minimal respiratory depression. It may be given by a loading dose then ongoing infusion. Load 1 µg/kg over 10 minutes then infuse in 0.9% saline at a rate of 0.2–0.7 µg/kg/min titrated to effect. Initial hypertension is common and can be attenuated by slow infusion. Subsequent fall in HR and slight fall in BP is normal and may be dose limiting. Myocardial oxygen demand may be reduced. It is not available in the United Kingdom.
- Remifentanil: Gaining in popularity. Useful when rapid neurological assessment is required. Provides profound analgesia rather than pure sedation.
- Anaesthesia involving large doses of opioid (≥10 µg/kg fentanyl), clonidine, heavy benzodiazepine premedication, or other similar long-acting agents may have no or little requirement for additional sedation.

Postop delirium

There is no magic bullet. Be guided by common practice in your institution. Treat only those who will cause or come to harm. Useful agents include:

- Haloperidol 0.5–1 mg increments titrated to effect. Onset is often slow. Beware of α-blockade-induced hypotension and the dysrhythmic effect of QT prolongation.
- Diazepam 2.5 mg increments. Beware respiratory depression, especially in the elderly and in combination with other agents. Paradoxical agitation can occur but seems less frequent than with midazolam.
- Propofol infusion at up to 150 mg/hr is used in some units in non-intubated patients. Respiratory depressant effects and tendency to suppress laryngeal reflexes give the potential for aspiration, sputum retention, and atelectasis. It is essential to restrict its use to those units with significant experience of this manner of administration.
- Alcohol.
- Olanzapine and risperidone. Note these are contraindicated in coronary artery disease.

Do not forget the basics of reassurance, nursing in a safe environment, and gentle and frequent reorientation to time and place.

Pain control

CABG performed via median sternotomy with open vein harvest from the lower limbs produces moderate to severe pain in the immediate postoperative period. Other access incisions may be more or less painful. Analgesic requirements fall sharply after the first 24–36 hours and after the removal of mediastinal drains. By day 3–4 many patients identify limb incisions as a greater source of discomfort.

Significance

Apart from humanitarian considerations there are a variety of undesirable sequelae of poor quality analgesia:

- Sympathetic activation, hypertension, tachycardia, increased bleeding, and perioperative ischaemia.
- Poor inspiratory effort and delays in weaning from ventilation.
- Delayed mobilization and atelectasis/sputum retention/respiratory infection.

Analgesia

Familiarize yourself with your unit's protocol/usual management and experience.

Intravenous opioid-based techniques

Most commonly morphine or similar agents by nurse-titrated infusion and boluses, or patient-controlled systems. For the first 12–24 hours most patients are reasonably comfortable on a morphine infusion at a rate of 1–3 mg per hour with boluses of 1–2 mg for breakthrough pain. Other opioids such as fentanyl, diamorphine, sufentanil, and remifentanil can all be used satisfactorily.

Adjuncts

There is routine use in most centres of paracetamol at 1 g every 4–6 hours. Tramadol at a dose of 50–100 mg every 4–6 hours is effective in moderate pain. Non-steroidal anti-inflammatory drug administration is controversial owing to the potential for platelet dysfunction/bleeding, renal dysfunction, and haemorrhage. These agents are used commonly in some centres. The NMDA antagonist ketamine can be added to PCA morphine at a dose of 1–5 mg/hr. At such a low dose delirium and sympathetic stimulant properties are minimal. Gabapentin, amitriptyline, and other agents are unusual, but occasionally have a role. Clonidine 75–300 µg by slow infusion may be uniquely useful in the agitated hypertensive patient.

Intrathecal opioid

This is usually morphine or diamorphine. Morphine doses have ranged widely from 0.1 to 1 or even 2 mg. Greater doses provide improved analgesia at the expense of increased risk of side effects. The main concern is respiratory depression, which may be profound and late – up to 36 hours post-administration. Analgesia is often excellent, but if supplemental analgesia is required, particularly in the first 24 hours, then opioid by other routes should be used only with caution and in a monitored environment. The older patient with respiratory comorbidity is at increased risk. Diamorphine, by virtue of shorter duration of action (lipophilicity), may be preferable but is not available in all countries.

Epidural analgesia

Usually a dilute local anaesthetic, e.g. ropivacaine 0.1% or bupivacaine 0.125%, and an opioid, e.g. fentanyl at 1–4 µg/ml. There are theoretical advantages to such techniques: high quality pain control; early extubation; coronary vasodilation/reduction in perioperative ischaemia; decreased inflammatory/stress response; and decreased incidence of atrial fibrillation. These must be offset against the risk of epidural haematoma in the setting of perioperative exposure to anticoagulation. These techniques are therefore not widely practised. Hypotension should be managed by judicious fluid and vasopressors with reduction in the epidural infusion rate if necessary. Progressive motor block should prompt reduction in the infusion rate and repeated assessments of motor function to identify epidural compression early. Nursing staff should record motor and sensory levels in addition to vital signs and sedation score.

Anaesthesia for coronary artery disease

Dr J Mackay

Pathology *332*
Pathophysiology of ischaemic disease *333*
Assessment *334*
Clinical presentation *336*
Preoperative investigations *337*
Haemodynamic goals *338*
Anaesthetic plan *340*
Adverse haemodynamics *342*
Therapeutic options *343*
Trans-oesophageal essentials *344*
Practice points *345*
Further reading *346*

Pathology

(📖 see also Chapters 4 and 11.)

Atherosclerosis

Definition

Degenerative disease of large and medium-sized arteries characterized by lipid deposition and fibrosis. Pathology of ischaemic heart disease is covered in more detail in Chapter 4.

The degenerative process occurs almost exclusively in the intima of all three coronary artery territories. Endothelial cells are particularly prone to 'wear and tear' at points of branching or bifurcation.

Nitric oxide (NO) activates guanylate cyclase and increases cGMP causing smooth muscle relaxation and arterial vasodilation. NO has a key role in endothelial cell homeostasis and inhibits processes causing early atherosclerosis.

Atherosclerosis begins with endothelial dysfunction from impaired bioavailability of NO.

There are three stages of atheromatous lesion:
- Early atherosclerosis – fatty streaks.
- Plaque formation – lipid-laden macrophages and necrotic material.
- Plaque rupture – platelet adhesion and thrombosis, plaque extension, and lumen occlusion.

Pathophysiology of ischaemic disease

Myocardial ischaemia may progress to infarction but not all elements of ischaemia are necessarily detrimental to myocardial function.

Infarction

Causes include incomplete revascularization, inadequate myocardial protection, emboli, and vasospasm.

Stunning

Transient contractile dysfunction that persists after reperfusion despite the absence of irreversible damage.

Hibernation

Chronic wall motion abnormalities in patients with ischaemic heart disease without infarction. The diagnosis requires reduced coronary perfusion, regional contractile dysfunction, and viable myocardium.

Ischaemic preconditioning

Ischaemic preconditioning describes the phenomenon whereby brief periods of ischaemia may reduce the subsequent injury from a prolonged ischaemic insult. Ischaemic preconditioning has been identified in many organs. Various physiological and pharmacological triggers can cause or mimic preconditioning.

Assessment (📖 see also Chapter 15)

The following should be considered:
- Surgical and associated illness.
- Functional status.
- Patient expectations.

Objective scoring systems such as Parsonnet and EuroSCORE are routinely used to calculate the risk of mortality in coronary artery surgery. General, cardiac, and operative factors all contribute to the projected risk of mortality. ASA status is subjective and of limited value in these patients.

Crude overall operative mortality is 2.0–2.5% for isolated coronary artery surgery. See www.cts.net for recent data.

EuroSCORE risk factors for CABG surgery (📖 see also p. 211)

General risk factors
- Age.
- Female sex.
- Chronic pulmonary disease.
- Extracardiac arteriopathy.
- Neurological dysfunction.
- Previous cardiac surgery.
- Renal dysfunction.
- Critical preoperative state.

Cardiac risk factors
- LV dysfunction.
- Presence of LV aneurysm.
- Unstable angina.
- Recent myocardial infarct.
- Pulmonary hypertension.
- Emergency surgery – operation carried out before the start of the next working day – is recognized to be a risk factor.

Non-EuroSCORE risk factors for CABG surgery

EuroSCORE is well validated and deliberately excludes risk factors that may be subject to bias or manipulation (📖 see also Chapter 15). Additional risk factors include:
- Morbid obesity.
- Diabetes – without end-organ dysfunction.
- Hypertension – without end-organ dysfunction.
- Severity of coronary artery disease.
- Left main stem disease.
- Size of coronary arteries.
- Intravenous nitrates.
- 'In-house urgent patients.'

Patients requiring operation during current admission – so-called 'in-house urgent patients' – need careful preoperative anaesthetic assessment. These patients do not attend a preadmission clinic and have an increased risk of suboptimal work-up.

Patients with permanent pacemakers and AICDs *in situ* should be managed according to the guidelines in Chapter 34.

Clinical presentation

Symptoms
- Angina:
  - Discomfort, tightness, or pain.
  - Stable vs. unstable.
- Breathlessness – may be difficult to distinguish pulmonary vs. cardiac.
- Other:
  - Palpitations.
  - Peripheral oedema.
  - Syncope.
- Asymptomatic.
- Functional status:
  - NYHA – New York Heart Association.
  - CCSC – Canadian Cardiovascular Society Classification.

Diagnoses
- Acute coronary syndromes.
- Non-ST segment elevation MI (NSTEMI).
- Acute MI with ECG changes.
- Unstable angina.
- Intermediate coronary syndromes.
- Arrhythmias.

Preoperative investigations

Clinical examination

The value of a thorough preoperative clinical examination should not be overlooked in the era of patient-care pathways. Results of blood tests and other investigations listed below should be checked.

Cross-match

Availability of blood should be confirmed before induction of anaesthesia, particularly when redo sternotomy is being performed.

CXR

- Cardiac:
  - Cardiothoracic ratio ≤50%.
  - Calcification of LV wall or pericardium.
  - Permanent pacing system.
- Mediastinum:
  - Calcification aorta.
- Lung fields:
  - Upper lobe blood diversion.
  - Pleural effusion(s).
  - Pulmonary disease.
- Pacing systems.
- Sternal wires and retrosternal space on lateral CXR (redo surgery).

ECG

Specific features to look for in patients undergoing CABG:

- Acute infarction or myocardial ischaemia.
- Chamber hypertrophy.
- Conduction abnormalities – AV and intraventricular.
- Arrhythmias.

Echocardigraphy (☐ see also Chapter 17)

- Systolic and diastolic:
  - LV function.
  - RV function.
- Concomitant valvular heart disease.

Angiography

- Angiography should be repeated if >1 year old.
- Left heart catheter:
  - Size, distribution, location, and degree of luminal obstruction.
- Left ventriculography:
  - Estimate of ejection fraction.
- Right heart catheter – if indicated.

Haemodynamic goals

The aims of anaesthesia for coronary surgery include:
- Prevention of perioperative ischaemia.
- Tight haemodynamic control.
- Early extubation.
- Avoidance of non-cardiac complications.
- Maintain preload – adequate filling is particularly important in dilated or impaired ventricles.
- Heart rate – avoid tachycardia to maximize the diastolic proportion of the cycle.
- Sinus rhythm – atrial contribution is important in the presence of diastolic dysfunction.
- Maintain MAP – avoid MAP <60, particularly in presence of left main stem disease.

Anaesthetic plan

Total intravenous anaesthesia or inhalational anaesthesia with mechanical ventilation is standard for patients undergoing CABG in the UK. The pros and cons of regional anaesthesia are discussed later.

Any anaesthetic plan must take into account intended surgical strategy and recent history of antiplatelet or anticoagulant drugs:
- Conventional on-pump or off-pump surgery.
- Intended surgical incision and conduit sites.

Routine CABG surgery

Intended conduit harvest sites (e.g. radial artery) may restrict placement of cannulae.

Drugs for induction of anaesthesia
- Induction agents:
  - Etomidate 0.15–0.3 mg/kg.
  - Propofol 1.0–1.5 mg/kg.
  - Midazolam 0.05–0.1 mg/kg.
- Muscle relaxants:
  - Pancuronium 0.1–0.15 mg/kg.
  - Vecuronium 0.1–0.2 mg/kg.

Pancuronium is still popular, particularly for β-blocked patients, although shorter-acting agents are used where 'fast-track' surgery is intended.

Drugs for maintenance of anaesthesia
- Propofol at 3–4 mg/kg/hr.
- Volatile agent at 0.5–2.0 MAC.
- Opioids:
  - Fentanyl 5–10 μg/kg at induction, 10–15 μg/kg total dose.
  - Remifentanil 0.2–0.5 μg/kg/min.

On-pump

Pre-bypass management, conduct, and separation of CPB are discussed in Chapter 18. Most anaesthetists agree that insertion of a pulmonary artery catheter adds little to the management of the low-risk patient undergoing CABG.

Off-pump surgery – 📖 see also Chapter 24

Possible benefits
- Avoids complications of bypass: possible decreased perioperative MI; stroke; renal failure; transfusion; atrial fibrillation.
- Less invasive.
- Reduced costs.

Possible disadvantages
- Technically challenging.
- Inadequate revascularization.
- Long-term graft patency concerns.

General considerations for off-pump surgery

- Heparinization required:
  - Full dose.
  - Partial anticoagulation.
- Heat conservation:
  - Theatre temperature.
  - Fluid warmers.
  - Heated mattress.
- Haemodynamic instability.
- Fluid management – higher postoperative fluid requirements.

MIDCAB

Single vessel LAD disease – not suitable for PTCA.

Advantages

- Limited left anterior short thoracotomy.
- Minimally invasive.
- Short hospital stay.

Disadvantages

- Technically surgically challenging.
- Limited resuscitation access.
- Increased postoperative analgesia requirements.
- Significant conversion rate requiring midline sternotomy.

Specific anaesthetic considerations for MIDCAB

- Apply external defibrillation pads before induction.
- Surgeon may occasionally ask for one lung anaesthesia.
- Postoperative analgesia.
- Consider:
  - Thoracic paravertebral block.
  - Regular non-steroidal anti-inflammatories.

Redo surgery – 📖 see also Chapter 14

- Represent 4% UK cases.
- Higher mortality 5–10%:
  - Older patients.
  - Poorer LV function.
  - More advanced comorbidities.
  - More severe surgical disease.
  - Increased risk on reopening.
  - Patent LIMA to LAD anastamosis.
  - RV, aorta, or grafts adherent to sternum.

Specific anaesthetic considerations for redo surgery

- Risk of dysrhythmias – apply external defibrillation pads before induction.
- Risk of catastrophic haemorrhage:
  - Confirm blood availability before sternotomy.
  - Substantial IV access – large-bore IV access useful.
  - Leave groin free for possible surgical cannulation for CPB.
- Strategies to reduce bleeding and transfusion requirements:
  - Consider aprotinin (📖 see also Chapter 6 p. 97).

Adverse haemodynamics

Adverse haemodynamics leading to myocardial ischaemia may occur in both on-pump and off-pump surgery.

Common causes of adverse haemodynamics

- Hypovolaemia.
- Impaired myocardial contractility.
- Dysrhythmias.
- Acidosis.
- Hypothermia.
- Extremes of SVR or PVR.
- Air embolus.
- Surgical manipulation.

Therapeutic options

The insertion of an epidural catheter or a spinal needle prior to full anticoagulation is less taboo than previously. Although it is feasible to undertake awake cardiac surgery, most anaesthetists do not consider it is rational and are put off by the significant conversion rate to general anaesthesia.

Regional anaesthesia

Pros of regional anaesthesia

- Cardiac sympathetic blockade T1-5:
  - Dilation coronary arteries.
  - Possibly fewer postop arrhythmias.
- Attenuation of stress response:
  - BP and HR response to surgery blunted.
  - Attenuation of increased catecholamine levels.
- Analgesia:
  - Excellent postoperative analgesia.
  - Early extubation.
  - Improved postoperative pulmonary function.

Cons of regional anaesthesia

- Risk of epidural haematoma.
- Risk of hypotension.
- Incomplete attenuation of stress response.
- Risk of unilateral block or missed segments.

Unanswered questions

1. What is incidence of epidural-associated spinal haematoma?
2. What is minimum interval between epidural insertion and heparinization?
3. What should be the response to a bloody tap?
4. Does epidural analgesia alter outcome? If so, where does the risk-benefit lie?

Trans-oesophageal essentials

According to the ACC TOE guidelines, life-threatening haemodynamic instability and patients with increased risk of myocardial ischaemia are category 1 and 2 indications for TOE, respectively.

Assessment of LV preload and contractility and detection of new regional wall motion abnormalities may be particularly useful in patients undergoing CABG with poor LV ± LV aneurysm.

Additional indications

• Screening for concomitant undiagnosed valve pathology – particularly in absence of preoperative TTE.
• Diagnosis and detection of aortic atheroma.
• Diagnosis and intraoperative assessment of LV aneurysm ± thrombus.

Limitations

• Monitoring of ischaemia is not feasible during anaesthetic induction.
• Aortic cannulation site is not visible due to presence of trachea between distal ascending aorta and TOE probe.
• Apical aneurysms and thrombus may be missed due to difficulty imaging the true LV apex.
• During OPCAB surgery, transgastric views may be unobtainable when the heart is elevated.

Practice points

- All patients should receive preoperative EuroSCORE.
- Urgent patients may have received recent antiplatelet therapy.
- Intended conduit harvest sites may restrict placement of monitors and cannulae.
- Permanent pacemakers and automated implantable defibrillators may need reprogramming before induction of anaesthesia.
- Presence of oesophageal pathology is a contraindication to TOE.

Further reading

1. Hansson G. Inflammation, atherosclerosis, and coronary artery disease. *NEJM* 2005; 352: 1685–1695.
2. Hueb W, Soares P, Gersh B, et al. The medicine, angioplasty, or surgery study (MASS-II): A randomized, controlled clinical trial of three therapeutic strategies for multivessel coronary artery disease. *Journal of the American College of Cardiology* 2004; 43: 1743–1751.
3. Lenzen M, Boersma E, Bertrand M, et al. Management and outcome of patients with established coronary artery disease: The Euro Heart Survey on coronary revascularisation. *European Heart Journal* 2005; 26: 1169–1179.
4. Libby P, Theroux P. Pathophysiology of coronary artery disease. *Circulation* 2005; 111: 3481–3488.
5. Moses J, Leon M, Popma J, et al. Sirolimus-eluting stents versus standard stents in patients with stenosis in a native coronary artery. *NEJM* 2003; 349: 1315–1323.

Off-pump surgery

Dr E Ashley

Background *348*
Managing the procedure *350*
Outcome *354*
Further reading *356*

Background

History and evolution of off-pump coronary artery bypass surgery (OPCAB)

Coronary artery bypass surgery without cardiopulmonary bypass was first performed in St Petersburg in 1964, but was abandoned with the rapid development of cardiopulmonary bypass. In the 1980s the technique was revived in South America, Turkey, and India, the renewed impetus being largely due to economic considerations.

Off-pump surgery lends itself well to minimally invasive techniques such as MIDCAB (minimally invasive direct coronary artery bypass), which involves anastomosing the left internal mammary artery to the left anterior descending coronary artery through a small anterior thoracotomy. Multivessel grafting is more commonly performed through a conventional median sternotomy, with the use of sophisticated tissue stabilizers and retractors.

Rationale for avoiding CPB

The perceived advantages behind the impetus for revisiting off-pump surgery and the technological innovations to assist the technique were reducing or eliminating some of the major complications of CABG surgery. The absence of aortic cannulation ought to reduce neurological embolic complications. There were expectations that inflammatory mediators would be reduced, postoperative renal failure would decrease, the utilization of blood and blood products would be reduced, and postoperative recovery would be rapid, with associated cost benefits.

Patient selection

Contraindications to OPCAB
- The presence of intracavity thrombus.
- Malignant ventricular arrhythmias.
- Deep intra-myocardial vessels.
- Inability to maintain cardiac output during grafting.
- Combined procedures with valve replacement or aneurysmectomy.

Relative contraindications
- Atrial fibrillation.
- Significant mitral regurgitation.
- Diffuse CAD with small vessels and poor targets for grafting.

Patients who may specifically benefit
- High-risk patients with significant comorbidities.
- The elderly.
- Patients with heavily calcified ascending aortas, in whom avoidance of aortic cannulation and cross-clamping may confer advantages for neurological outcome.
- Patients with poor ventricular function.
- Patients with renal or liver dysfunction.
- Patients with respiratory disease.

Managing the procedure

Stabilizers and other devices

Off-pump CABG can be carried out using a variety of stabilizing devices and methods. The simplest is a **broad tape with swabs**, which is sutured to the posterior pericardium. Traction is applied to the tape to elevate and position the heart for grafting and the tape is then snared. This technique is associated with the most cardiovascular instability.

Pressure stabilizers are fork-shaped rigid metal retractors that stabilize the area being grafted by pressing down. They stabilize the heart less well than suction devices and cause more haemodynamic compromise as they squash and distort the ventricle.

Various **suction devices** have been developed to position the heart whilst minimizing haemodynamic changes. A two-pronged device with suction cups and a flexible arm (e.g. Medtronic Octopus) is used to stabilize the segment of myocardium where the distal anastomosis is being carried out. The retractor can be adjusted to optimize positioning and is screwed on to the sternal retractor. The suction can also be adjusted by the surgeon to minimize myocardial bruising. In addition there are cup-shaped devices that attach to the apex of the heart by a similar suction mechanism and elevate the heart away from the pericardium into a vertical position (also known as 'heel to the sky' position), to allow grafting of lateral and posterior vessels. These sometimes cause acute mitral regurgitation and haemodynamic instability (e.g. Medtronic Starfish and Urchin).

Intracoronary shunts are flexible, disposable intracoronary shunts, which consist of an atraumatic round-ended tube and are inserted into the distal arteriotomy. They have several advantages including diversion of blood away from the operative field and maintenance of distal myocardial perfusion. They are removed immediately prior to the final sutures and completion of the distal anastomosis. Their ability to cause endothelial damage is controversial.

Blower-Misters improve visibility in the operative field by blowing away blood with a fine jet of gas. They use humidified carbon dioxide, which minimizes the risk of air embolus due to its solubility.

Positioning the heart and grafting

Proximal anastomoses to the ascending aorta are carried out using a conventional side-biting clamp. This necessitates careful control of arterial blood pressure to prevent damage to the aorta and displacement of the side-biting clamp. This provides a source of particulate emboli in off-pump CABG, despite the avoidance of aortic cannulation and aortic cross-clamping. A systolic blood pressure below 100 mmHg is desirable during this phase. Some surgeons elect to perform all the proximal anastomoses first, with subsequent blood pressure and heart rate elevation to maintain cardiac output during the suturing of distal anastomoses.

Conventionally the distal LAD anastomosis is performed next, to achieve maximal revascularization and improvement in cardiac contractility, prior to displacement of the heart for posterior and inferior grafts. This aims to minimize the concomitant compromise in cardiac output. The intermediate or obtuse marginal grafts are performed next and finally the right coronary artery or posterior descending grafts are performed. These can be the most challenging, as the 'heel to the sky' position severely compromises cardiac output and ischaemia in the RCA territory leads to bradycardia and hypotension.

Anaesthesia for off-pump CABG

Excellent communication and cooperation between the surgeon, anaesthetist, and theatre team is essential.

Induction of anaesthesia

see also Chapter 23 on induction of anaesthesia for CABG. OPCAB lends itself well, through the absence of CPB and profound temperature changes, to early extubation ('fast-track' techniques). Therefore short-acting opioids and muscle relaxants are preferred.

Anticoagulation

Full anticoagulation is not required as blood will not come into contact with an extra-corporeal circuit. The activated coagulation time is kept to approximately 300 seconds, with a half-dose of heparin of approximately 10–20 IU/kg. This should be administered before division of the internal mammary artery, checked at 30 minute intervals during grafting, and topped up as required. The heparin may be reversed at the end of the procedure with an appropriate dose of protamine, although this is not universal practice. The reduced degree of anticoagulation and decreased platelet activation is beneficial from the point of view of bleeding complications and transfusion requirements, but may have thrombotic implications and implications for graft patency. For this reason aspirin and clopidogrel are commenced in the early postoperative period and low molecular heparin prophylaxis is advisable.

Maintenance of haemodynamic stability

Regional ischaemia, cardiac manipulation, displacement of the heart, and ventricular compression by tissue stabilizers cause rapid haemodynamic changes during grafting. This is most marked during lateral and posterior grafting, when the heart is lifted out of the pericardium and the apex stabilized vertically, requiring blood to flow upwards into the ventricles and causing A-V valve incompetence.

Management involves maintenance of a reasonable myocardial perfusion pressure with a MAP >65 mmHg, and low myocardial oxygen consumption. Trendelenberg position, increased filling pressures, and vasoconstrictors such as metaraminol, phenylephrine, or norepinephrine are used. Tachycardia increases myocardial oxygen consumption and makes surgical conditions difficult. However, a profound bradycardia is more worrying and can severely compromise cardiac output. Chronotropic drugs such as atropine or isoprenaline are useful, or temporary epicardial pacing is employed.

Arrhythmias will compromise the technique and therefore potassium should be maintained at >4.5 mmol/l. Magnesium supplementation may also decrease the risk of arrhythmias.

Maintenance of temperature

This is one of the major problems associated with OPCAB surgery without bypass and a heat exchanger. The patient can rapidly lose heat from both the chest and the legs during vein harvesting. It is important to commence active warming of the patient prior to induction of anaesthesia, encourage the swift closure of leg wounds to minimize heat and blood loss, and employ all passive and active warming devices available. These include: a silver hat; warming mattress; humidification of the anaesthetic circuit; a fluid warmer; and a sterile forced-air warming blanket for the legs and lower body when vein harvesting is completed. The theatre temperature must also be elevated, despite protests from cardiac surgeons!

Monitoring

Monitoring is as for conventional CABG surgery. Conventional five-lead ECG monitoring can be compromised by positioning of the heart, resulting in axis changes and changes in the shape and amplitude of the trace. ST segment analysis may also be difficult to interpret, making detection of ischaemia problematic. The use of epicardial ECG electrodes has been reported. CVP readings are unreliable when the heart is manipulated or the patient placed in the Trendelenberg position. Similarly, pulmonary artery pressures may be erroneous due to the vertical position of the heart and mitral regurgitation during grafting. Indeed, a pulmonary artery flotation catheter may actually induce arrhythmias during manipulation of the heart. Pulse contour cardiac output monitoring may be very useful.

TOE can also be difficult to interpret during grafting, due to displacement of the heart. High-quality images are hard to obtain in the presence of air in the pericardium and swabs behind the heart. TOE is useful when grafting is complete to detect new segmental regional wall motion abnormalities.

Cell salvage

The use of a cell saver allows the processing and retransfusion of suctioned blood and limits transfusion of donor blood.

Emergence and extubation

The use of moderate doses of opiates and short-acting anaesthetic agents can accelerate emergence and extubation, especially if temperature has been successfully maintained. Postoperative analgesia can be multimodal using opiates, intravenous paracetamol, and non-steroidal anti-inflammatory drugs if no contraindications exist. Some groups use thoracic epidural analgesia, which confers other benefits including dilation of epicardial arteries and decreased myocardial oxygen consumption.

Postoperative care

This is similar to care of conventional CABG patients. Patients may require active warming and increased filling compared to conventional CABG patients, as they have not received the extra fluid volume comprising the bypass prime. They may be oliguric and acidotic. The acidosis reflects hypoperfusion during grafting and usually resolves rapidly when normal blood pressure is maintained in the postoperative period. As the patients have not been fully anticoagulated during surgery, it is prudent to commence thromboprophylaxis with low molecular weight heparin on the first postoperative day, as well as aspirin and clopidogrel.

Outcome

Following early enthusiasm for off-pump CABG, results have not matched expectations and its popularity may be waning. Inflammatory markers (C3a, C5a, TNF-alpha, and interleukins 6 and 8) are reduced in OPCAB patients. However, this does not appear to translate into statistically significant improved clinical outcomes. A large meta-analysis evaluating 37 randomized-controlled trials and 3369 patients was published in 2004. It compared off-pump coronary artery surgery versus conventional surgery.

The meta-analysis described the following advantages:
- AF decreased in the OPCAB group by 42%.
- Blood transfusion decreased by 57%.
- Respiratory infections decreased by 59%.
- Inotrope usage decreased by 52%.
- Duration of ventilation decreased by 3.4 hours.
- ICU stay decreased by 0.3 days.
- Hospital stay decreased by one day.
- Consequent reduction in hospital costs in the OPCAB group.

The following complications were not reduced in the OPCAB patients:
- IABP usage.
- Acute MI, although there were decreased troponin levels in the OPCAB group.
- Renal dysfunction.
- Cerebrovascular accidents, although there were decreased S100 protein levels in the OPCAB group.
- Mediastinitis and wound infection.
- Re-exploration for bleeding.
- Re-intervention.

These results were similar across single-vessel and multivessel groups and in trials using ventricular assist devices. The lack of neurocognitive and cerebrovascular outcome benefits is particularly disappointing, since this formed a main impetus to the technique.

A recent large randomised trial of over 2000 patients (2009) showed worse graft patency and outcome at 1 year.

Neurocognitive dysfunction

Improvements in neurocognitive function have been demonstrated in the OPCAB group between two and six months postoperatively. However, this benefit is not sustained in the medium- to long-term. This may be due to the fact that gaseous emboli, which are more prevalent on bypass, are less harmful than particulate emboli arising from manipulation of diseased aortas, which may not be substantially reduced by OPCAB techniques.

Graft patency

Early outcomes, 30-day mortality, and short-term (one-year) graft patency rates were initially comparable in off-pump and on-pump groups, but recent information suggests potentially worse graft patency outcome.

Conclusions

It is difficult to define the advantages of off-pump techniques in younger patients with moderate cerebral and aortic atheromatous disease. OPCAB surgery may be beneficial in terms of morbidity and mortality in elderly high-risk patients with significant comorbidity and severely diseased aortas. It poses a significant haemodynamic challenge for the cardiac anaesthetist.

Further reading

1. Alston R. Pumphead – or not! Does avoiding cardiopulmonary bypass for coronary artery bypass surgery result in less brain damage? *BJA* 2005; 94: 699–702.
2. Kelleher A, Gothard J. Anaesthesia for off-pump coronary artery surgery. *BJA* 2004; 92: 324–325.
3. Cheng D and The Evidence-based Perioperative Clinical Outcomes Research Group. Does off-pump coronary artery bypass reduce mortality, morbidity, and resource utilization when compared with conventional coronary artery bypass? A meta-analysis of randomized trials. *Anesthesiology* 2005; 102: 188–203.
4. Nathoe H, van Dijk D, Jansen W, et al. A comparison of on-pump and off-pump coronary bypass surgery in low-risk patients. *NEJM* 2003; 348: 394–402.
5. Puskas J, Williams W, Duke P, et al. Off-pump coronary artery bypass grafting provides complete revascularization with reduced myocardial injury, transfusion requirements, and length of stay: A prospective randomized comparison of two hundred unselected patients undergoing off-pump versus conventional coronary artery bypass grafting. *Journal of Thoracic and Cardiovascular Surgery* 2003; 125: 797–808.
6. Widimsky P, Straka Z, Stros P, et al. One-year coronary bypass graft patency: A randomized comparison between off-pump and on-pump surgery angiographic results of PRAGUE-4 trial. *Circulation* 2004; 110: 3418–3423
7. Shroyer A, Grover F, Hattler B et al. On pump versus off pump coronary artery bypass surgery. *NEJM* 2009; 361:1827–1837.

Aortic valve surgery

Dr M Barnard and Dr B Martin

Aortic stenosis 358
Aortic regurgitation (AR) 362
Surgical essentials and therapeutic options 366
TOE essentials 370
Practice points 374
Further reading 375

Aortic stenosis

Pathology
- Congenital: subvalvar, supravalvar, valvar – bicuspid (most common).
- Acquired: degenerative calcification (most common), rheumatic.

Pathophysiology
- Wall stress = pressure × radius/2 × wall thickness.
- Increased pressure due to outflow obstruction increases wall stress, although this is alleviated by an increase in wall thickness (concentric hypertrophy). The hypertrophy causes diastolic dysfunction and elevated left ventricular end diastolic pressure.
- Coronary perfusion: Hypertrophy and increased wall tension increase myocardial oxygen requirements. Coronary perfusion pressure (aortic diastolic pressure – left ventricular end-diastolic pressure) is decreased due to elevated left ventricular end-diastolic pressure. Coronary vasculature does not increase proportionally with myocyte hypertrophy. *Patients with severe AS can develop coronary ischaemia even in the absence of coronary artery disease.*
- Fixed stroke volume: In moderate and severe stenosis, stroke volume is limited by obstruction. Blood pressure is therefore dependent on vascular tone, since cardiac output cannot be increased by contractile reserve (blood pressure = cardiac output × systemic vascular resistance).

Severity assessment
- Mean gradient (mmHg):
  - Mild 0–20.
  - Moderate 20–50.
  - Severe >50.
- When assessing the gradient, ask yourself – *which gradient am I considering?* (Figure 25.1). Peak left ventricle to peak aortic gradient can be measured at cardiac catheterization, but this is uncommon (can be dangerous in severe stenosis). Peak instantaneous gradient is estimated (not measured directly) from Doppler ultrasound, which quantifies the maximum instantaneous blood flow velocity across the stenotic valve. Catheter and ultrasound can both give mean gradients that calculate the average throughout cardiac ejection. Mean gradients are useful as they are less influenced by extremes of ventricular loading (pregnancy, anaemia, hypovolaemia).
- Gradients diminish with ventricular failure and low gradients do not exclude severe stenosis in the presence of significant LV impairment. Low gradient aortic stenosis can be assessed with dobutamine stress echocardiography. An increase in stroke volume (and calculated valve area) after dobutamine administration implies contractile reserve and is associated with improved outcome. Conversely, although high gradients can be dangerous, they provide the reassurance that ventricular function is preserved. One paper showed that in patients with valve area <0.8 cm^2 and ejection fraction <45%, those with mean gradients above 30 mmHg had 81% one-year survival compared with 63% in those with gradients below 30 mmHg.

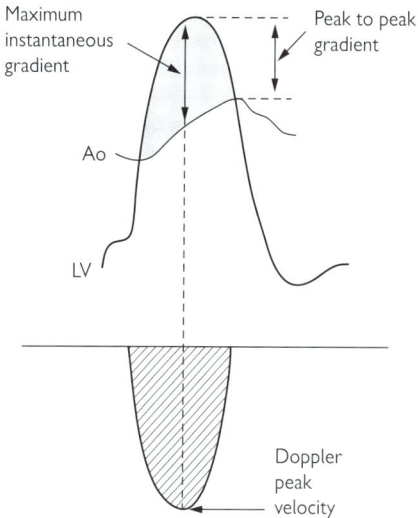

Figure 25.1 Aortic and left ventricle pressures and gradients.

- Valve area is useful as it is not influenced by loading conditions or ventricular function. It is usually derived from 2D and Doppler echo (📖 see also TOE Essentials, p. 370) measurements of left ventricle outflow tract diameter and velocity of blood flow at left ventricle outflow tract and aortic valve.
- Aortic valve area (cm^2):
  - Mild 1.5–2.0.
  - Moderate 0.8–1.5.
  - Severe <0.8.

Clinical presentation
- Angina – usually on exertion.
- Syncope – first symptom in 30%.
- Shortness of breath – indicating left ventricular failure.

Preoperative investigations
- ECG – LV hypertrophy, bundle branch block.
- Chest X-ray – heart size.
- Echocardiography – valve morphology, calcification (surgical difficulty, likelihood of postoperative heart block), ventricular function, aortic root morphology, aortic annular dimensions, other valvar lesions.
- Angiography – coronary anatomy in patients >40 years, ventricular function.

Haemodynamic goals

- Maintain systemic vascular resistance* – stroke volume fixed, therefore blood pressure dependent on vascular resistance.
- Avoid tachycardia* – to avoid cardiac ischaemia and maintain cardiac output (stroke volume limited).
- Sinus rhythm – important in hypertrophied, low compliant ventricles. Adds 30 to 40% to stroke volume.
- Avoid bradycardia – stroke volume is fixed and therefore cardiac output reduced at low heart rates. Can cause sudden cardiac arrest.
- Maintain preload – ventricle stiff, non-compliant. Therefore dependent on high filling pressure.

(* = key goal.)

Anaesthetic plan and adverse haemodynamics

- Blood pressure must be measured continuously from arrival in anaesthetic area. Place arterial line and large intravenous drip prior to induction. Central line not essential prior to induction but can be placed at same time. *Very slow* intravenous induction with agents least likely to cause vasodilation/myocardial depression. Etomidate or high-dose fentanyl are common. Propofol also used – but cautiously. Consider ketamine if absolutely critical. Maintenance with volatile agent (isoflurane) is fine. Aim for haemodynamic goals, adjusting intravenous and inhalational agents accordingly.
- During induction treat vasodilation with anticipation. As soon as the blood pressure starts to fall from baseline, even by a few mmHg, increase fluid transfusion and administer pure vasoconstrictor – phenylephrine bolus or start noradrenaline infusion. Easy administration of vasoconstrictor – dilute 1 mg of phenylephrine in 20 ml syringe and give 50 microgram boluses each time the blood pressure starts to dip. Duration of clinical action is usually a few minutes. Avoid bradycardia at all cost as may cause sudden cardiac arrest. Aim to keep heart rate between 50 and 90 bpm. Atropine or Epinephrine (adrenaline) boluses are useful. Give 1 ml of 1:100,000 epinephrine (equates to 10 microgram boluses).
- If haemodynamic collapse or cardiac arrest occurs, resuscitation will be difficult. External cardiac massage is usually ineffective in the presence of severe stenosis. The only effective course is to perform immediate sternotomy and internal cardiac massage and institute emergency cardiopulmonary bypass. *An experienced cardiac surgeon and perfusionist must be immediately available in the operating theatres to perform this.*
- Following valve replacement, prepare for weaning from bypass. Rhythm and ventricular function should be considered. The hypertrophied heart is susceptible to problems with myocardial preservation. A temporary period of 'stunning' or impaired ventricular function is possible. Assess the LV directly and with echo, and have an inotrope infusion ready to administer. Alternatively, those patients with good, preserved contractile function who have had their obstruction relieved may manifest significant systemic hypertension. This can be treated with beta-blockers, labetalol, or vasodilator infusions such as glyceryl trinitrate or sodium nitroprusside.

- 1% of patients will develop complete heart block requiring a permanent pacemaker. Transient heart block or sinus arrest also occurs and is probably due to oedema or trauma to the conducting system. It requires epicardial pacing. It is preferable to use atrial and ventricular epicardial leads with sequential A-V pacing due to the importance of atrial contribution. Check all the pacing leads and thresholds before closing the chest. Postoperatively, check the pacing thresholds and underlying rhythm at least once per day. If pacing requirements continue beyond 72 hours, refer to a cardiologist for assessment regarding permanent pacemaker.

Postoperative morbidity

General

- Bleeding/tamponade.
- Perioperative myocardial injury.
- Sternal wound infection.
- Prolonged ventilation.
- Cerebrovascular accident (higher than other types of cardiac surgery – 3% in isolated valve replacement).
- Organ dysfunction.

Specific

- Complete heart block.
- Prosthetic endocarditis.
- Thromboembolism.
- Paraprosthetic leak.

Aortic regurgitation (AR)

Pathology
Acute/chronic
- Acute – aortic dissection, endocarditis.
- Chronic – rheumatic (uncommon), degenerative, aortic dilation (connective tissue disease, infection), congenital (Marfan syndrome, cystic medial necrosis).
- Chronic aortic regurgitation can accompany calcific degenerative aortic stenosis when the leaflets are unable to completely close.

Pathophysiology
- Diastolic regurgitant flow.
- Increased systolic stroke volume.
- Increased systolic pressure.
- Widened pulse pressure.

The degree of regurgitation is dependent on the pressure gradient between aorta and ventricle (during diastole), the size of the regurgitant 'orifice', and the duration of regurgitation (length of diastole, and therefore heart rate). 'Eccentric' left ventricle hypertrophy implies increased ventricular volume. Wall stress is reduced by an increase in wall thickness. Stroke volume is increased (end-diastolic volume increases disproportionately to end-systolic volume). Aortic diastolic pressure is lowered due to the low pressure run-off during diastole.

Acute/chronic
Acute and chronic AR have different effects on ventricular volume and pressures. Contractility is more likely to be impaired in (severe) chronic regurgitation. This leads to an alteration in ventricular compliance, which means that end-diastolic pressure is not greatly elevated relative to the increase in chamber size. In acute regurgitation there is inadequate time for adaptation, compliance is not changed, and ventricular diastolic pressures are significantly elevated. *Acute massive AR is one of the most haemodynamically challenging lesions.* Forward flow is compromised due to the large regurgitant fraction with each stroke volume. Equally important, coronary perfusion pressure is compromised by the large increase in left ventricle end-diastolic pressure and reduction in aortic diastolic pressure. In severe cases coronary perfusion pressure (aortic diastolic pressure – left ventricular end-diastolic pressure) can approach zero.

Clinical presentation
- 5–10% prevalence, 0.5% to 3% moderate or severe.
- Affects more men than women.
- Presentation increases with age.
- Chronic – asymptomatic, dyspnoea, fatigue, palpitations. Angina usually late.
- Acute – hypotension, cardiac ischaemia, shock.

Investigations
- Echocardiography – valve morphology and pathology, ventricular function, aortic root dimensions, ventricular dimensions.

- Angiography – coronary anatomy in patients over 40 years, ventriculography.

Severity assessment
- New York Heart Association class III–IV symptoms are associated with increased postoperative mortality (8% vs. 1% in class I–II).

Echocardiographic assessment (📖 see also TOE Essentials, p. 370):
- Left ventricle dimensions:
  - End-diastolic diameter >80 mm.
  - End-systolic diameter >55 mm.
  - Uncorrected diameter criteria are biased against women. End-systolic diameter indexed to body surface area probably best predictor of severity (>25 mm/m^2 = severe).
- Left ventricle function:
  - Ejection fraction below 45–50% is a sign of LV dysfunction in moderate to severe AR.
  - Ejection fraction predicts postoperative outcome.
- Width of regurgitant jet origin compared to LV outflow tract jet width.
- Continuous-wave Doppler with pressure half-time measurement.
- Calculation of regurgitant orifice size and regurgitant fraction (using continuity equation).
- Diastolic flow reversal in descending aorta. The more distal in the aorta (nearer abdominal), the greater the likelihood of severe regurgitation.
- Criteria for assessing the requirement for intervention have evolved (Table 25.1).

Table 25.1 Criteria for assessing requirement for intervention

	Historical criteria	New criteria
Symptoms	Class III–IV	Class II
LV dilation	LVD >80 mm, LVS >55 mm	LVS/BSA >25 mm/m^2
LV function	EF <45–50%	EF <55%
Severe AR	–	ERO >30 mm^2
		VC >6 mm

LV: Left ventricle; LVD: left ventricular end-diastolic diameter; LVS: left ventricular end-systolic diameter; BSA: body surface area; EF: ejection fraction; AR: aortic regurgitation; ERO: effective regurgitant orifice area; VC: vena contracta.

Haemodynamic goals ('full, fast, forward')
- Maintain preload – adequate filling is important.
- Heart rate slightly elevated – to minimize diastolic proportion of cardiac cycle and regurgitation duration.
- Sinus rhythm – atrial contribution important, particularly when left ventricular diastolic pressure is elevated.
- Maintain contractility – which may be impaired in both acute and late chronic regurgitation.

- Vascular resistance decrease – reduces the regurgitant pressure gradient. Aortic diastolic pressure must not decrease unduly.

Anaesthetic plan

Place arterial line and large-bore intravenous cannula prior to induction. In most patients commence moderately rapid fluid infusion with induction. Slow intravenous induction is usual with agents such as etomidate or high-dose fentanyl (10–20 µg/kg). Propofol can be used, although it should be administered slowly. Monitor arterial blood pressure continuously – usually decreases can be tolerated due to the associated reduction in regurgitation (vasodilation). However, keep a close eye on diastolic blood pressure. If it falls too low, coronary perfusion will be compromised. Paradoxically, small doses of vasoconstrictors (phenylephrine 50 µg) can be given to restore vascular tone when diastolic pressure is too low. After bypass inotropic support may be required. This is influenced by the pre-existing ventricular function.

Adverse haemodynamics

As mentioned above, severe acute aortic regurgitation can be very difficult to manage. Dobutamine infusion possesses the correct haemodynamic goals but will not be effective in a catastrophic state. Intra-aortic balloon pumping is contraindicated as it worsens the regurgitation. In the most severely affected patients, the only effective treatment is to proceed to immediate valve replacement. High-dose inotropic support is employed until cardiopulmonary bypass is established.

Surgical essentials and therapeutic options

Aortic stenosis

Percutaneous balloon valvoplasty
Useful in children with congenital bicuspid valves. Rarely used in adults due to calcification and risk of severe regurgitation.

Surgical commissurotomy
Uncommon in adults due to nature of calcific degenerative leaflets.

Surgical valve replacement
Symptomatic patients and those with severe stenosis (assessed by gradient or valve area) should be offered surgery. Hospital mortality is 3–5%.

Mechanical:
- Requires anticoagulation; 2% risk of thrombosis per patient year.
- Durable, lasting >30 years.
- Higher gradient in smaller sizes.
- Common examples – bi-leaflet (St Jude Medical, CarboMedics, Sorin Bicarbon); tilting disc (Bjork-Shiley, Medtronic-Hall) (Figure 25.2).

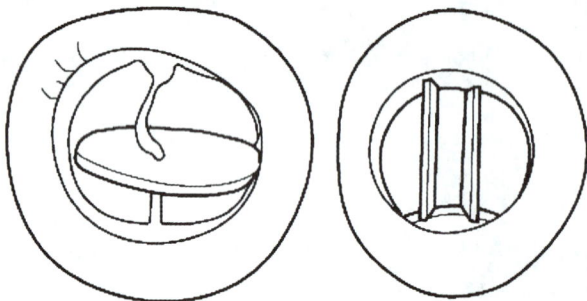

Figure 25.2 Bi-leaflet and tilting disc mechanical valves.

Bioprosthetic:
- Avoids anticoagulation.
- More prone to calcification, particularly in renal failure.
- Previously less durable, current generation better: over 90% free from failure at 12 years. They may last longer in older patients.
- Some are (surgically) more technically demanding.

Types:
- Xenograft (Heterograft): Stented on metal frame or stentless.
- Homograft: Human cadaveric aortic root. Less common as lower durability. Low risk of infection/endocarditis.

- Autograft ('Ross procedure'): Replacement of the aortic valve with patient's own native pulmonary valve. Pulmonary valve is replaced with pulmonary homograft. Excellent haemodynamics for aortic substitute. Good durability. Pulmonary homograft likely to need replacing within patient's lifetime. Risk of autograft dilation and failure, thereby transforming single valve problem into dual valve pathology.
- Aortic root replacement: Mechanical valve, tissue valve, or re-implantation of the native aortic valve, proximal aortic replacement, and coronary artery re-implantation – see also Chapter 27.

Aortic regurgitation

Surgery is indicated in the presence of symptoms or left ventricular dysfunction (ejection fraction <55%) and left ventricular dilation (end-systolic diameter >25 mm/m^2).
- Aortic valve replacement.
- Aortic valve repair.

Surgical technique

- Cardiopulmonary bypass – usually 28°C or 32°C.
- Aortic cross-clamping with cardioplegia (antegrade/retrograde).
- In aortic regurgitation either fibrillate heart and give cardioplegia directly into coronary ostia, or give retrograde cardioplegia via coronary sinus.

Transcutaneous aortic valve implantation – TAVI

- Surgical replacement remains the gold standard.
- Transcutaneous valve implantation has been developed to address the high morbidity and mortality in the elderly with comorbidities.
- Two models:
  - Balloon expandable prosthesis (Edwards Lifesciences – Cribier-Edwards valve, replaced with Edwards-Sapiens valve).
  - Self-expandable prosthesis (CoreValve Inc – CoreCalve).
- Both devices incorporate porcine bioprostheses in a stainless steel or nitinol tubular stent.

Valves can be inserted via:
- Transfemoral approach (artery or vein):
  - A special deflectable guiding catheter (RetroFlex catheter) is steerable and facilitates placement around the arch and through the valve.
  - The device is deployed during rapid ventricular pacing.
- Transapical approach (apex of left ventricle):
  - The prosthesis is introduced under direct vision into the left ventricle via a mini-thoracotomy without cardiopulmonary bypass, through a ventricular puncture and guided with fluoroscopy.
  - This removes the difficulties of vascular access with large sheaths and catheters through tortuous or diseased ilio-femoral and aortic vessels.

Initial reports report moderate success, although with high morbidity. This is expected as so far they have been restricted to high-risk patients deemed not suitable for surgery. Long-term data and randomized trials are awaited.

Anaesthesia for these procedures is challenging. The patients are old, unwell, with multiple serious comorbidities. The haemodynamic changes during implantation are profound. The procedures are carried out in interventional cardiology suites or 'hybrid' rooms, where access and space are limited, but facilities for emergent cardiopulmonary bypass must be available.

TOE essentials

The role of TOE in aortic valve surgery includes:
- Verifying diagnosis and modifying surgery.
- Assessing surgical results; detecting complications, valve dysfunction, and paraprosthetic leak.*
- De-airing.*
- Assessing left and right ventricular function.

(* = key role.)

Anatomic components of the aortic root
- Aortic annulus.
- Sinuses of Valsalva.
- Aortic cusps.
- Sinotubular junction.

Aortic annulus diameter is greater than sinotubular junction in young adults, equal in middle age, and less in the elderly. The base of a cusp is 1.5 times the free margin.

Echo assessment before cardiopulmonary bypass (Figures 25.3–25.5)

Aortic regurgitation
- Anatomy – root, valve leaflets (number, type).
- Jet – origin, direction.
- Grade – pressure half-time, colour flow jet, diastolic flow reversal in thoracic aorta, proximal isovolumic surface area (PISA), effective regurgitant orifice (ERO), and effective regurgitant volume (RVol).
- Mechanism – root, valve (prolapse, retraction, calcification, perforation, vegetation).

Aortic stenosis
- Gradient – transgastric long axis with continuous wave Doppler.
- Aortic valve area – by planimetry or continuity equation.
- Calcifications.
- Contractility – fractional shortening, fractional area change, regional abnormalities.

Regurgitation and stenosis
- Aortic root diameters – size of annulus, sinuses, sinotubular junction.

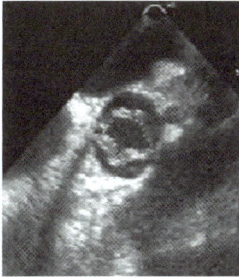

Figure 25.3 Planimetry of bicuspid aortic valve. The maximum systolic orifice area is traced out on a frozen image. This method can give reliable results with normal valves, and non-calcified bicuspid valves – but is difficult to perform accurately with a calcified degenerative valve.

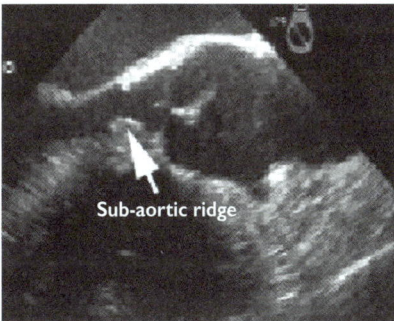

Sub-aortic ridge

Figure 25.4 Long axis view of sub-aortic stenosis, demonstrating discrete ridge just below aortic valve.

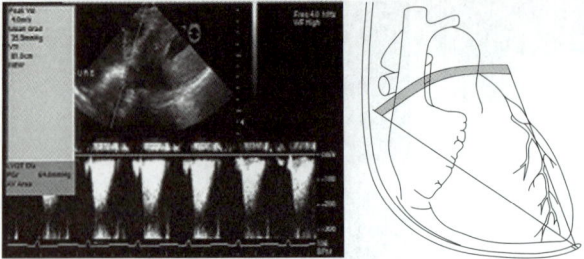

Figure 25.5 Transgastric long axis continuous wave Doppler examination of aortic valve. The illustration on the right demonstrates the path of the Doppler signal from the apex towards the axis of the left ventricular outflow tract. The peak velocity of the red blood cells is measured from the Doppler signal, and a gradient is derived from this using the modified Bernoulli equation. The gradient will be underestimated if the Doppler signal is not closely aligned with blood flow. Deviation more than 30° from the true direction of flow will lead to important errors.

Post-bypass

Repair/stentless valve

- Residual aortic incompetence – grade, jet origin and direction, mechanism.
- Gradient/valve area.
- Coaptation – length, plane.
- Root dimensions.

Mechanical

- Gradient
- Paravalvular leak.
- 'Built-in' regurgitation.

Practice points

- Patients with severe aortic stenosis can develop coronary ischaemia even in the absence of coronary artery disease.
- In aortic stenosis low gradients do not exclude severe stenosis if the LV is impaired.
- Valve area is generally more useful than pressure gradients.
- In aortic stenosis avoid tachycardia and maintain SVR as priorities.
- In aortic stenosis treat the blood pressure as soon as it starts to fall (or even before).
- Fluid administration and 50 µg boluses of phenylephrine are useful in maintaining blood pressure in aortic stenosis.
- A cardiac surgeon and perfusionist must be immediately available to institute emergency cardiopulmonary bypass.
- Aortic stenosis patients may require temporary pacing after valve replacement.
- Aortic regurgitation patients are more likely to have compromised ventricles.
- Acute aortic regurgitation can be life-threatening and difficult to improve. Immediate transfer to the operating theatre is occasionally the only available therapeutic manoeuvre.

Further reading

1. Bonow RO, Carabello BA, Chatterjee K, et al. ACC/AHA 2006 Guidelines for the management of patients with valvular heart disease: A report of the American College of Cardiology/ American Heart Association Task Force on Practice Guidelines (Writing Committee to Develop Guidelines for the Management of Patients With Valvular Heart Disease). *Circulation* 2006; 114: e84–e231.

2. Edmunds L. Evolution of prosthetic heart valves. *American Heart Journal* 2001; 141: 849–855.

3. Stein PD, Alpert JS, Bussey HI, et al. Antithrombotic therapy in patients with mechanical and biological prosthetic heart valves. *Chest* 2001; 119: 220S–227S.

4. Vahanian A, Baumgartner H, Bax J, et al. Guidelines on the management of valvular heart disease: The Task Force on the Management of Valvular Heart Disease of the European Society of Cardiology. *European Heart Journal* 2007; 28: 230–268.

5. Zajarias A, Cribier A. Outcomes and safety of percutaneous aortic valve replacement *JACC* 2009; 53:1829–1836.

Surgery of the thoracic aorta

Dr K Grebenik

Introduction *378*
Thoracic aneurysms *380*
Ascending aortic aneurysms and aortic arch surgery *382*
Descending thoracic aneurysms *386*
Aortic dissection *390*
Practice points *395*
Further reading *396*

Introduction

Thoracic aortic surgery deals with two main pathologies, aneurysm and dissection, which may be acute or chronic, and which may coexist. Anaesthetic management varies according to the urgency and type of procedure, rather than the pathology.

Thoracic aneurysms

- Ascending – proximal to the innominate artery.
- Arch – between the innominate and the origin of the left subclavian.
- Descending – from the left subclavian to the diaphragm.

Pathology

In true aneurysm there is dilation of the aortic wall of at least 50% greater than normal. False aneurysms contain no component of the arterial wall and occur after penetrating trauma or transection when haemorrhage is contained by overlying structures. Thoracic aortic aneurysms are more prone to rupture than abdominal aneurysms. 10–20% of patients will have associated abdominal aneurysms – usually the thoracic aneurysm should take surgical priority.

Aetiology is multifactorial but the majority are degenerative:

- Atheromatous – in association with hypertension and smoking.
- Infective – syphilis or mycotic infection.
- Connective tissue disorders, e.g. Marfan's or Ehlers Danlos syndromes.
- Inflammatory arteritis.
- Mechanical – post-aortic stenotic dilation, or following blunt aortic trauma.

Clinical presentation

- Sudden death due to free rupture.
- Asymptomatic – picked up as incidental finding.
- Pain – due to aneurysmal expansion or erosion of bony structures.
- Hoarseness (stretching of recurrent laryngeal nerve).
- Cough or dyspnoea due to atelectasis or pneumonitis from tracheo-bronchial compression.
- Haemoptysis – pulmonary parenchymal erosion.
- Dysphagia – oesophageal compression.
- Sudden onset of severe chest or back pain implies impending or contained rupture or dissection.

Preoperative investigations

High-quality imaging of the aneurysm is vital to define the vascular anatomy and allow the surgical approach to be planned. Comorbidities are common and may significantly affect outcome, or alter surgical management. The need for immediate surgery limits preoperative investigation in the emergent situation.

Investigations

- Routine blood tests – full blood count, urea and electrolytes, and clotting.
- Creatinine clearance in those with elevated creatinine.
- Chest X-ray (CXR).
- Lung function tests, including arterial gases, in those with obstructive airways disease.
- Carotid duplex scanning in those with a bruit, history of stroke, or transient ischaemic attack (TIA).
- ECG and coronary angiography where indicated.

- Echo to assess left ventricular and valve function.
- CT scanning with detailed 3D reconstruction will give adequate information, but image quality and resolution is better with MRI.
- Aortography provides accurate information about location and branch anatomy, but does not demonstrate the aortic wall and peri-aortic tissues, and is unhelpful in delineating complex aneurysms with intraluminal thrombosis. It may be combined with coronary angiography.

Ascending aortic aneurysms and aortic arch surgery

Indications for surgery
- Acute dissection.
- Aneurysm diameter >5 cm.
- Moderate to severe aortic regurgitation in association with aneurysm.

Arch replacement is needed when the aortic arch is affected by aneurysm or dissection.

Anaesthetic plan
- A standard anaesthetic technique is suitable but maintenance of haemodynamic stability is of paramount importance.
- Avoid surges in blood pressure that could precipitate rupture in the pre-bypass period and increase bleeding post-bypass.
- Prepare for possible large blood loss — several large-bore peripheral lines or a 12 FG sheath with rapid infusion blood warmer.
- Use of cell saver is recommended.
- Monitor coagulation carefully and correct clotting defects appropriately as guided by the thromboelastogram (TEG).
- Adequate rewarming on bypass to avoid afterdrop in temperature and postoperative hypothermia. Vasodilators may help to produce more thorough rewarming. Forced air rewarming is needed after bypass to maintain body temperature during chest closure.
- Postoperative myocardial dysfunction is a major risk when bypass and cross-clamp times are prolonged.

Deep hypothermic circulatory arrest (DHCA) (📖 see also Chapter 19)
- Involves whole body cooling on bypass and intentional arrest of the circulation.
- Used during ascending aorta and arch surgery to allow re-implantation of the head and neck vessels, or anastomosis of the ascending aorta to the arch.
- Safe duration uncertain; 30–45 minutes is usually tolerated at nasopharyngeal temperatures of 16–18°C. Longer periods may be necessary but the risk of delayed awakening or overt neurological damage increases.

Cerebral protection during DHCA
- Hypothermia is the mainstay of brain protection: aim to cool for at least 20 minutes before circulatory arrest. The best outcome will be obtained if cooling is uniform throughout the tissues and not concentrated in the core (nasopharyngeal temperature) area.
- pH-stat (temperature adjusted) blood gas regulation during cooling phase increases $PaCO_2$ and therefore vasodilates the cerebral circulation, leading to luxury brain perfusion and more even brain cooling. The approach to temperature adjustment (alpha-stat vs. pH-stat) varies between units.

- Haemodilution to a haematocrit of 20–25% reduces the inevitable increase in blood viscosity with cooling.
- Avoid hyperglycaemia, which is associated with adverse cerebral outcome. Start an insulin infusion and check blood glucose every 20–30 minutes.
- Pack head in ice to reduce brain rewarming during arrest.
- Antegrade or retrograde cerebral perfusion is used by some surgeons to extend the safe period of circulatory arrest. Antegrade perfusion implies forward flow through cannulation of head and neck vessels; retrograde perfusion involves reverse flow via venous cannulation through to the arterial system. Retrograde perfusion appears to be clinically safe, but animal studies have produced conflicting results. It is possible that the major effects are maintenance of brain cooling and flushing of air and debris from the cerebral circulation.
- Intermittent reperfusion may be useful when a long duration of circulatory arrest is anticipated.
- Pharmacologic protection – evidence for effectiveness of pharmacologic protection is extremely limited, but a variety of strategies are described and used clinically. The variety of agents used reflects the lack of first choice agent:
  - Steroids (methylprednisolone 1 g).
  - Barbiturates (sodium thiopental 10 mg/kg five minutes before circulatory arrest) were commonly used previously, but lack of evidence of efficacy means they are no longer employed.
  - Mannitol – may act as a free radical scavenger.
  - Nimodipine.
  - Glutamate receptor blockers.
  - Calcium channel blockers.
- Cold reperfusion for 5–10 minutes before slow rewarming.
- Avoid postoperative hyperthermia – rewarm to a nasopharyngeal temperature of 36°C.

Surgical essentials

- Operative mortality for elective ascending aortic aneurysm is 2–10%. Involvement of the arch increases difficulty and complexity and increases mortality (5–20%). Mortality is related to the experience and skill of the surgeon and team.
- Surgery of the aortic root and ascending aorta requires the use of CPB with moderate or profound hypothermia.
- If there is sufficient length of normal aorta, the aortic cannula may be placed in the proximal arch. Alternatively bypass is instituted by femoro-caval or femoro-femoral cannulation. Alternatively the subclavian or axillary artery can be used (usually via a prosthetic tube graft). The aortic cannula may be transferred to the ascending aorta at a later stage in the procedure.
- Surgical procedure consists of excision of the aneurysmal section of the aorta. This is replaced with a tube graft on to a relatively normal section of aorta. Occasionally an aortic homograft may be used. Aortic root replacement involves aortic valve replacement with re-implantation of the coronaries into the graft. Alternatively, the patient's own valve may be resuspended if it is functionally normal.

- For aneurysms extending into the aortic arch, a period of DHCA is required to allow the distal anastomosis to be made with the aorta wide open and bloodless. This permits assessment of the interior of the transverse arch and arch vessels and facilitates the accurate attachment of the graft to the underside of the arch.
- Aneurysms that extend into the descending aorta may be managed by a two-stage 'elephant trunk' procedure in which the ascending aorta and arch are initially replaced and a length of Dacron tube graft is left extending into the descending aorta ready for the second procedure.
- Bleeding problems are an important cause of morbidity and mortality – good surgical technique with reinforcement of fragile suture lines and use of tissue glue sealants helps to reduce haemorrhage.

TOE essentials

- Dilation of the aorta involving the aortic sinuses is a common cause of aortic regurgitation.
- It is important to distinguish between morphologically normal and abnormal aortic valves, since the former may be amenable to valve-sparing surgery.
- Following re-implantation of the coronaries, the flow pattern in the coronary ostia should be checked. New segmental wall motion abnormalities are suggestive of problems with the coronary anastomoses.

Descending thoracic aneurysms

Surgical mortality is 10–20% and is increased by comorbidities, particularly chronic respiratory disease. The risk-benefit balance for asymptomatic patients should be carefully considered.

Indications for surgery

- Progressive increase in aneurysmal size.
- Compromise of a major aortic branch.
- Haemorrhage.
- Pain from compression of surrounding structures.

Anaesthetic management

- Use of a double lumen endotracheal tube or a combined endotracheal tube and bronchus blocker will allow the left lung to be deflated to facilitate surgical access. Distortion of the left main stem bronchus may make positioning of the tube difficult. Recheck the tube position with fibre-optic bronchoscope after turning the patient lateral.
- Use lung protective ventilation – small tidal volumes (5–6 ml/kg) and low peak airway pressure during one lung ventilation.
- A nasogastric tube will keep the stomach empty.
- The right radial artery should be used for pressure monitoring, as occasionally the aortic cross-clamp may be applied proximal to the left subclavian artery. It may be helpful to monitor distal arterial pressure from the femoral artery.
- External defibrillator paddles should be applied as access to the heart with internal paddles may be difficult.
- Facilities for rapid transfusion are required. Use of antifibrinolytics and a cell saver is strongly recommended. Careful attention should be paid to factors likely to contribute to coagulopathy – hypothermia, acidosis, excessive dilution, and reversal of anticoagulation.
- If cardiopulmonary bypass is not being used, 5000–10,000 units of heparin should be given prior to aortic cross-clamping.
- During the clamping phase of thoracic aortic surgery there is likely to be severe proximal hypertension – arterial pressure rises by about 40%, whilst distal pressure beyond the clamp falls by about 80%. Vasodilators may be needed to reduce proximal pressure but should be used with caution as they may compromise flow to the tissues distal to the cross-clamp. Alternatively, increasing the volatile anaesthetic agent or using a short-acting beta-blocker will help to control hypertension.
- With proximal descending aortic cross-clamping, adequate spinal cord perfusion requires collateral circulation to the cord and sufficient spinal cord perfusion pressure. Theoretically, decreasing cerebrospinal fluid (CSF) pressure by inserting a spinal drain should improve spinal perfusion pressure (spinal artery pressure minus CSF pressure). The protective effect of this technique may be limited, however, as it increases arterial perfusion pressure by only 8–10 mmHg and results from comparative studies are conflicting. CSF drainage has been used successfully to increase spinal cord perfusion pressure when somatosensory-evoked potentials (SSEPs) have changed or motor

function has deteriorated in the lower limb of patients postoperatively. Similarly, epidural cooling using an infusion of normal saline at 4°C further reduces the risk of spinal cord ischaemic injury.

- Removal of the cross-clamp often causes profound hypotension from a combination of myocardial depression, hypovolaemia, and decreased vascular resistance. Washout of vasodilator metabolites and reactive hyperaemia will contribute.
- Maintain body temperature with forced air rewarming, but ensure that lower body warming is switched off during the period of aortic cross-clamping.
- At the end of the procedure the endobronchial tube should be replaced with a single-lumen endotracheal tube.
- Good preoperative planning and communication between surgeon and anaesthetist are vital.

Surgical techniques

- Descending thoracic aortic surgery is performed through a left lateral thoracotomy, which may be extended to allow access to the abdominal aorta. The patient is positioned with the hips rotated to allow access to the left groin for cannulation.
- The operation may be performed on:
  • Full bypass with cooling.
  • Partial left heart bypass.
  • No bypass, with or without a shunt.
- If the anastomosis can be completed within 20–30 minutes, then simple cross-clamping with normothermia is frequently employed. Many different surgical techniques have been described – suggesting that none is entirely successful – and each brings their own problems.
- Simple aortic cross-clamping is not suitable for patients with any degree of aortic incompetence as severe left ventricular distension will occur. Similarly, patients with impaired left ventricular function will tolerate cross-clamping poorly.
- Selective visceral and renal perfusion can be performed using partial left heart bypass with drainage from the left atrium, a centrifugal pump, and heparin-bonded tubing to perfuse the femoral artery or distal aorta.
- Distal retrograde perfusion decreases the ischaemic time to gut and kidney and may be protective to the spinal cord, but the value of shunt procedures in reducing the risk of paraplegia remains a personal decision.
- The surgical technique can be modified to limit the number of intercostal arteries that are sacrificed, and if necessary re-implant them into the replacement graft. Some centres sacrifice intercostal arteries gradually prior to institution of bypass (the clamp-and-sew technique), monitoring the effect on SSEPs. If there is a change in SSEPs when an artery is clamped it is preserved if at all possible. In addition, preoperative radiological imaging may ensure that appropriate anastomosis of critical intercostal vessels and the rapid re-establishment of the blood supply to the spinal cord is achieved.

Complications

- Death (5–10%).
- Neurologic deficit (3–10%).
- Renal failure (8–30%).
- Pulmonary complications (30–40%).
- Postoperative paraplegia – the risk of paraplegia is increased by the following:
  - Advanced age.
  - Preoperative renal impairment.
  - Emergency surgery.
  - Prolonged aortic cross-clamp time.
  - Thoraco-abdominal aneurysm.
  - Previous aortic surgery.

TOE essentials

- TOE is useful in monitoring cardiac function during repair, when the heart cannot be visualized directly.
- Any degree of aortic incompetence is likely to be poorly tolerated and may induce ventricular dilation.

Thoracic aortic stents

Some patients with descending aortic pathology may be suitable for endoluminal stenting – a considerably less invasive procedure than surgery. Indications for stent rather than surgery include multiple comorbidities or advanced age with prohibitive surgical mortality. Stenting can only be performed where there is a sufficient length of normal aorta above and below the pathology to allow the stent to be anchored.

Anaesthetic management for aortic stents

- Despite increasing experience and improved endovascular device technology, the technique is not free from serious and unexpected complications. Where there are technical challenges or where complicated vascular anatomy makes stent deployment difficult, it is prudent to set up anaesthesia as for invasive surgery, with endotracheal intubation and full monitoring. However, many cases have been performed using regional anaesthetic techniques, with or without sedation in hybrid theatres.
- Positioning and deployment of the stent may take a considerable time and it is necessary to stop ventilation for image acquisition and stent positioning.
- Rapid blood pressure control may be required.
- Postoperatively, patients should be nursed in an ICU/HDU facility (for at least a few hours) to allow rapid detection and treatment of any complications.

Complications of stenting
- Death (MI, rupture).
- Stroke.
- Paraplegia.
- Organ ischaemia.
- Endoleaks (failure to exclude the aneurysm from the circulation).
- Retroperitoneal bleeding.
- Bleeding from access sites.
- Retrograde aortic dissection.

Aortic dissection

Aortic dissection may occur within a chronic aneurysm or in a previously normal aorta.

Pathology

A tear in the intima of the aorta, which may be due to cystic medial necrosis or rupture of the vaso vasorum, allows a column of blood driven by aortic pressure to track beneath the intima, destroying the media of the vessel and stripping the intima from the adventitia for a variable distance. This may be blind-ending, producing a haematoma in the aortic wall, or may rupture back into the true lumen of the aorta, creating a false passage. Rupture into the pericardium will cause tamponade. Stretching of the aortic annulus can cause acute aortic regurgitation. Aortic dissection may present as an acute emergency or as a chronic problem.

Causes

- Hypertension.
- Connective tissue disorders, e.g. Marfan's syndrome, Ehlers-Danlos syndrome.
- Pregnancy.
- Aortopathy associated with bicuspid aortic valve.
- Iatrogenic (following aortic cannulation/cross-clamping, or introduction of intra-aortic balloon pump).

Pathophysiology

Severe acute aortic regurgitation into a normal-sized left ventricle will cause a precipitate rise in left atrial pressure and pulmonary venous congestion with pulmonary oedema.

Assessment

- Diagnosis must be confirmed prior to surgery with suitable imaging.
- Chest X-ray.
- Transthoracic echo may demonstrate dissection, but equivocal findings need to be confirmed by other means.
- CT scan – spiral CT with intravenous contrast is the most commonly used imaging technique to show the extent of dissection. It may also show pericardial fluid, intramural haematoma, or thrombosis of the false lumen.
- MRI scan – the most sensitive and specific imaging, but not always available. MRI produces images of the aorta in multiple planes and gives information on flow properties within the aorta. Current technology can distinguish blood from thrombus, differentiate between true and false lumens, show location and extent of dissection, and define origins of aortic branch vessels. MRI may also be used to evaluate ventricular function and identify aortic regurgitation.
- Aortography – now outmoded as a diagnostic method. Expensive, time-consuming, and requires transport to a catheter lab that may not be staffed out of hours. Standard brachial or femoral cannulation may not give access to the true lumen of the aorta and runs the risk of extension of the dissection or displacement of thrombotic material.

Angiography only gives information about vessels in which there is still intraluminal flow.
- Trans-oesophageal echo – safer if performed after induction of anaesthesia in suspected dissection. TOE is now the method of choice for diagnosis of acute aortic dissection and its complications.

The distinction must be made between type A dissection (any involvement of the ascending aorta regardless of the site of the intimal tear) and type B dissection (dissection limited to the descending aorta), since currently the majority of patients with type B dissection will be managed medically (Figure 26.1).

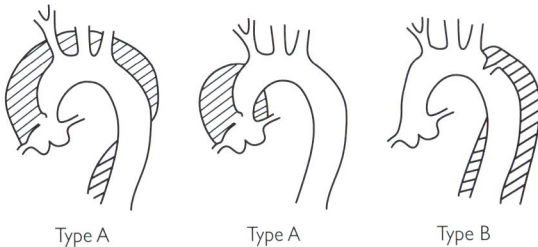

Type A   Type A   Type B

Figure 26.1 Classification of aortic dissection.

Type A dissection

A surgical emergency; mortality is said to be 1–2% per hour in the first 24–48 hours. Hence surgery should be expedited once the diagnosis has been confirmed. Surgical mortality is around 10–30%, except in the elderly (over 80s) in whom mortality and morbidity is much higher – heroic surgery is often not appropriate in this group. The presence of preoperative haemodynamic instability, renal failure, stroke, paraplegia, or limb or visceral ischaemia will greatly increase surgical risk. Five-year survival is around 50–80%. There is a high incidence of co-existing disease – hypertension, IHD, diabetes, COPD, and renal impairment.

Clinical presentation
- Sudden onset tearing central chest or back pain, which can be confused with myocardial infarction. Occasionally painless.
- 30% of patients will die almost immediately from free rupture, stroke, myocardial infarction, or tamponade.
- Creation of a false lumen can cause obliteration of flow in branches of the aorta, presenting with a cold pulseless limb, stroke, impaired consciousness, paraplegia, or symptoms of renal or mesenteric ischaemia.
- Retrograde extension of the dissection may cause myocardial ischaemia with ECG changes (that may complicate the diagnosis), or acute aortic regurgitation with pulmonary oedema.
- Rupture into the pericardium can produce tamponade.

Preoperative investigations
- Creatinine and troponin may be elevated if diagnosis has been delayed.
- The ECG should be inspected for signs of ischaemia.
- Coronary angiography prior to acute dissection surgery is hazardous and delays definitive surgery so is rarely indicated. 64-slice CT may be an alternative for those with a history of ischaemic heart disease or signs of acute ischaemia.
- Trans-oesophageal echo should be performed after induction of anaesthesia to confirm the diagnosis and to assess the extent of dissection, aortic and mitral valve morphology, and left ventricular function.

Haemodynamic goals
Initially the aims of haemodynamic management are to reduce the shear forces on the aorta by lowering blood pressure, whilst maintaining vital organ perfusion. Beta-blockers can be administered with vasodilators to decrease arterial pressure and dP/dT. Examples include:
- Esmolol bolus 5–50 mg IV, followed by infusion 25–300 µg/kg/min.
- Sodium nitroprusside infusion 0.5–2.0 µg/kg/min.
- Labetalol bolus 10–80 mg, followed by infusion 0.5–2.0 mg/min.

Transfer from other hospitals
Some patients will require transfer from units without cardiac surgical facilities. Invasive arterial and CVP monitoring should be set up prior to transport, and antihypertensive treatment commenced. Results of investigations and cross-matched blood should be transferred with the patient.

Anaesthetic management
- Arterial cannulation should preferably be in the left radial artery because of the possibility of cross-clamping the innominate artery during surgical repair.
- Avoidance of hypertension during induction is crucial to reduce the risk of free rupture.
- Modified rapid sequence induction is recommended where necessary.
- Induction of anaesthesia in the presence of tamponade may be accompanied by haemodynamic collapse, and therefore should be performed in the operating theatre with a surgeon standing by.
- Relief of tamponade may cause a significant blood pressure surge.
- Femoral cannulation may be performed prior to sternotomy to reduce the risk of rupture on opening the chest.
- Postoperative myocardial dysfunction is a risk and may be exacerbated by preoperative myocardial ischaemia or acute ventricular dilation secondary to acute aortic regurgitation, as well as long CPB and cross-clamp times.
- Haemorrhage is a common complication, and necessitates adequate venous access. Two wide-bore peripheral lines or a 12 FG sheath in the jugular vein will allow rapid transfusion. Rapid transfusion fluid warmers and a cell saver should be used.
- The use of antifibrinolytics is recommended. Six units of blood should be cross-matched initially.
- Use of thromboelastography allows rational use of clotting products.

Surgery

- Arterial cannulation can be established in the femoral artery, taking care to ensure that the true lumen is cannulated. A single venous cannula is placed in the right atrium. Cooling to 28–30°C is used to protect against ischaemic injury.
- Surgical management for acute dissection aims to replace the dissected aorta with an interposition tube graft and to re-establish flow into the true lumen of the aorta, thus reperfusing key organs. Where there is dissection within a chronic aneurysm, the entire aneurysmal segment should be resected, and the tube graft joined to relatively normal aorta. Resuspension of an otherwise normal aortic valve may be possible when there is dilation of the sinotubular junction. If the aortic valve is abnormal or the coronary arteries are involved, a root replacement with re-implantation of the coronaries may be required.
- Deep hypothermic circulatory arrest (DHCA) is frequently needed to allow the distal anastomosis to be done open and the arch to be inspected. Complete or hemi-arch replacement may sometimes be required.
- Haemostasis is frequently difficult; meticulous expedite surgical technique is required. Tissue glue may be used to reduce oozing from suture lines.

TOE findings (Figures 26.2 and 26.3)

- Imaging of the distal ascending aorta and proximal arch is limited by shadowing from the trachea and left main bronchus.
- There is separation of the normal single discrete echo signal from the aortic wall into two discrete echoes, the flap of the intima being seen to move in unison with the aortic wall.
- Entry and exit points of the false lumen may be detected by colour flow Doppler. Flow in the false lumen may be sluggish and may show spontaneous echo contrast.
- The true lumen tends to be smaller than the false lumen.
- If there is clot within the false lumen, a clear dissection flap may not be visualized, but the aortic wall appears thickened.
- Related pathology to assess includes:
  - Presence and severity of aortic regurgitation.
  - Presence of pericardial effusion/tamponade.
  - Coronary involvement.
  - Ventricular function.
- Following repair, TOE is used to assess any residual aortic incompetence or regional wall motion abnormalities and to check flow within the coronary ostia.

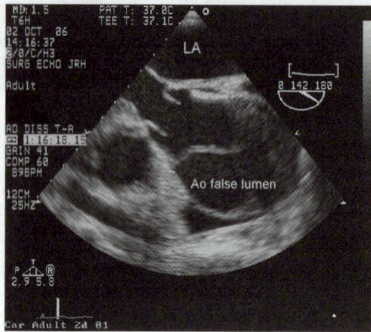

Figure 26.2 Long axis view showing dissection flap in ascending aorta.

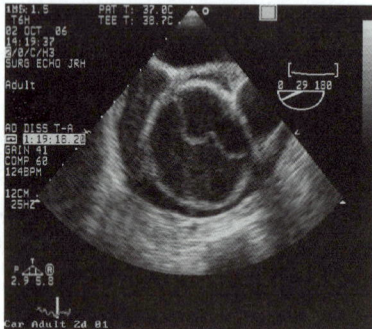

Figure 26.3 Short axis view to show dissection flap.

Complications of surgery
- Haemorrhage.
- Low cardiac output.
- Stroke.
- Renal failure.
- Visceral ischaemia.
- Sepsis.
- Respiratory failure.

Type B dissection

This is initially treated medically with beta-blockers and antihypertensive medication. Surgical repair may be indicated if there is continued expansion of the dissection – the principles of management are those relating to descending thoracic aortic aneurysm.

Practice points

- Anaesthetic management for aortic surgery is challenging; optimal outcome requires good cooperation and teamwork.
- High-quality imaging is important when planning surgery.
- Make sure you understand the operative plan.
- Patients frequently have multiple comorbidities.
- Patients may present for emergency surgery in hypovolaemic shock and may be haemodynamically unstable.
- Massive blood loss may occur.

Further reading

1. Patel H, Deeb M. Ascending and arch aorta: Pathology, natural history, and treatment. *Circulation* 2008; 118: 188–195.
2. Swee W, Dake M. Endovascular management of thoracic dissections. *Circulation* 2008; 117: 1460–1473.
3. Kohl BA, McGarvey ML. Anesthesia and neurocerebral monitoring for aortic dissection. *Seminars in Thoracic and Cardiovascular Surgery* 2005; 17: 236.
4. Neri E, Toscano T, Massetti M, et al. Operation for acute type A aortic dissection in octogenarians: Is it justified? *Journal of Thoracic and Cardiovascular Surgery* 2001; 121: 259–267.
5. Hagan PG, Nienaber CA, Isselbacher EM, et al. The International Registry of Acute Aortic Dissection (IRAD). New insights into an old disease. *JAMA* 2000; 283: 897–903.
6. Cohn L. *Cardiac Surgery in the Adult.* Third edition. New York, McGraw-Hill Professional 2007, pp. 1193–1394.

Mitral valve surgery

Dr B Martin and Dr M Barnard

Introduction *398*
Mitral regurgitation *400*
Mitral stenosis (MS) *404*
Mixed mitral valve disease *408*
Practice points *409*
Further reading *410*

Introduction

'**The mitral valve is the left ventricle and the left ventricle is the mitral valve.**'

(Steve Bolling, personal communication)

Consequently, repair rather than replacement is preferred wherever possible to minimize disrupting this relationship and compromising left ventricular function. Operative mortality and long-term outcome is much improved if this is achieved – it is the standard of care.

Mitral regurgitation

The commonest type of mitral valve surgery in the developed world is for mitral regurgitation. The mitral valve apparatus is a complex saddle-shaped structure made up of the two leaflets, chordae, papillary muscles, and the left ventricle. Failure of any single component is likely to lead to regurgitation.

Pathology

Primary valve failure:
- Prolapse of leaflets above the annulus (most common).
- Myxomatous degeneration; a floppy valve with excess tissue.
- Endocarditis with leaflet perforation.
- Rheumatic regurgitation, combined with MS.

Secondary failure:
- Ischaemia with shortening of papillary muscles and LV dilation of the annulus (30% of patients for CABG).
- Dilated cardiomyopathy.

Pathophysiology

Acute
- Disruption of chordae from an MI or ischaemia.
- Perforation of leaflet from endocarditis.
- Both lead to sudden increase in LA and PA pressures causing acute pulmonary oedema, often with fatal outcome.

Chronic
- LA dilation.
- Gradual dilation and hypertrophy of the LV from volume overload.
- Increasing PA pressures with RV hypertrophy and eventual failure.

Once the regurgitant fraction reaches >60%, congestive heart failure occurs with a spiralling deterioration in LV function as progressively less blood moves 'forward'. The regurgitant orifice acts as a 'low pressure, blow-off valve' into the pulmonary circulation. This encourages the blood to flow backwards, rather than forwards against the higher systemic pressure.

Severity assessment

There are several methods of grading the severity of MR using 2D and Doppler echocardiography:
- Colour Doppler of regurgitant area and 2D changes (most common and easiest).
- Measurement of proximal width of regurgitant jet, the 'vena contracta'. More than 6 mm indicates severe MR.
- Pulmonary venous Dopplers looking for systolic flow reversal.
- Regurgitant volume calculations as percentage of stroke volume.
- Proximal isovelocity surface area to calculate the regurgitant orifice area.

Clinical presentation

Acute
- Sudden pulmonary oedema, typically pink frothy sputum in a pale, sweaty, distressed patient.

Chronic
- Fatigue.
- Congestive cardiac failure.

Clinical findings
MR is found in 30% of patients at the time of CABG. There is a strong association with ischaemic heart disease.
- Pansystolic murmur.
- Signs of chronic congestive heart failure.
- Most chronic MR patients develop AF.

Preoperative investigations

- FBC and INR (warfarin for AF).
- U/E and LFTs: right heart failure with hepatic and renal congestion.
- CXR: increased heart size and Kerley B lines.
- ECG: AF, ischaemia, LVH, RVH.
- TOE: 2D and Doppler echo essential part of the diagnoses, as above.
    - Beware the LV that is said to have a good EF. Even a poor, dilated LV will look 'great' if most of the EF is going backwards into the low pressure pulmonary circulation! It is a very different story when this route is removed with a good repair and the LV has to eject entirely against systemic pressure.
- Angiography: a high incidence of significant CAD.

Haemodynamic goals

The main plan is to encourage forward flow of blood and avoid the factors that make backward flow more likely during systole – 'Keep full and off-loaded':
- **Maintain preload** to make sure there is adequate LV filling. Augment with caution if the left heart is very dilated; this could increase annular dilation and therefore regurgitation. Most patients are in AF.
- **Maintain heart rate and avoid bradycardia**. The slower the heart rate, the longer diastole and the time for LV filling. This may cause more dilation, which can increase regurgitation.
- **SVR reduction**: 'off-loading' is beneficial, encouraging forward blood flow. Fortunately general anaesthesia achieves this. The opposite is true of alpha-agonists, which should therefore be used with caution. If BP is a problem, increasing the heart rate and preload are usually better options to try first.
- **Inotropy** increases contraction and can reduce regurgitation by reducing annular dilation, thus increasing forward flow. The type III phosphodiesterase inhibitors, e.g. enoximone and milrinone, can achieve this and have the advantage of 'off-loading' both ventricles by reducing the SVR and pulmonary resistance (inodilators).

- **Pulmonary vascular resistance** should not be exacerbated in patients with pulmonary hypertension. Hypercapnoea and hypoxia must be avoided, as well as drugs that may cause pulmonary vasoconstriction.

Anaesthetic plan and adverse haemodynamics

A large-bore intravenous cannula and smaller radial arterial line are placed peripherally before induction. The patient is pre-oxygenated and slow intravenous induction is achieved with high-dose fentanyl and propofol/etomidate. A long-acting muscle relaxant is used such as pancuronium; intubation and the siting of a central line follow. Maintenance is usually with a volatile agent such as isoflurane in oxygen and air.

If the patient is relatively bradycardic before induction, an anticholinergic such as atropine or glycopyrronium bromide can be used, as the fentanyl can slow the heart further. If bradycardia becomes a problem, 1 ml of 1 in 100,000 epinephrine into a fast running IV will improve chronotropy and inotropy.

Following CPB and valve repair or replacement, we commonly use an inodilator such as enoximone, a type III phosphodiesterase inhibitor, to come off bypass. This is usually required as the LV may take some time to adjust to ejecting against an unfamiliar systemic pressure. LV failure may be immediately apparent, as soon as separation from CPB is attempted, or more likely some hours later. The ventricle will tire, CO reduces, and the patient becomes increasingly acidotic. An alpha-agonist such as norepinephrine is also used to counteract some of the off-loading. If additional inotropy is required, low-dose epinephrine works well in combination with enoximone. Pacing is also usually required.

In the immediate post-CPB phase an inodilator infusion is useful for the poor LV, which has just had its 'low pressure blow-off' valve closed and now has to work hard against systemic pressure for the first time in years.

ITU management is guided by cardiac output measurement and echocardiography.

'DDD': **D**ilators, **D**iuretics, and **D**igoxin in the postoperative period, the latter for AF rate control, and some inotropy if required.

These infusions are usually continued until the patient is extubated, off-loaded, and dilated with an oral ACE inhibitor, a diuretic such as furosemide, and/or spironolactone. These are usually continued long term.

Therapeutic options and surgical essentials

Repair or replacement is the main question.

Repair is more likely
- Posterior leaflet involved.
- Posterior chord rupture.
- Myxomatous degeneration.

Replacement is more likely
- Anterior leaflet problem.
- Rheumatic valve disease with MR and calcification.
- Endocarditis.

A mechanical bi-leaflet metallic valve is used in patients with a life expectancy of greater than ten years and those able to manage warfarin anticoagulation.

A bovine or porcine tissue valve is used in elderly patients and those not able to take warfarin. A tissue valve will need replacing in approximately ten years but anticoagulation is unnecessary.

Surgical approach

- Midline sternotomy.
- Right thorocotomy, i.e. useful in redos.
- Minimally invasive surgery, via ports through right chest.

There are various techniques for leaflet repair, which involve resection of the leaflet and sliding plasty, chordal transfer, shortening or replacement of chordae with GorTex, papillary muscle re-implantation, and annuloplasty with a ring.

In most cases valve repair is supported with an annuloplasty ring, which strengthens the repair and reduces the size of the annulus, increasing leaflet apposition and making the valve more competent. The annuloplasty ring is sutured around the superior surface of the posterior leaflet, being flexible or rigid, a complete or an incomplete ring.

Trans-oesophageal essentials

Pre-surgery

- Colour Doppler to assess regurgitant area and width of vena contracta.
- 2D echo showing the valve anatomy, a dilated LA, and possibly LV dilation.
- Pulmonary venous Dopplers looking for systolic flow reversal.

Post-surgery

- Assessment of repair or replacement valve for peri-valvular leak.
- Characteristic regurgitant 'washing jets' with mechanical valves.
- LV filling and function.
- RV filling and function.

Mitral stenosis (MS)

Pathology
- Acquired:
  - Rheumatic, post-group A *Streptococcal* infection (most common).
  - Lupus.
  - Rheumatoid arthritis.
  - Carcinoid syndrome.
- Congenital: very rare paediatric presentation.

Pathophysiology
- Progressive fusion with calcification of leaflets and chordae, obstructing the left atrial outflow.
- Left atrial distension causing atrial fibrillation and thrombus formation.
- Pulmonary hypertension.
- Right ventricular hypertrophy and eventual failure.
- Left ventricular function usually preserved but chronic under-filling may cause cardiomyopathy in end-stage disease.
- TOE characteristics.

Fixed cardiac output
- Because of obstruction to flow through the left heart, much like aortic stenosis (🔲 see also Chapter 25), cardiac output and consequently coronary perfusion are relatively fixed. Maintenance of SVR is therefore most important as it is the one variable that can easily be manipulated with the use of an alpha-agonist.
- Cardiac output and the importance of optimizing stroke volume is reliant on the duration of diastole for left ventricular filling; by avoiding tachycardia this allows more time for filling.
- Pulmonary hypertension is a consequence of obstruction to flow from the right to left heart at the mitral valve. This causes the right ventricle to work harder, become hypertrophied, and ultimately fail, reducing left ventricular ejection further. This makes assessment of filling/preload difficult and occasionally in end-stage disease may require inotropic support once anaesthesia is achieved, as this tends to reduce the SVR.

Clinical presentation
Patients are usually asymptomatic for up to 40 years following a group A *Streptococcal* throat infection as a child. Presentation is bimodal, with peaks under the age of 40 and over 50 years, with the younger age group having the more aggressive disease. Dyspnoea on exertion is the commonest symptom, precipitated by tachycardia or a higher demand for cardiac output. This is not usually apparent until the valve area is moderate to severe (<1.5 cm) and pulmonary hypertension is established.

Precipitating factors for symptoms

- Atrial fibrillation.
- Pregnancy.
- Anaemia.
- Thyrotoxicosis.

Presenting features

- Dyspnoea – sudden onset with modest exertion (commonest).
- Fatigue.
- Angina.
- CVA.

Clinical findings

- 'Frail, flushed, and fibrillating.'
- Tapping apex with left parasternal heave from RVH.
- Delayed mid-diastolic murmur, loud first HS, and opening snap.
- Signs of right heart failure, raised JVP, peripheral oedema, liver congestion/ascites.

Preoperative investigations

- FBC and INR (warfarin for AF).
- U/E and LFTs: renal and hepatic congestion.
- CXR: increased heart size, annular calcification, and Kerley B lines in late stage.
- ECG: AF, notched P waves if in SR, and right axis deviation with RVH.
- TOE: 2D echo showing dilated LA with spontaneous contrast and restriction of calcified mitral orifice.
- Classical 'hockey stick' bowing, with thickened tip leaflet deformity. Doppler echo, PW or CW depending on velocities, showing loss of A wave due to AF, a high gradient, and calculation of small valve area using P1/2t (📖 see also Chapter 17).
- Angiography: 25% of patients have significant CAD.

Haemodynamic goals

- MS is a relatively rare condition in the developed world; it is much more of a problem in patients from the developing world.
- As a general rule the LV function is usually well preserved and the RV, although hypertrophied, also functions well. It is usually only in end-stage patients that RV and LV failure become a problem and inotropes are required once anaesthesia is established.
- Type III phosphodiesterase inhibitors are used frequently for separation from CPB.
- **Avoid tachycardia** by maintaining normal heart rate to allow time in diastole for left ventricular filling and coronary perfusion.
- **Maintain SVR**, as with a relatively fixed cardiac output, BP is maintained through vascular tone. Cautious use of alpha-agonists such as phenylephrine; this may occasionally have an adverse effect on pulmonary hypertension.
- **Inotropes** such as epinephrine pre-CPB may be required occasionally for RVF in end-stage disease pre-CPB.
- **Preload** is not usually an issue with obstructed high right-sided pressures.

Anaesthetic plan and adverse haemodynamics

- A large-bore intravenous cannula and a smaller arterial line are placed before induction; the central line can be placed post-induction. Consider a pulmonary artery catheter; with any right or left heart dysfunction, it may be very useful postoperatively. ICU management is facilitated by cardiac output measurement and echocardiography.
- IV induction is usually with high-dose fentanyl and etomidate to maintain cardiovascular stability. Avoid tachycardia and vasodilation as much as possible, with careful use of an alpha-agonist such as phenylephrine to maintain SVR.
- Cardiac arrest at induction is fortunately unusual, but as with AS (📖 see also Chapter 25) requires immediate CPR and emergency cardiopulmonary bypass. The surgeon, perfusionist, and heparin need to be close at hand.
- Post-bypass most cases of MS have preserved, good LV function; if an inotrope is required a type III phosphodiesterase inhibitor such as milrinone or enoximone with norepinephrine (an alpha-agonist) may be necessary. Using an inodilator will 'drive' the ventricles, as well as 'off-load' both the pulmonary and systemic circulations, making it easier for the heart to eject.
- An infusion of these inotropes, if used, will probably be continued for at least the first 24–48 hours. It is usual practice for temporary pacing wires to be placed because of surgical interference and oedema to the conducting pathways.

Therapeutic options and surgical essentials

Closed
- Balloon valvotomy if no significant MR or atrial thrombus present.
- High recurrence and MR is a significant risk.
- Useful in early disease to delay surgery, e.g. during pregnancy and in the young.

Open
- Commisurotomy if no significant MR or atrial thrombus; 30% recurrence in five years, again with the risk of MR.
- Valve replacement required if severe MR, fibrosis, or heavy calcification of the valve.

Trans-oesophageal essentials

- Dilated LA >4.5 cm with spontaneous contrast 'smoke'.
- Calcified, restricted mitral leaflets with doming and 'hockey stick' deformity.
- Enlarged RV with hypertrophy.
- Inodilators occasionally required to come off CPB.

Mixed mitral valve disease

This is almost always as a result of rheumatic mitral stenosis with a varying degree of progressive MR. Management is based on following a plan for the dominant lesion, after careful echo and angiographic assessment, as above.

It is less likely that valve repair will be feasible and replacement is the likely outcome.

Haemodynamic goals
- Maintain the SVR.
- Maintain a stable HR.
- Maintain filling and contractility.

Anaesthetic plan

A large-bore venous cannula and a radial arterial line, awake, with a standard intravenous induction following pre-oxygenation. The idea is to **maintain cardiovascular stability** as much as possible and treat any changes as for the dominant valve lesion. These can be difficult cases to manage.

Practice points

Mitral regurgitation
- Repair is far preferable to replacement.
- A thorough knowledge and application of TOE is essential.
- Assume the LV is always poor, despite the echo report.
- Inodilators to come off CPB.
- 'Dilators, Diuretics, Digoxin' in the postoperative phase.

Mitral stenosis
- Consider a pulmonary artery catheter to aid postoperative management if complicated with ventricular failure.
- TOE essential for perioperative period.

Mixed mitral valve disease
- Manage the dominant lesion.
- Maintain CV stability.
- Valve replacement likely.
- Difficult case!

Further reading

1. Bonow RO, Carabello BA, Chatterjee K, et al. ACC/AHA 2006 Guidelines for the management of patients with valvular heart disease: A report of the American College of Cardiology/American Heart Association Task Force on Practice Guidelines (Writing Committee to Develop Guidelines for the Management of Patients with Valvular Heart Disease). *Circulation* 2006; 114: e84–e231.
2. Fedak P, McCarthy P, Bonow R. Evolving concepts and technologies in mitral valve repair. *Circulation* 2008; 117: 963–974.
3. Gillinov A, Cosgrove D. Current status of mitral valve repair. *American Heart Hospital Journal* 2007; 1: 47–54.
4. Savage E, Bruce Ferguson T, DiSesa V. Use of mitral valve repair: Analysis of contemporary United States experience reported to the Society of Thoracic Surgeons National Cardiac Database. *Annals of Thoracic Surgery* 2003; 75: 820–825.
5. Vahanian A, Baumgartner H, Bax J, et al. Guidelines on the management of valvular heart disease: The Task Force on the Management of Valvular Heart Disease of the European Society of Cardiology. *European Heart Journal* 2007; 28: 230–268.

Other valve disease

Dr M Barnard and Dr B Martin

Mixed valve lesions *412*
Tricuspid regurgitation *414*
Tricuspid stenosis *416*
Pulmonary stenosis and regurgitation *418*
Further reading *420*

Mixed valve lesions

Many patients present with mixed valve lesions. The general approach is to determine which is the predominant pathology and most significant, and apply treatment principles for that lesion. Haemodynamic goals can be opposite for each lesion, and so maintaining normal haemodynamic conditions and treating for the predominant lesion are important.

Aortic stenosis and mitral stenosis

- Not a good combination! These patients can be difficult as forward flow is limited at two separate points.
- Pathology similar to severe mitral stenosis with pulmonary hypertension and right heart failure.
- Aortic stenosis may be underestimated due to low gradient caused by inadequate LV filling.
- Increase preload, normal to low heart rate, and maintain contractility.
- If diastolic pressure falls, coronary perfusion at risk – increase SVR.
- Avoid increases in PVR ($PaCO_2$ and FiO_2).

Aortic stenosis and mitral regurgitation

- Mitral regurgitation can be exacerbated by LV dysfunction due to aortic stenosis. This may improve after aortic valve replacement, without replacing the mitral valve.
- Haemodynamic goals for each lesion are opposite.
- Aortic stenosis is more dangerous and should generally be given priority.
- Increase preload, and maintain coronary perfusion by maintaining SVR.
- Avoid tachycardia and maintain contractility.

Aortic stenosis and aortic regurgitation

- Not well tolerated as LV is subjected to both volume and pressure loads.
- Myocardial oxygen consumption significantly increased. Ischaemia is a risk.
- Maintain preload.
- Heart rate and afterload goals are contradictory. In general treat for aortic stenosis, as this is the more dangerous lesion when compromised. Maintain afterload and normal heart rate.

Aortic regurgitation and mitral regurgitation

- This is a common combination.
- Keep SVR relatively low (although without compromising coronary perfusion).
- Augmented preload and increased heart rate are beneficial.

Mixed mitral valve disease

- Consider which lesion is predominant.
- In general normal heart rate, afterload, and contractility are useful.
- Increase preload and avoid increases in PVR.

Tricuspid regurgitation

Pathology
- Endocarditis.
- Carcinoid.
- Trauma.
- Congenital.
- Secondary:
  - RV failure.
  - Pulmonary hypertension.
  - Mitral/aortic valve disease.

Pathophysiology
- RV volume overload.
- RV is better accustomed to volume load rather than pressure load. Increased afterload can readily lead to RV failure.
- Atrial arrhythmias.
- Severity:
  - Echocardiography, with Doppler colour flow.
  - Grade 1: Jet <5 cm^2.
  - Grade 2: Jet 5–10 cm^2.
  - Grade 3: Jet >10 cm^2.
  - Grade 4: Jet >10 cm^2 + hepatic vein flow reversal.
- CVP shows V waves. Size is determined by changes in atrial compliance.

Therapeutic options
- Surgery is indicated at time of aortic or mitral surgery if TR is severe and there is pulmonary hypertension.
- Valve plication or annuloplasty is preferred to replacement.
- The 'Cone' repair has become popular in congenital Ebstein's. This involves detaching leaflets and reattaching them higher.

Haemodynamic goals
- Preload: maintain or increase.
- Heart rate: normal or increased.
- Contractility: maintain. Mechanical ventilation and elevated PVR can cause RV decompensation.
- SVR: Maintain, but has little effect.
- PVR: Decrease.

Anaesthetic plan
- PA catheters can be difficult to place, and can give inaccurate cardiac output measurements (retrograde injectate flow).
- Prosthetic valve replacement mandates increasing preload, with a small resting gradient.
- Impaired RV at risk of acute failure when tricuspid valve made competent, if it is unable to cope with PVR. Inotropes will be necessary; enoximone or milrinone are agents of choice (lusitropy, decreased PVR).

Tricuspid stenosis

Pathology
- Rheumatic – primary acquired cause. Rare and almost always associated with rheumatic mitral valve disease.
- Systemic lupus erythematosus.
- Endomyocardial fibrosis.
- Fibroelastosis.
- Tumour.
- Carcinoid.
- Congenital.

Pathophysiology
- Hepatomegaly, hepatic dysfunction, peripheral oedema, elevated venous pressures.
- Normal gradient 1 mmHg. Valve area 7–9 cm^2.
- Valve area <1.5 cm^2 and gradient >3 mmHg impair cardiac output.
- Right atrial dilation.
- Reduced cardiac output with severe lesions.

Assessment
- Cardiac catheterization and echocardiography.
- Severe – valve area 1 cm^2, gradient >5 mmHg.

Therapeutic options
- Medical therapy with diuretics and digoxin.
- Most surgical patients are undergoing simultaneous operation on other valves.
- Commissurotomy is preferred to valve replacement.

Haemodynamic goals
- Preload – maintain or increase.
- Heart rate – maintain sinus rhythm. Urgent treatment of supraventricular arrhythmias.
- Contractility – maintain to compensate for decreased filling. Depressed contractility poorly tolerated.
- SVR – maintain or increase to avoid hypotension (limited stroke volume).
- PVR – little effect, maintain.

Anaesthetic plan
- Main goals are to maintain high preload, high afterload, and contractility.
- PA catheters difficult to place and would interfere with surgery. Discuss with surgeon if you are considering placement.
- Ensure adequate SVC drainage from caval cannula during cardiopulmonary bypass.
- Post-bypass, maintain increased preload. Inotropes if RV is impaired.

Pulmonary stenosis and regurgitation

Pulmonary stenosis

Pathology
- Most are congenital.
- Rare: rheumatic, carcinoid, extrinsic compression (tumour, aneurysm).

Pathophysiology
- Frequently asymptomatic.
- Normal pressure gradient <5 mmHg.
- Mild: <50 mmHg.
- Moderate: 50–100 mmHg.
- Severe: >100 mmHg.
- Causes concentric RV hypertrophy.
- As hypertrophy progresses, RV subendocardial blood flow is compromised.
- Ultimately subendocardial blood flow only occurs during diastole (normally 30% in systole), similar to LV.
- Coronary perfusion pressure therefore important.
- PA upstroke slow rising.
- Prominent 'a' wave in CVP trace.

Therapeutic options
- Intervention indicated for severe pulmonary stenosis (RV pressure >100 mmHg).
- Surgical options are valvotomy or replacement.
- Balloon valvuloplasty or percutaneous valve insertion are interventional cardiological alternatives.

Haemodynamic goals
- Preload – maintain or increase. RV function is very preload-dependent in the face of increased afterload.
- Heart rate – maintain or increase (forward flow occurs during systole). Atrial contraction important.
- Contractility – maintain. RV is hypertrophied, which maintains RV pressure in the face of increased afterload. However, very large increases in afterload will lead to RV failure and necessitate inotropic support. Enoximone and milrinone are preferred.
- SVR – maintain to provide adequate coronary perfusion pressure.
- PVR – relatively little effect. Keep low/normal, especially in mild or moderate stenosis, where PVR has more effect.

Pulmonary regurgitation
- Annular dilation secondary to left heart disorders or pulmonary hypertension.
- Connective tissue disorders, carcinoid, infective endocarditis, rheumatic.
- Congenital heart disease – commonly adult tetralogy of Fallot, with previous valve interventions.

- RV dilation and ultimately RV failure.
- RV distension increases risk of ventricular arrhythmias.
- Treatment is valve replacement:
  - Often with tissue prosthesis or human cadaveric homograft.
  - Mainly performed in congenital heart patients.

Further reading

1. Bonow RO, Carabello BA, Chatterjee K, et al. ACC/AHA 2006 Guidelines for the management of patients with valvular heart disease: A report of the American College of Cardiology/American Heart Association Task Force on Practice Guidelines (Writing Committee to Develop Guidelines for the Management of Patients with Valvular Heart Disease). *Circulation* 2006; 114: e84–e231.
2. McCarthy P, Bhudia S, Rajeswaran J, et al. Tricuspid valve repair: Durability and risk factors for failure. *Journal of Thoracic and Cardiovascular Surgery* 2004; 127: 674–685.
3. Vahanian A, Baumgartner H, Bax J, et al. Guidelines on the management of valvular heart disease: The Task Force on the Management of Valvular Heart Disease of the European Society of Cardiology. *European Heart Journal* 2007; 28: 230–268.

Paediatric congenital heart disease

Dr A McEwan

Foetal circulation *422*
Neonatal physiology *424*
Preoperative assessment and premedication *426*
Drugs used in paediatric cardiac anaesthesia *428*
Equipment and monitoring *429*
Management of cardiopulmonary bypass in children *430*
Coagulopathy after cardiac surgery in children *432*
Classification of congenital heart lesions *433*
'Simple' left to right shunts *434*
'Simple' right to left shunts *435*
Atrial septal defect *436*
Patent ductus arteriosus (PDA) *438*
Tetralogy of Fallot (TOF) *440*
Transposition of the great arteries (TGA) *442*
Truncus arteriosus *444*
Anomalous pulmonary venous connections *446*
Hypoplastic left heart syndrome *448*
Ventricular septal defect (VSD) and atrioventricular septal
    defect (AVSD) *452*
Interrupted aortic arch *454*
Aortic stenosis (AS) *456*
Coarctation of the aorta *458*
Three common paediatric cardiac surgical procedures *460*
Cardiac catheterization and interventional cardiology *462*
Paediatric cardiac transplantation *464*
Further reading *467*

Foetal circulation

- The foetal circulation is arranged so that blood with the highest oxygen saturation flows to the developing brain and less saturated blood is diverted to the lower body.
- Foetal gas exchange takes place in the placenta. The vascular resistance in the placenta is low and it receives 50% of the foetal cardiac output. The placenta receives oxygenated blood from the maternal uterine arteries, and this blood flows into the intervillous sinusoids. Deoxygenated blood from the foetus reaches the placenta through umbilical arteries, which form capillaries that protrude into the sinusoids. This blood–blood interface is relatively inefficient at gas exchange and blood leaving the placenta has a PO_2 of only 4 kPa.
- Oxygenated umbilical vein blood flows via the ductus venosus into the inferior vena cava and on to the right atrium. The majority of the oxygenated IVC blood is then directed through the foramen ovale into the left atrium and then to the aorta, coronary arteries, and brain.
- Deoxygenated blood from the right ventricle is directed through the ductus arteriosus into the descending aorta (PO_2 = 2.9 kPa). Pulmonary vascular resistance is high because of vasoconstriction of the small muscular pulmonary vessels mediated by low PO_2, and therefore only a small amount of right ventricular blood (10%) flows to the lungs. Pulmonary vascular resistance falls near birth, associated with the production of surfactant.
- Cardiac output increases late in the third trimester. The right ventricle pumps about two thirds and the left ventricle about one third of the combined cardiac output.
- The foetal ventricle is less compliant even than the neonatal ventricle as a result of the proportions of contractile and non-contractile elements.

Neonatal physiology

The cardiovascular system

- Neonatal myocardium is less compliant than in the adult because it contains less contractile tissue and more supporting tissue. This results in a relatively fixed stroke volume and cardiac output is heart rate dependent.
- Reduction in myocardial compliance and high oxygen consumption predispose neonates to heart failure.
- Reduced contractility reflects immature myofibrils and sarcoplasmic reticulum. Calcium regulation is immature and makes the neonatal myocardium sensitive to hypocalcaemia and calcium channel blocking drugs (including inhalational anaesthetics).
- Cardiac output is high: 300–400 ml/kg/min. This is *2-3 times* that of adults and reflects the relatively high oxygen consumption.
- SVR is low, which means low blood pressure despite a high cardiac output.
- At birth the right ventricle (RV) mass is greater than that of the left ventricle (LV). However, the LV mass increases rapidly and by about four months the LV:RV ratio has assumed adult proportions.
- Heart rate (HR) is 100–170 bpm (average 120). HR decreases with growth. HR is 110 bpm at two years and 90 at eight years.
- Blood pressure varies with age and gestation and increases gradually with age. It is much lower in neonates and children than adults (Table 29.1).

Table 29.1 Normal blood pressure

Age	Systolic BP (mmHg)
Preterm	49
Full term	60
3–10 days	70–75
6 months	95
4 years	98

Pulmonary circulation

Neonatal pulmonary vascular resistance (PVR) is high but falls in the first weeks of life. High foetal PVR is due to smooth muscle in the media of peripheral pulmonary arterioles. This muscle regresses gradually after birth but until regression is complete; the pulmonary vasculature remains reactive and periods of pulmonary hypertension are possible. PVR is raised by hypoxia, hypercapnia, and acidosis.

Respiratory system

- Alveolar growth accelerates after birth, reaching adult values by about eight years of age.
- Ribs are horizontal and therefore contribute little to breathing because there is no 'bucket handle' effect. The diaphragm is flatter, poorly developed, and less efficient.
- Chest wall is very compliant. Low functional residual capacity (FRC) because the lungs are relatively stiff at birth and tend to draw the chest wall inwards during expiration. This is even more marked in premature infants with low levels of alveolar surfactant, which further reduces compliance.
- Airway closure is common during normal tidal breathing.
- Periods of apnoea are common, particularly in preterm neonates. Hypoxia initially stimulates respiration but after a few minutes respiratory depression results, leading to prolonged apnoeas and possibly bradycardia.

The kidney

- The foetal kidney produces dilute urine and contributes to amniotic fluid volume.
- Renal blood flow increases in the first few weeks of life from 6% of cardiac output at birth to 20% at one month. GFR increases to a similar extent.
- At birth the kidney has limited concentrating ability and therefore requires adequate water to excrete a solute load.
- Excess water is poorly handled.

Central nervous system

Pain

- Myelination is incomplete.
- Cerebral cortex is less developed.
- Neonates, including preterm infants, are capable of experiencing pain.

CBF

- Autoregulation impaired in ill neonates.
- Fragile capillaries (prone to intraventricular haemorrhage).

Temperature regulation

- Prone to hypothermia.
- Large surface area to weight ratio.
- Little subcutaneous fat.
- Primarily non-shivering thermogenesis utilizing brown fat (increased VO_2).

Preoperative assessment and premedication

Preoperative assessment

Aims of the preoperative visit include:
- Medical assessment.
- Providing information.
- Creating a relationship with the child and family.
- Formulating an anaesthetic plan, including premedication.

Medical assessment (Box 29.1)

- Determine diagnosis and nature of the planned surgery and understand the pathophysiology.
- Detailed diagnostic information obtained from the medical records, particularly echocardiographic, catheter, and MRI data. Review joint cardiology/surgical planning meetings, previous operation reports, anaesthetic records, or discharge summaries.
- Review chest X-ray, ECG, and blood results.
- Directed history and physical examination.

Box 29.1 Indices of significant impairment in CHD

- Chronic hypoxaemia (arterial saturation <75%).
- Pulmonary to systemic blood flow ratio >2:1.
- Left or right ventricular outflow tract gradient >50 mmHg.
- Elevated pulmonary vascular resistance.
- Polycythemia (Hct >60%).

Premedication

- Practice varies but sedative premedication can be very useful.
- It is probably unnecessary in infants less than four weeks but is not contraindicated.
- Avoid sedative premedication in children with severe heart failure.
- Cyanotic patients such as those with tetralogy of Fallot often benefit from sedative premedication because crying and struggling worsen cyanosis. Older children are frequently very anxious. Suggested sedative drugs and doses are outlined in Table 29.2.
- Prescribe local anaesthetic cream even if inhalational induction is planned as cannulation is possible at a lighter plane of anaesthesia.

Table 29.2 Suggested premedication for cardiac surgery

Age/weight	Drug	Dose	Comments
<4 weeks	No premed		EMLA® or Ametop®
4 weeks to 6 kg	Triclofos	50–75 mg/kg	
6–15 kg	Triclofos	50–75 mg/kg	
>15 kg	Midazolam	0.5–1.0 mg/kg	Max 15 mg
	Temazepam	0.5–1.0 mg/kg	Max 20 mg

Giving information

- Give information about premedication, starvation times, time of surgery, mode of induction, monitoring and lines to be used, ventilation in the intensive care unit (ICU), likely length of stay, and the use of blood and blood products. Questions about risk often arise and should be answered honestly.
- Preoperative fasting times:
  - Food and milk 6 hours.
  - Breast milk 4 hours.
  - Clear fluids 3 hours.

Drugs used in paediatric cardiac anaesthesia

- Induction: Intravenous or inhalational. In older children it is most appropriate to use an IV induction. In small infants gas induction is often preferred.
- **Etomidate** is a safe drug with a LD50:ED50 of 26. It has little effect on the cardiovascular system in both health and cardiac disease. A single dose of etomidate causes adreno-cortical suppression but the effect on outcome is unlikely to be important.
- **Ketamine** increases blood pressure, heart rate, and cardiac output. The exact mechanism is unknown but it may stimulate the release of endogenous stores of catecholamines. It is a negative inotrope in the denervated heart. It may be a poor choice in patients with pre-existing maximal catecholamine stimulation (cardiomyopathy) and when tachycardia is undesirable (aortic stenosis). Uniquely, it can be administered intramuscularly.
- **Fentanyl** has a potency 50–100 times that of morphine and is relatively haemodynamically stable. In high doses it may cause bradycardia and chest wall rigidity. It is seldom used as a sole agent for induction of anaesthesia but is frequently used in combination with other agents.
- **Propofol** is used in older children with stable haemodynamics. It causes pain on injection and a dose-dependent decrease in arterial pressure and systemic vascular resistance. It should be used with care in patients with fixed cardiac output such as severe aortic stenosis or mitral stenosis.
- **Thiopental** causes a decrease in blood pressure due to a reduction in SVR, and like propofol should be used with great care in patients with a fixed cardiac output. Small infants and neonates are particularly sensitive.
- **Midazolam** is a short-acting water-soluble benzodiazepine. It provides cardiovascular stability and has a wide margin of safety.
- **Sevoflurane** is an agent of choice for induction as it is rapidly acting, non-irritant to the airway, and causes less myocardial depression than halothane.
- After intubation a low-dose volatile agent is used to maintain anaesthesia in combination with air and oxygen. Nitrous oxide is generally avoided as there is always a risk of air entering the circulation during surgery, and because of its negative inotropic effects and increased pulmonary vascular resistance.
- A number of different muscle relaxants can safely be used. **Pancuronium** is still used if early extubation is not planned.

Equipment and monitoring

Monitoring

Monitoring commences prior to induction of anaesthesia. This includes ECG, pulse oximetry, and non-invasive blood pressure.

- **ECG**: A five-lead monitor is preferred.
- **Pulse oximeter**: The algorithms on which oximeters rely become less reliable below a saturation of 80%.
- **End-tidal CO_2**.
- **Central venous pressure**: Sites include internal jugular, femoral, subclavian, or umbilical veins. Generally multi-lumen lines; either 4 or 5 French gauge (FG) double or triple lumen lines. Heparin-bonded lines reduce the risks of sepsis and venous thrombosis. Ultrasound-guided placement of central lines is becoming more widespread. Some units in USA and Europe avoid percutaneous central access, preferring to use surgically-placed atrial lines.
- **Pulmonary artery flotation catheters** are seldom used in paediatric practice. Left atrial lines or pulmonary artery catheters may be directly placed during surgery.
- **Arterial line**: Radial, femoral, or axillary arteries are commonly used. The brachial artery should be avoided as this is an end artery. In neonates 24 FG cannulae are generally used for the radial artery. 22 FG can be used at other sites. Avoid injection of air when flushing arterial lines and use small volumes and slow rates of injection.
- **Temperature**: Nasopharyngeal temperature and skin temperatures are measured.
- **Urinary catheter**.
- **Trans-oesophageal echocardiography** is increasingly being used in paediatric cardiac surgery.
- **Near infra-red spectroscopy** (NIRS) is a method of measuring cerebral oxygenation. Its use is limited since normal levels of cerebral oxygenation have not been determined in neonates and small infants, and nor have levels that are critical in terms of cerebral damage.
- **Transcranial Doppler (TCD)**: TCD measures cerebral blood flow and is able to detect microemboli. Like NIRS it is limited by the lack of normative data during bypass. However, it is likely to prove useful in detecting inadequate flow during bypass.
- **Bi-spectral analysis monitor (BIS)**: BIS is used to determine depth of anaesthesia. It may be useful in monitoring depth of anaesthesia during CPB in children.

Management of cardiopulmonary bypass in children

Cardiopulmonary bypass in children is similar to adults (📖 see also Chapter 18) but with certain important differences:

- The bypass circuit is smaller than that used for adults.
- Although the volume of the circuit is smaller, it is large relative to the child's blood volume. This is most significant in neonates and results in significant haemodilution with dilution of coagulation factors and drugs.
- The use of modified ultrafiltration post-bypass.

Prior to the commencement of CPB

- Baseline ACT and blood gas.
- Heparin. Usually 300–400 IU/kg. ACT after heparin should be at least three times baseline or greater than 400 seconds. Neonates may be relatively resistant to heparin because of low levels of antithrombin III and may require higher doses. Recently, it has been suggested that ACT correlates poorly with heparin levels in infants and that measuring heparin levels may be more reliable.
- Antibiotics according to local protocols.
- Additional fentanyl, midazolam (0.2 mg/kg), and muscle relaxant is given. Propofol with or without remifentanil is used by some for maintenance of anaesthesia during CPB.

Aspects of CPB

- Ventilation is discontinued during CPB.
- Hypotension after the start of bypass may be due to haemodilution, or the presence of collateral shunts to the lungs, PDA, or surgical shunt. A PDA or surgical shunt should be ligated as soon as possible after the start of bypass. A vasoconstrictor such as phenylephrine (1–5 µg/kg) or metaraminol (1–10 µg/kg) may be required to increase perfusion pressure.
- Hypertension may indicate inadequate anaesthesia and should be treated accordingly. If hypertension persists a vasodilator such as phentolamine (1–5 µg/kg) may be required.
- Cardioplegia: Some operations are performed on the beating heart but it is often necessary for the heart to be stopped to allow surgery. This is achieved by the infusion of a cold cardioplegic solution into the aortic root after cross-clamping the aorta. This causes the solution to flow into the coronaries and perfuse the heart. This is repeated every 20–30 minutes. If aortic regurgitation is present, flow into the coronaries will be inadequate and will result in poor myocardial preservation. In this case it is sometimes necessary to open the aorta and perfuse the coronaries under direct vision.
- ACT and blood gases assessed regularly by perfusionist.
- Potassium, bicarbonate, calcium, and magnesium are given as required.
- Temperature: Usually temperature is maintained at 28–32°C. For complex surgery lower temperatures are used; occasionally deep hypothermic circulatory arrest (DHCA) requiring a core temperature of 16–18°C. There is an increasing tendency towards CPB at warmer temperatures.

Surgery requiring DHCA (📖 see also Chapter 19)

- Interrupted aortic arch.
- Total anomalous venous drainage.
- Aortic arch repair associated with the Norwood procedure.

DHCA is used for as short a time as possible because it is associated with adverse neurological outcomes. Thirty minutes seems to be the duration of DHCA at which neurodevelopmental changes, including lower IQ, become significant in later life. Factors that improve outcomes after DHCA are maintaining haematocrit at 30% and adequate cooling. There is no good evidence that steroids improve neurological outcome after DHCA.

Prior to separation from bypass, ventilation is re-established, inotropes are started if required, blood products are available, blood gases are reviewed, and rewarming is satisfactory.

Coagulopathy after cardiac surgery in children

- Bleeding after cardiac surgery in children contributes to postoperative morbidity.
- The coagulopathy that occurs during and after bypass in children is more severe than that which occurs in adults.
- Coagulopathy and the extent of bleeding after surgery are related to the patient's size and weight. Patients less than 8 kg can be expected to have a more severe coagulopathy and bleed more in the postoperative period.
- The primary defect that occurs in children is a result of haemodilution and this is most important in neonates.
- In neonates, on initiation of bypass, coagulation factors including fibrinogen and antithrombin III are reduced by 50% and platelets are reduced by 70%. Coagulation factors and platelets are further reduced during bypass as a result of consumption and this is stimulated by activation of the inflammatory response.
- Risk of postoperative bleeding in children increases with:
  - Decreasing age.
  - Decreasing size (8 kg thought to be important).
  - Preoperative cyanosis.
  - Preoperative heart failure.
  - Length of CPB.
  - Degree of hypothermia.
  - Redo sternotomy.
- Methods to reduce postoperative bleeding:
  - Aminocaproic acid EACA and tranexamic acid TA. These have been shown to reduce bleeding after cardiac surgery in children. Doses for use in paediatric cardiac surgery have not been clearly established.
  - The use of aprotinin in children is controversial. Many reports have documented that aprotinin is effective in reducing bleeding, length of time on the ventilator, and ICU stay in children. A large study in adults undergoing revascularization surgery reported significantly increased risks of adverse cardiovascular events. There is no evidence to date to suggest that this is true in children. Doses used in children vary widely but if a prime dose is used that is based on the size of the pump prime rather than on the size of the child, plasma aprotinin levels are similar to those seen in adults. Aprotinin is expensive and there is a risk of anaphylaxis, particularly if the patient has been previously exposed. Its use within a year of previous exposure is contraindicated.
  - Ultrafiltration significantly reduces bleeding after cardiac surgery in children.
  - Blood products. Platelets and cryoprecipitate are first-line treatment of coagulopathy in neonates and small infants. Cryoprecipitate contains high levels of fibrinogen, factor VIII, and von Willebrand factor, all of which are essential for clotting. There is no evidence that fresh frozen plasma is of benefit.

Classification of congenital heart lesions

There are a number of different ways in which congenital heart disease can be classified. The following is a simple, easily understood classification.

'Simple' left to right shunt: Increased pulmonary blood flow

- Atrial septal defect (ASD).
- Ventricular septal defect (VSD).
- Patent ductus arteriosus (PDA).
- Endocardial cushion defect, e.g. atrioventricular septal defect (AVSD).
- Aortopulmonary window (AP window).

'Simple' right to left shunt: Results in cyanosis

- Tetralogy of Fallot (TOF).
- Pulmonary atresia.
- Tricuspid atresia.
- Ebstein's anomaly.

Complex shunts: Mixing of pulmonary and systemic blood flow with cyanosis

- Transposition of the great arteries (TGA).
- Truncus arteriosus.
- Total anomalous pulmonary venous drainage (TAPVD).
- Double outlet right ventricle (DORV).
- Hypoplastic left heart syndrome (HLHS).

Obstructive lesions

- Aortic stenosis.
- Mitral stenosis.
- Pulmonary stenosis.
- Coarctation of aorta.
- Interrupted aortic arch.

'Simple' left to right shunts

These shunts result in increased pulmonary blood flow resulting in volume loading of the right side of the heart with right atrial enlargement and right ventricular hypertrophy, perhaps associated with tricuspid and pulmonary regurgitation. This combination results in cardiac failure. Clinical features of cardiac failure in children include:

- Failure to thrive.
- Difficult feeding.
- Breathlessness.
- Recurrent chest infection.
- Tachycardia.
- Cardiac murmur.
- Hepatomegaly.
- Cardiomegaly.
- Pulmonary plethora.
- Wheezing.

Medical management of these children includes the use of diuretics, sometimes in combination with digoxin.

If pulmonary blood flow is high, pulmonary vascular disease begins to develop. In the early stages the changes are reversible but in time the changes may become irreversible. Eisenmenger's syndrome refers to the situation in which severe pulmonary vascular disease results in supra-systemic pulmonary artery pressures leading to shunt reversal and cyanosis; at this point the patient becomes inoperable. Increasingly, definitive surgery is being performed at a younger age to reduce the risk of pulmonary vascular disease. If early definitive surgery is not possible, a pulmonary artery band is applied to reduce pulmonary blood flow. This gives the baby the opportunity to grow and for definitive surgery to be postponed without the risk of developing pulmonary hypertension. In the presence of significantly increased pulmonary blood flow, pulmonary vascular disease is often severe and irreversible by the age of one year and definitive surgery should take place before six months.

'Simple' right to left shunts

This results in cyanosis because deoxygenated blood is mixing with oxygenated blood. Prolonged cyanosis results in polycythemia. The shunt may be dynamic as with tetralogy of Fallot and this results in varying degrees of cyanosis.

Atrial septal defect

Occurs 1:1500 (10% of CHD).

Several types exist

- Patent foramen ovale (PFO): Normal foetal communication between the two atria, which usually closes soon after birth. Remains patent in 30%.
- Secundum ASD (Figure 29.1): This is found in the region of the fossa ovalis and results from a deficiency in the septum secundum.
- Primum ASD (Figure 29.2): Located at the inferior part of the atrial septum close to the atrioventricular (AV) valve. (A variant of AVSD.)
- Sinus venosus ASD (Figure 29.3): Occurs high in the atrial septum close to the opening of the SVC. Associated with partial anomalous pulmonary venous drainage.
- Coronary sinus ASD (unroofed coronary sinus): A defect in the atrial wall allows blood to flow from the left atrium to the right atrium through the coronary sinus.
- Common atrium: A complete absence of the atrial septum. The AV valves may be abnormal or unaffected.

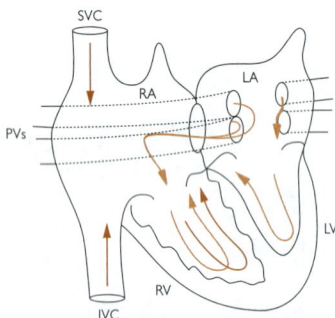

Figure 29.1 Secundum atrial septal defect (great vessels removed).

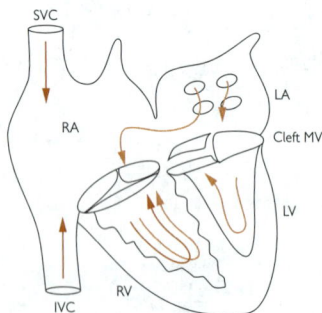

Figure 29.2 Primum atrial septal defect (great vessels not shown).

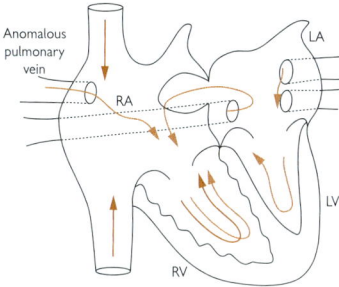

Figure 29.3 Sinus venosus atrial septal defect.

Pathophysiology
- Left to right shunt.
- Volume-loaded right heart.

Anaesthetic considerations
- Many ASDs are now closed using percutaneous, transcatheter devices in the angiography suite.
- If catheter closure is not possible, closure requires surgery with CPB.
- Usually well, older children.
- These patients can frequently be extubated on the operating table or early in the ICU and smaller doses of opioid can be used. Alternatively, short-acting drugs (remifentanil) by infusion, possibly in combination with propofol, are useful if early extubation is planned.
- The problems of postoperative pulmonary hypertension are seldom encountered.

Patent ductus arteriosus (PDA)

Occurs in 1 in 2500 live births (10% of CHD).

Pathophysiology

- The ductus arteriosus is part of the foetal circulation. It extends from the descending aorta to the main pulmonary artery and usually closes after birth (Figure 29.4).
- Left to right shunt with volume loading of right heart and heart failure.
- Common in premature babies and contributes to ongoing requirement for mechanical ventilation.

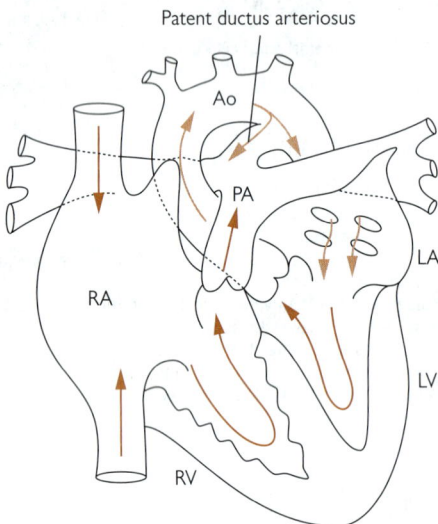

Figure 29.4 Patent ductus arteriosus.

Management

- Medical management with indomethacin.
- In small babies a left thoracotomy is required to ligate PDA.
- Also occurs in older children but these cases are usually managed by transcatheter closure.

Anaesthetic management of neonate with PDA

- In many centres PDA closure in small premature babies is undertaken in the neonatal intensive care unit (NICU). This avoids transferring very small infants to the operating theatre and all the associated problems, particularly hypothermia.
- Blood cross-matched.
- Antibiotics (risk of endocarditis).
- Vitamin K.

Particular perioperative risks

- Difficult ventilation or desaturation during lung retraction.
- Tearing of PDA with massive haemorrhage.
- Inadvertent ligation of aorta or pulmonary artery.
- Endocarditis.
- Paradoxical air embolism.

Anaesthesia

- Standard monitors but in addition two pulse oximeters, one on the right hand, one on a lower limb. If the pulse is lost from the lower limb during a test clamping of the duct, this indicates that the aorta has been clamped inadvertently.
- Invasive blood pressure is helpful if already established or if it can be placed reasonably quickly but is not absolutely necessary.
- A dedicated IV for fluids and drugs with long (100–150 cm) extension to allow access from a distance. (Space around cot is limited if performed in NICU.)
- Opioid-based technique.
- Muscle relaxation.
- The endotracheal tube should have only a small air leak. A large leak will make ventilation difficult during lung retraction.
- Intercostal nerve block by surgeon on completion of surgery.
- Maintain glucose-containing fluids.

Tetralogy of Fallot (TOF)

6% of CHD.

Pathophysiology

- The four features of the tetralogy are (Figure 29.5):
  - VSD.
  - Overriding aorta.
  - Right ventricular outflow tract obstruction (RVOTO).
  - Right ventricular hypertrophy.
- Level of the obstruction varies but commonly a dynamic sub-pulmonary infundibular obstruction is present.
- The relationship between the RVOTO and the systemic vascular resistance determines the degree of right to left shunting and thus the degree of cyanosis.
- TOF may be associated with a large number of other cardiac and extracardiac anomalies.
- Hypercyanotic 'spells':
  - Occur in 20–70% of untreated patients. Often initiated by crying or feeding and may occur during anaesthesia.
  - Contributing factors include: metabolic acidosis, increased pCO_2, circulating catecholamines, and surgical stimulation are implicated.
  - Due to dynamic infundibular obstruction in the RVOT.
- Management of hypercyanotic 'spells':
  - 100% oxygen.
  - Hyperventilation.
  - IV fluid bolus (10 ml/kg).
  - Sedation, e.g. fentanyl.
  - Sodium bicarbonate.
  - Vasoconstriction.
  - Norepinephrine 0.5 μg/kg bolus then 0.1–0.5 μg/kg/min.
  - Phenylephrine 5 μg/kg bolus then 1–5 μg/kg/min.
  - Beta-blockers to relax infundibular spasm and reduce heart rate.
  - Propranolol 0.1–0.3 mg/kg bolus.

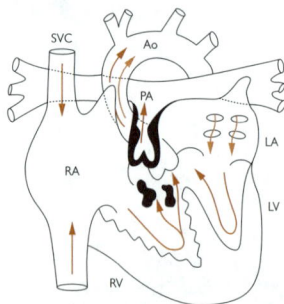

Figure 29.5 Tetralogy of Fallot. The RV outflow obstruction can be subvalvular, valvular, or supravalvular. The aorta is overriding both ventricles and there is a VSD.

Surgical management

- The choice is between initial palliation with a systemic to pulmonary shunt followed by a complete repair when the baby is older, versus early complete repair.
- Complete repair involves closure of the VSD and relief of the RVOTO utilizing a trans-annular patch, which involves a right ventriculotomy.
- Right ventricular dysfunction is a particular problem after repair and a degree of pulmonary regurgitation is almost always present.
- Junctional ectopic tachycardia (JET) is a particular risk after complete correction.

Anaesthetic considerations for repair

- Patients may or may not have previously had a systemic to PA shunt.
- If presenting for complete correction with no systemic pulmonary shunt, likely to be a neonate or small infant.
- Presence of a shunt reduces the risk of hypercyanotic spell during anaesthesia.
- Sedative premedication is more helpful in those at risk of a hypercyanotic episode.
- Both IV and inhalational induction are appropriate.
- Right ventricular dysfunction as well as pulmonary regurgitation may be postoperative problems.
- Excessive use of inotropes may worsen RVOTO postoperatively by dynamic narrowing of RVOT.
- Milrinone may be particularly useful as it promotes diastolic relaxation of the stiff right ventricle.
- Pyrexia and excessive ß-adrenergic stimulation may contribute to development of JET postoperatively.
- Perioperative echocardiography is useful in assessing repair and RV function.

Transposition of the great arteries (TGA)

6% of CHD.

Pathophysiology

- Usually an isolated lesion and is rarely associated with extra-cardiac anomalies.
- Aorta arises from the right ventricle and the pulmonary artery arises from the left ventricle. This is described as ventriculo-arterial (V-A) discordance.
- Parallel circulations rather than normal series circulation, therefore babies are cyanosed (Figure 29.6).
- Some mixing of circulations does occur through the PDA or through a VSD, which is present in approximately 25% of cases.
- If mixing is inadequate, balloon atrial septostomy is performed in the neonatal period.
- Pulmonary vascular disease develops early.
- At risk of developing pulmonary hypertensive crises in the postoperative period.
- Untreated, most will die in the first year of life from hypoxia and heart failure.

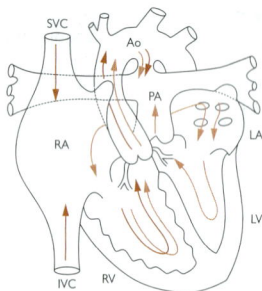

Figure 29.6 Transposition of the great arteries. The aorta arises from the RV and the PA arises from the LV, creating two parallel circuits. Mixing of the two circuits occurs via the PDA in this figure.

Surgical options

- In TGA with intact ventricular septum the left ventricle is exposed to the low pressure of the pulmonary circulation and becomes deconditioned. In this situation arterial switch operation (ASO) is performed early in the neonatal period, to minimize this deconditioning.
- An unrestrictive VSD exposes both the left and right ventricles to systemic blood pressure and the left ventricle is better conditioned to perform the work of the systemic ventricle after ASO. Surgery is less urgent although is still performed early.

Arterial switch operation (ASO) (Figure 29.7)

- Operation of choice if anatomy allows.
- Transection of main arterial trunks distal to their respective valves and 'switching' them to produce ventricular-arterial concordance.
- Origins of the coronary arteries are moved from the 'old' aorta to the neo-aorta.
- Normal anatomy and physiology is therefore restored.
- Good coronary transfer is the major determinate of outcome.
- Children with a good repair can expect a normal life.

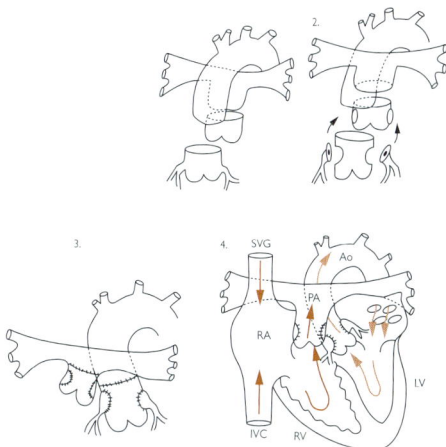

Figure 29.7 Arterial switch operation. The main arterial trunks are transected. The PA is moved anterior to the aorta. The coronary buttons are attached to the neo-aorta.

Anaesthetic considerations

- Neonate.
- Inhalational or IV induction.
- Invasive arterial and central venous lines required.
- Post-CPB myocardial dysfunction:
  - Inherently poor LV.
  - Poor myocardial protection.
  - Inadequate coronary transfer.
  - Coronary air.
- Risk of postoperative pulmonary hypertension.
- Inotropes are almost always required. Commonly enoximone or milrinone and dopamine or epinephrine.
- A left atrial monitoring line is placed after CPB.
- Left ventricle poorly compliant postoperatively. Fluid given slowly.
- Post-bypass coagulopathy common.

Truncus arteriosus

Rare; 1% of CHD (0.7 per 1000 live births).

Pathophysiology (Figure 29.8)

- Common arterial outlet for the aorta and pulmonary artery associated with a single truncal valve that is usually incompetent and may be stenotic, plus a VSD.
- Three types described depending on how the PAs arise from the aorta and on the size of the aorta.
- Mixing of blood at the arterial level with a resultant high pulmonary blood flow, heart failure, and high risk of pulmonary vascular disease.
- Surgery performed early to prevent pulmonary vascular disease from becoming irreversible.
- Associated with DiGeorge syndrome and irradiated blood products should be used and calcium levels carefully monitored.

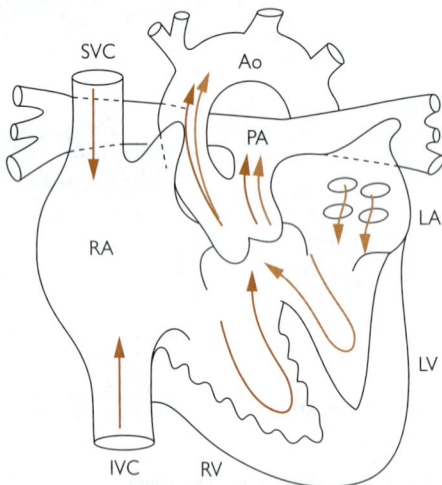

Figure 29.8 Truncus arteriosus. A common truncal valve gives rise to both aorta and PA.

Surgical management

- Separation of systemic from pulmonary circulation and closure of the VSD with disconnection of pulmonary arteries from aorta and repair of truncal valve.
- Right ventricle is connected to PAs with a valved conduit.
- Deep hypothermic circulatory arrest often required.
- High perioperative mortality (5–25%).
- Risk factors include truncal valve stenosis, coronary abnormalities, and low birth weight.

Anaesthetic considerations

- Small neonate in the first month of life.
- High-risk procedure.
- Presence of heart failure.
- Risk of postoperative pulmonary hypertension.
- Often intubated and ventilated preoperatively and may already be on inotropic support.
- If not ventilated, premedication is probably best avoided.
- Invasive lines required.
- Circulatory arrest may be required.
- Post-bypass coagulopathy common.
- Postoperative inotropic support.

Anomalous pulmonary venous connections

2.5% of CHD.

Pathophysiology

- Either total anomalous pulmonary venous connection (TAPVC) or partial anomalous pulmonary venous connection (PAPVC).
- Anomalous veins may be obstructed leading to high pulmonary venous pressure.
- Three types of TAPVC exist: supracardiac, cardiac, and infracardiac.
- Supracardiac TAPVC (Figure 29.9): The pulmonary veins connect to the SVC via an ascending vertical vein.
- Cardiac TAPVC (Figure 29.10): The pulmonary veins connect to the right atrium via the coronary sinus.
- Infracardiac TAPVC (Figure 29.11): Pulmonary veins connect to the IVC via a common vein, which traverses the diaphragm.
- An ASD is always present.
- These infants are usually cyanosed and may be in heart failure. Pulmonary hypertension and pulmonary oedema may be present.

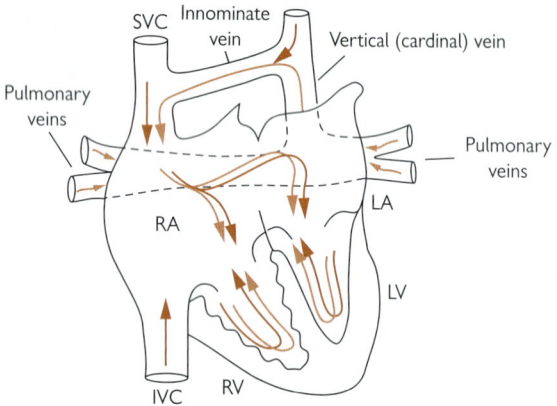

Figure 29.9 Supracardiac TAPVC (great vessels removed). Oxygenated blood from the pulmonary veins drains to RA via the innominate vein.

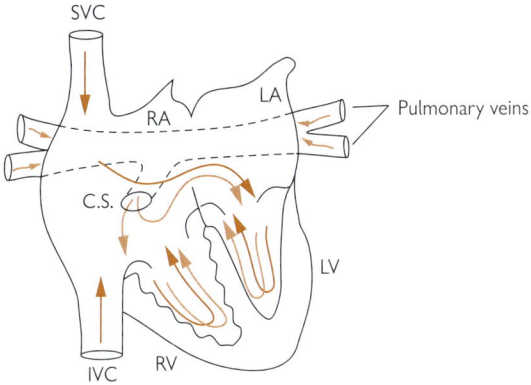

Figure 29.10 Cardiac TAPVC (great vessels not shown). Oxygenated blood from the pulmonary veins drains via coronary sinus to the RA.

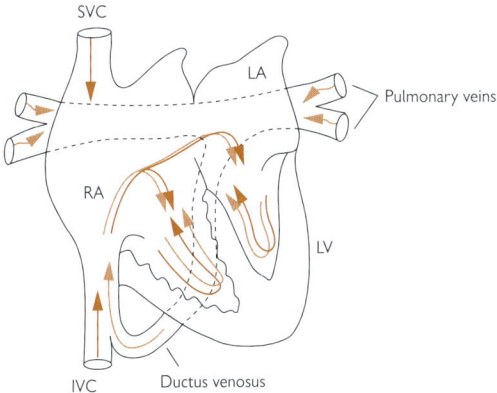

Figure 29.11 Infracardiac TAPVC (great vessels not shown). Oxygenated blood from the pulmonary veins drains to RA via ductus venosus.

Anaesthetic considerations

- May be a neonate.
- Heart failure present.
- Pulmonary oedema may be present.
- Risk of pulmonary hypertension both pre- and postoperatively. Nitric oxide may be required after surgery.
- Deep hypothermic circulatory arrest often required.
- Post-bypass coagulopathy.

Hypoplastic left heart syndrome

Incidence of hypoplastic left heart syndrome (HLHS) in the United States is about 2 per 10,000 live births. In Europe this figure is lower as termination is more common.

The prognosis of patients with HLHS has improved dramatically in recent years. Previously, virtually all babies died, whilst today in the better centres many children survive into childhood. The longer-term outlook has not been fully determined but many hurdles remain.

Pathophysiology

Anatomical features of HLHS include (Figure 29.12):
- Hypoplastic left ventricle.
- Mitral stenosis or atresia.
- Aortic stenosis or atresia.
- Hypoplastic aortic arch.
- Duct-dependent circulation.
- Atrial septal defect.
- Pulmonary venous blood returns to the left atrium and the majority passes through the ASD to RA, mixes with systemic venous blood, and then proceeds to RV and PA. The aorta is supplied from the PDA as there is very little antegrade flow from the LV.
- A fall in pulmonary vascular resistance (PVR) causes systemic hypoperfusion and acidosis whilst an increase in PVR results in low pulmonary blood flow and increasing cyanosis.

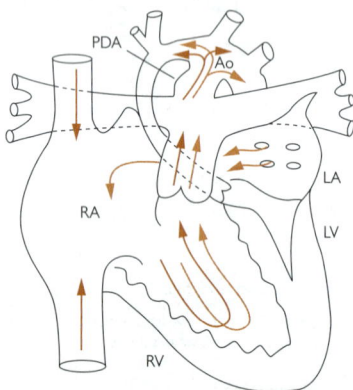

Figure 29.12 Hypoplastic left heart syndrome. The LV, mitral valve, aortic valve, and aorta are all hypoplastic. Systemic blood flow is provided via the PDA.

Diagnosis

Prenatal diagnosis is common but may be difficult and is occasionally missed. Infants present with tachypnoea, tachycardia, and cyanosis, and a systolic murmur can be heard.

Surgical management

The aim of surgical treatment is to convert the anatomy into a single ventricle-type circulation in which the right ventricle becomes the single systemic ventricle and the pulmonary blood flow is supplied passively from the SVC and IVC (Fontan circulation). This is done by a series of three operations known as the Norwood stage I, Norwood stage II (Glenn shunt), and Norwood stage III (Fontan).

Norwood Stage I (Figure 29.13)

Performed in the neonatal period. The main PA is transected just below the bifurcation. The aortic arch is reconstructed so that it arises from the transected pulmonary trunk. The pulmonary valve becomes the neo-aortic valve. The pulmonary blood supply is provided from either a shunt from the subclavian artery (BT shunt) or from a conduit arising from the right ventricle (Sano modification).

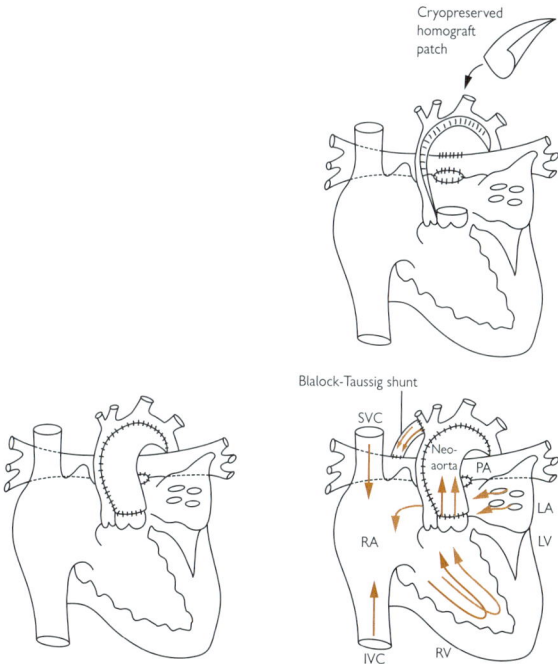

Figure 29.13 Steps in the Norwood Stage I operation. The main PA is transected. The aortic arch is reconstructed using pulmonary homograft tissue. The ASD is enlarged to allow unobstructed flow of blood from LA to RA. Pulmonary blood supply is via a BT shunt from subclavian artery to PA.

Anaesthetic implications

- Understanding HLHS physiology is essential.
- Aim to maintain the balance between systemic and pulmonary circulation by manipulating PVR and SVR.
- Prior to anaesthesia babies are best managed breathing spontaneously in air. If ventilation required, maintain normal/high arterial CO_2 and low oxygen concentrations, usually air.
- Prostaglandin infusion to maintain ductal patency pre-surgery.
- Air should be available for transfer to theatre or a self-inflating bag can be used.
- High-dose opioid technique is preferred.
- Central venous access via the femoral veins or umbilical veins. The internal jugular is avoided as narrowing of the SVC would jeopardize the Glenn shunt (Stage II Norwood).
- Deep hypothermic circulatory arrest may be required.
- Postoperative myocardial dysfunction is common and inotropes are required. Milrinone and epinephrine are commonly used.
- Balancing systemic and pulmonary blood supply is also important post-bypass.
- Post-bypass coagulopathy usual.
- The sternum is frequently left open and closure delayed for several days.

Ventricular septal defect (VSD) and atrioventricular septal defect (AVSD)

VSD (Figure 29.14)

- Most common congenital defect in children, occurring in 1.5–3.5 per 1000 live births and accounting for 20% of CHD.
- Many VSDs now closed using a percutaneous, transcatheter device.

Pathophysiology

- Four types are described: subarterial (5%), perimembranous (80%), inlet (5%), and muscular (10%).
- 'Restrictive' if flow through the VSD is small and 'unrestrictive' if flow is large.
- The haemodynamic effects associated with VSD include left to right shunting at ventricular level resulting in high pulmonary blood flow, volume-loaded right heart, heart failure, and the risk of pulmonary vascular disease.

Anaesthetic considerations

- May be in heart failure.
- Hyperventilation and high oxygen concentrations reduce PVR and can increase blood flow to the lungs.
- Inotropic support may be required postoperatively.
- Postoperative pulmonary hypertension may be a problem.

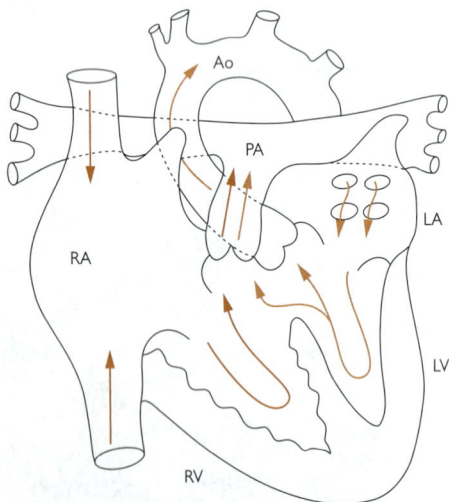

Figure 29.14 Ventricular septal defect. The shunt is usually left to right resulting in increased pulmonary blood flow.

AVSD

- 0.2 per 1000 live births (3% of CHD).
- May be associated with other cardiac lesions and DiGeorge syndrome.

Pathophysiology

- Also known as AV canal defects or endocardial cushion defects and are commonly associated with trisomy 21.
- Two common types of AVSD exist:
  - Partial AVSD. A primum ASD with a cleft in the anterior mitral valve leaflet.
  - Complete AVSD. A large septal defect with both atrial and ventricular components and a common AV valve (Figure 29.15).
- The haemodynamic effects associated with AVSD include shunting at atrial or ventricular level resulting in heart failure, and the risk of pulmonary vascular disease and AV valve regurgitation.

Anaesthetic considerations

- If the patient has trisomy 21 the anaesthetic implications of this need to be managed.
- May be in heart failure.
- Hyperventilation and high oxygen concentrations reduce PVR and can increase blood flow to the lungs.
- Inotropes are frequently required.
- Postoperative pulmonary hypertension may occur.
- TOE is useful in assessing repair, particularly of left A-V valve.

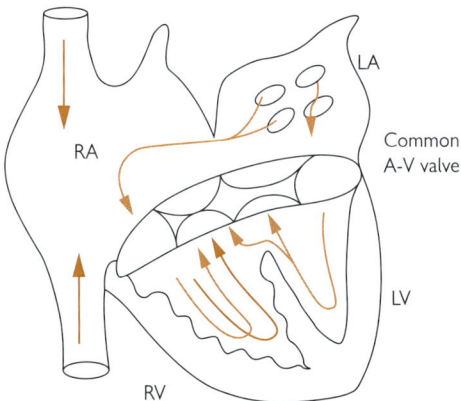

Figure 29.15 Atrioventricular septal defect (AVSD) (great vessels removed). There is a common AV valve, an ASD, and VSD.

Interrupted aortic arch

1% of CHD.

Pathophysiology

- Disruption of the aorta between the ascending and descending aorta.
- Three types exist, depending on the level at which the disruption takes place. A PDA is present supplying the descending aorta (Figure 29.16).
- VSD usually present.
- Commonly associated with 22q11 deletion resulting in the DiGeorge syndrome.
- Prostaglandin infusion required to maintain ductal patency.
- Babies are sick with progressive acidosis and poor cardiac output.
- Surgical repair.
- One- or two-stage repair depending on the associated lesions, particularly the presence or absence of a VSD.
- The single-stage repair involves reconstruction of the arch and closure of the VSD.
- A two-stage repair involves repair of the aortic arch and banding of the PA to limit pulmonary blood flow. The VSD is closed later.
- Deep hypothermic circulatory arrest is used for the arch reconstruction. Some centres use selective regional perfusion to try and limit neurological injury.
- Surgical mortality is high and is increased with small size, preoperative acidosis, and associated cardiac lesions.
- Later reoperation likely to deal with recurrent LVOTO.
- Later restenosis of the repaired aortic arch can be dilated with a transluminal balloon.

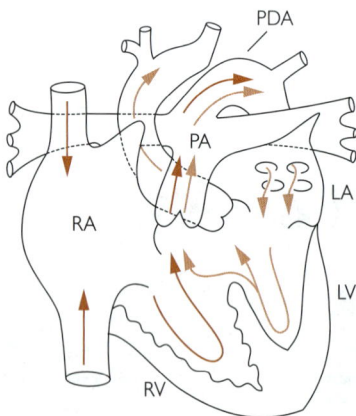

Figure 29.16 Example of interrupted aortic arch with VSD (type B). Blood to the descending aorta is via the PDA.

Anaesthetic implications
- Sick neonate, often small for dates and/or premature.
- DiGeorge syndrome (particularly hypocalcaemia and need for irradiated blood products).
- High-dose narcotic technique usual.
- Ideally monitor blood pressure above and below interruption. Often difficult in practice.
- Deep hypothermic circulatory is used.
- Post-bypass coagulopathy common.
- Anticipate poor renal function postoperatively.
- Risk of postoperative pulmonary hypertensive crises.

Aortic stenosis (AS)

- 10% of CHD.
- Severe critical aortic stenosis in neonates occurs in about one in ten of cases of aortic stenosis and requires urgent treatment.

Pathophysiology

- Obstruction to the left ventricular outflow tract (LVOT) can occur either at the valvular, subvalvular, or supravalvular area.
- There is an imbalance between oxygen supply and demand.
- Risk of left ventricular hypertrophy and LV failure. Risk of sudden death.
- Age of presentation is a risk factor, with younger children being most at risk.
- Two thirds of those presenting in the first three months of life will require either inotropic or ventilatory support before treatment.
- Supravalvular aortic stenosis is commonly associated with William's syndrome.

Treatment options

- Depends on age, severity, and type of lesion.
- Critical aortic stenosis in the neonate requires urgent valvuloplasty. Options include: surgery with CPB, or transluminal balloon angioplasty.
- In older children various surgical approaches are used depending on the anatomy.
- Transluminal balloon valvuloplasty is also common in the older age group.
- Valve replacement either with mechanical valves or bioprosthetic valves is delayed as long as possible because of long-term problems associated with anticoagulation needed with mechanical valves and because of inevitable calcification of bioprosthetic valves.
- Another option, the Ross procedure, involves using the pulmonary valve in the aortic position, and using a homograft in the pulmonary position. The need for reoperation with the Ross procedure is reduced because the systemic valve (neo-aortic valve) grows with the patient and calcification of the homograft in the pulmonary position is slow. In addition there is no need for anticoagulation.
- The most common complications of valvuloplasty are aortic incompetence or residual aortic stenosis.

Transluminal balloon valvuloplasty

- Crossing the aortic valve with a balloon catheter often results in dramatic cardiovascular changes, with myocardial ischaemia and bradycardia.
- Urgent resuscitation may be required.
- Post-procedure ventilation may be required and ventricular function may be poor.
- Invasive arterial monitoring is useful.

Anaesthetic considerations

- Principal aim of anaesthesia is to maintain the oxygen supply and demand balance:
  - Maintain normal heart rate.
  - Maintain SVR to preserve coronary perfusion.
  - Avoid hypertension (increased oxygen consumption).
  - Avoid myocardial depression.
- Anaesthesia for neonates having surgery with CPB is similar to other neonatal cardiac surgery.
- Post-bypass myocardial dysfunction common. Inotropic support usually required.

Coarctation of the aorta

5% of CHD.

Pathophysiology

- Discrete narrowing of the aorta.
- May be preductal, juxtaductal, or postductal depending on the relationship to the ductus arteriosus (DA). The most common form presenting in the neonatal period is the preductal type.
- Preductal coarctation is associated with minimal collateral circulation below the coarctation and requires prostaglandin in order to maintain ductal patency.
- Both juxtaductal and postductal coarctation are characterized by the development of collateral vessels that supply the area below the coarctation. This is important as the spinal cord is supplied by these collaterals and it is these vessels that supply the spinal cord during aortic cross-clamping.
- In practical terms these children fall into two groups. One group presents in the neonatal period with preductal coarctation with few collaterals and very poor LV function. The second group present later and have well-developed collaterals and better LV function.

Anaesthesia for neonatal repair

- These infants are usually sick, with poor LV function, heart failure, and progressive acidosis.
- Some babies may be intubated and ventilated and may be on an inotropic support.
- IV access will often already be established in order to give prostaglandin. This can be used for induction. It is the authors' preference to give incremental doses of fentanyl (up to 5 µg/kg), then muscle relaxant, and supplement this with a very low dose of isoflurane (0.3–0.5%). This can be omitted if hypotension ensues.
- Inotropes may be required prior to surgery.
- Ideally, the arterial line should be situated in the right arm to allow blood pressure measurement during arterial cross-clamping. The left subclavian may be partially obstructed during the repair. Some have advocated an arterial line below the coarctation as well, to measure perfusion pressure during cross-clamping, but this may be very difficult in practice as femoral pulses are usually absent.
- Surgery usually takes place through a left thoracotomy without the use of CPB. The lung will be retracted and ventilation may be problematical. The endotracheal tube should have no leak because a tube with a large leak will make ventilation very difficult during lung retraction.
- Paraplegia is a risk and is thought to be due to hypoperfusion during aortic cross-clamping. To reduce the chance of spinal cord damage, babies should be cooled to about 34°C before the cross-clamp is applied, ventilated to normocarbia, and upper limb blood pressure maintained. Low-dose anticoagulation may also be used. A short cross-clamp time is also thought to be important.

- Epidural anaesthesia has been used but its use is not widespread.
- Postoperative hypertension may be a problem and a vasodilator such as sodium nitroprusside may be required.

Anaesthesia in the older child

- Usually these children are not as sick as the neonates.
- Right arm arterial line and CVP.
- A careful IV induction with a combination of fentanyl and an induction agent of choice is usual. Etomidate is a good agent because of its cardiovascular stability.
- Although a collateral blood supply is present the spinal cord is at risk and cooling to 34°C is advised.
- An oral cuffed tube is useful as early extubation is the norm.
- Postoperative hypertension is a frequent problem and good analgesia combined with sodium nitroprusside and ß-blockers is often required. Many children, perhaps up to 30%, will go on to have long-term hypertension that will require therapy.
- Increasingly some of these cases are dealt with by balloon angioplasty with or without stent placement. Rupture of the aorta is a risk in these patients and the institution in which the procedure is undertaken should be in a position to deal with this if it were to occur.

Three common paediatric cardiac surgical procedures

- Blalock-Taussig shunt.
- Glenn shunt.
- Fontan operation (total cavo-pulmonary connection or TCPC).

Blalock-Taussig shunt (BT shunt) (Figure 29.17)

- The BT shunt is used to improve pulmonary blood supply and alleviate severe cyanosis.
- A GoreTex tube is anastamosed between the subclavian artery and one of the main PAs. This can be done on either the left or right side.
- It is usually a short-term palliation before a more definitive repair is undertaken.
- It is most commonly undertaken in the neonatal period.
- It may be performed through a thoracotomy or via a median sternotomy and does not require cardiopulmonary bypass.

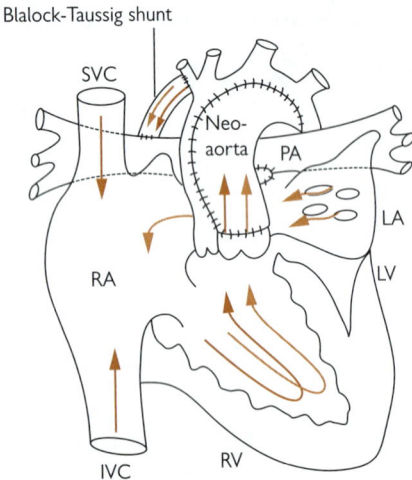

Figure 29.17 Blalock-Taussig shunt (in this case as part of Norwood I repair).

Glenn shunt (Figure 29.18)

- This is a connection between the SVC and the PA.
- It provides pulmonary blood flow but the blood flow to the lungs is entirely passive and at systemic venous pressure.
- It is essential that the PA pressures are low.
- It is performed via a median sternotomy and does require cardiopulmonary bypass.

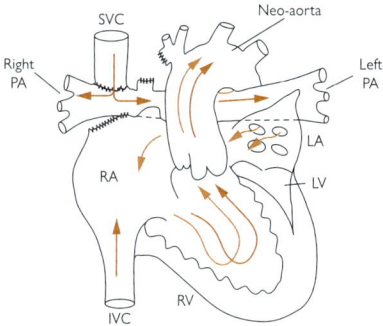

Figure 29.18 Glenn shunt. The SVC is connected to the RPA.

Fontan circulation (TCPC, Figure 29.19)

- The Glenn shunt may have previously been performed.
- The IVC is connected to the PA via a conduit. The conduit commonly runs from extracardiac although intracardiac conduits are also performed.
- This results in a single ventricle physiology where the systemic blood supply is from a functional or actual single ventricle.
- The pulmonary blood is now all passively supplied via the SVC and IVC. This circulation depends on a low pulmonary pressure for success as all the flow to the lungs is passive.
- Surgery is performed through a median sternotomy and requires cardiopulmonary bypass.

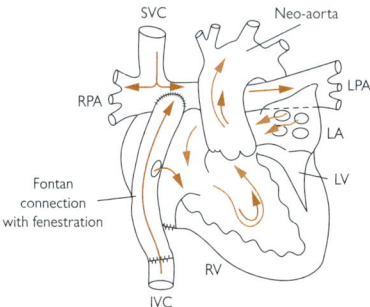

Figure 29.19 Fontan circulation. The SVC is connected to the RPA and the IVC is also connected to the PA. In this example there is a small fenestration between the conduit and the RA. This allows shunting of blood if the PA pressures rise and cardiac output is thus maintained, albeit with increased cyanosis because of right to left shunt.

Cardiac catheterization and interventional cardiology

- Cardiac catheterization was until quite recently the mainstay of cardiac imaging.
- Diagnostic cardiac catheterization is used to acquire anatomical images, pressures, and pressure gradients and to measure oxygen saturation to calculate shunts and cardiac output.
- Advances in echocardiography and MRI imaging have reduced the number of diagnostic cardiac catheterizations.
- The number of interventional procedures is increasing.

Interventional cardiac catheterization (ICC)

- First reported ICC was the atrial balloon septostomy in 1966.
- Since then the repertoire of the interventional cardiologists has increased dramatically.

Interventional procedures

Balloon atrial septostomy:

- Performed in neonates with transposition of the great arteries.
- Balloon-tipped catheter is passed across the atrial septum and the balloon is inflated and then pulled back across the atrial septum. This creates an ASD, allowing better mixing and improving arterial saturation.

Occlusion procedures

- These include the closure of PDAs, ASDs, and some VSDs.
- Balloon dilation of valves:
  - The pulmonary and aortic valves are most commonly dilated using a balloon, but the mitral valve can also be treated in this way.
  - One of the most challenging balloon procedures is the dilation of the aortic valve in neonates with critical aortic stenosis. These patients are frequently very ill and already ventilated in ICU with inotropic support. Surgical treatment of these neonates has poor results and balloon valvotomy is the palliation of choice.

Balloon dilation of arteries with and without stents

- Dilation of pulmonary arteries is most common.
- Dilation of obstructions to the aorta, particularly after previous surgery (coarctation repair or arch reconstruction).
- Dilation of native aortic coarctation is controversial because of the high incidence of recurrence and because of the risk of rupture during dilation. However, the ballooning of re-coarctation of the aorta is more successful. The indication for stent placement in these patients is still being debated.

Embolization procedures

These procedures are carried out to occlude unwanted vascular connections such as aortopulmonary collaterals or previously placed BT shunts.

Risks

- The overall rate of adverse events is in the order of 8–10%.
- Closure of a PDA or ASD had the lowest event rate (4%).
- Highest event rate (11.6%) is in other interventional procedures.
- Diagnostic cardiac catheters have a rate of about 9%.
- A higher complication rate of 14% exists for those under one year compared with those over a year (7%).
- Adverse events include:
  - Arrhythmias.
  - Myocardial perforation.
  - Hypotension.
  - Air embolism.
  - Reaction to contrast or other drugs.

Anaesthetic considerations

- General anaesthesia most common in UK.
- Sedation common in USA. Often administered by cardiologist following guidelines.
- Cardiac catheterization suites are frequently in remote sites.
- Careful preoperative review to understand pathophysiology.
- Premedication if indicated.
- Induction can be inhalational or IV.
- Endotracheal intubation with positive pressure ventilation most commonly used.
- Secure IV access.
- Active warming for small infants and temperature monitoring.
- Antibiotics according to local protocols.
- Arms frequently positioned above the head (care of brachial plexus).
- Standard monitors. Some require invasive monitoring. $ETCO_2$ is particularly useful because it quickly reflects changes in cardiac output and pulmonary blood flow.

Paediatric cardiac transplantation

Outcomes in children receiving heart transplants has improved in recent years to such an extent that heart transplantation has become an acceptable form of treatment. The majority of transplants take place in children over the age of one year but 25% are carried out in the under-ones.

The indications for transplantation are:
- Congenital heart disease that cannot be repaired and cardiomyopathy.
- In those less than a year the majority of transplants are carried out for CHD, usually HLHS.
- In those over one year of age the main indication is cardiomyopathy.

Cardiomyopathy
- Cardiomyopathy is rare and affects around 1:100,000 children per year.
- Classified either as dilated, hypertrophic cardiomyopathy (HCM) or restrictive cardiomyopathy.
- Pulmonary hypertension is common because of increased pulmonary venous congestion secondary to high LA pressure.

Contraindications for transplantation
- Pulmonary vascular resistance greater than 6 wood units/m^2 that is unresponsive to pulmonary vasodilators (oxygen, nitric oxide, and intravenous agents).
- Active malignancy.
- Multiple organ failure.
- Severe systemic disease.
- Severe sepsis.

Matching donor to recipient
Several criteria used:
- Blood type.
- Size of donor compared with recipient. This does not need to be an exact match and frequently the donor organ is large for the recipient.
- Urgency of recipient's need and length of wait, including need for mechanical support.

Donor shortage
- There is a critical shortage of donor organs in paediatrics.
- Difficult decisions about the use of 'marginal donor organs'.
- The use of high-dose inotropic support or a history of prolonged cardiac arrest would not necessarily mean that organs would not be considered.

Organizational aspects
- Logistics surrounding heart transplantation are considerable.
- Transplant co-ordinator is responsible for the logistics.

- Challenges include:
  - Coordinating retrieval of the organ.
  - Arranging admission of the recipient and ensuring that the recipient is in theatre at a time that allows the retrieved organ to be implanted without delay.
  - Ischaemic times for the donor heart are increasing as better myocardial preservation techniques are used. Four hours was once used as the limit for cold ischaemic time but this has been challenged and ischaemic times of as much as ten hours have been reported. There does appear to be evidence that ischaemic times of up to eight hours are not associated with adverse outcomes.

Anaesthetic management

- Many patients are very unwell and may be ventilated or on inotropic support.
- A small number of these patients will be on extracorporeal membrane oxygenation (ECMO) or other mechanical support such as a left ventricular assist device (LVAD). Moving these patients to theatre from the ICU can be challenging.
- Careful preoperative review is important. It is essential that the anaesthetist has a clear understanding of the pathophysiology of the recipient.
- Close liaison with the transplant co-ordinator is important.
- Monitoring should include central venous and arterial catheters.
- Induction depends on the individual patient. Etomidate is frequently chosen as the IV induction agent.
- Anaesthesia is usually based on a high-dose narcotic technique.
- Local protocol for immunosuppression and antibiotics.
- Inotropes usually required post-bypass. Milrinone is frequently used in combination with a ß-adrenergic drug such as dopamine or adrenaline.
- The transplanted heart is denervated and will have a relatively slow heart rate. Isoprenaline or atrial pacing is usually employed to increase the heart rate to a desirable level. The use of atrial pacing is usually preferred as the use of isoprenaline in combination with milrinone may lead to hypotension.
- Pulmonary hypertension may be a problem post-bypass and good ventilation is essential to optimize arterial PCO_2 and PO_2. Nitric oxide may be required.
- TOE is useful in assessing post-bypass cardiac function and optimizing fluid and inotrope management.

Postoperative problems

- Bleeding.
- Pulmonary hypertension.
- Renal failure. Some renal impairment can be expected in up to 20% of patients post-transplant.
- Poor ventricular function.

Outcomes after heart transplantation

- Early morbidity and mortality is related to preoperative condition and age.
- Causes of death after transplantation include acute rejection, graft failure, and infection. Later, coronary artery disease becomes a problem along with an increased risk of malignancy.
- Survival is constantly improving as immunosuppression therapy improves.

Further reading

1. Abdul-Khaliq H, Uhlig R, Bottcher W, Ewert P, exi-Meskishvili V, Lange PE. Factors influencing the change in cerebral hemodynamics in pediatric patients during and after corrective cardiac surgery of congenital heart diseases by means of full-flow cardiopulmonary bypass. *Perfusion* 2002; 17: 179–185.

2. Bennett D, Marcus R, Stokes M. Incidents and complications during paediatric cardiac catheterisation. *Paediatric Anaesthesia* 2005; 15: 1083–1088.

3. Berman EB, Barst RJ. Eisenmenger's syndrome: Current management. *Progress in Cardiovascular Diseases* 2002; 45: 129–138.

4. Elkins RC, Lane MM, McCue C. Ross operation in children: Late results. *Journal of Heart Valve Disease* 2001; 10: 736–741.

5. Freed DH, Robertson CM, Sauve RS, et al. Intermediate-term outcomes of the arterial switch operation for transposition of great arteries in neonates: Alive but well? *Journal of Thoracic and Cardiovascular Surgery* 2006; 132: 45–52.

6. Hein R, Buscheck F, Fischer E, et al. Atrial and ventricular septal defects can safely be closed by percutaneous intervention. *Journal of Interventional Cardiology* 2005; 18: 515–522.

7. Jonas RA. Deep hypothermic circulatory arrest: Current status and indications. *Seminars in Thoracic and Cardiovascular Surgery* 2006; 5: 76–88.

8. Kang N, Cole T, Tsang V, Elliott M, de Leval M. Risk stratification in paediatric open-heart surgery. *European Journal of Cardiothoracic Surgery* 2004; 26: 3–11.

9. Kloth RL, Baum VC. Very early extubation in children after cardiac surgery. *Critical Care Medicine* 2002; 30: 787–791.

10. Maron BJ. Hypertrophic cardiomyopathy in childhood. *Pediatric Clinics of North America* 2004; 51: 1305–1346.

Adult congenital heart disease

Dr M Barnard and Dr B Martin

Introduction *470*
Assessment *471*
Terminology *472*
Classification *474*
Pathophysiology *476*
Specific lesions *478*
Sequelae *486*
Management *488*
Endocarditis *490*
Further reading *491*

Introduction

In the future there will be more adults than children with congenital heart disease – this already applies to tetralogy of Fallot, which is the commonest of the cyanotic lesions. Fewer than 20% of patients with congenital heart disease would survive to adult life without treatment. There is an increasing population of patients with adult congenital heart disease who require long-term follow-up.

Completely normal cardiovascular anatomy and physiology is rarely achieved by corrective surgery during childhood. One important principle is that patients have had their cardiac lesions *repaired – not cured*. Many patients will continue to manifest residua of their underlying pathology and/or sequelae of therapeutic interventions.

Assessment

A simple pathophysiologic approach involves four questions:

1) Is cyanosis present?

This implies right to left shunting, although pulmonary blood flow is not necessarily reduced. Systemic oxygen saturation is determined by pulmonary venous saturation, systemic venous saturation, and the relative proportion of both types of venous blood represented in the arterial blood. In contrast to the normal circulation, factors that influence systemic venous saturation will affect arterial saturations.

2) If there is shunting of blood, what are its consequences?

Shunting may be left to right, right to left, or mixing in a common chamber. This causes volume overload, chamber enlargement, hypertrophy, and decreased cardiac reserve. Pulmonary blood flow may be excessive or inadequate.

3) Is the pulmonary circulation dependent upon a shunt or connection?

Such a connection may be a limiting factor when cardiac output or demand is increased. Systemic saturations will depend on pulmonary to systemic flow ratio and mixed venous oxygen saturation.

4) What are the structure and function of the systemic and pulmonary ventricles?

There may be congenital and acquired abnormalities of ventricular structure and function. The systemic ventricle may be morphologically right or left.

Risk

- Higher perioperative risk is probably conferred by:
  - Chronic hypoxaemia.
  - Pulmonary to systemic blood flow ratio greater than 2:1.
  - Elevated pulmonary vascular resistance.
  - Secondary erythrocytosis.
  - Ventricular outflow tract obstruction with a gradient more than 50 mmHg.
- Recent heart failure, syncope, or substantial deterioration in exercise tolerance are concerns.
- Pulmonary hypertension carries significant risks.
- Endocarditis is a risk in nearly all corrected and uncorrected lesions, and appropriate antibiotic prophylaxis should be employed.

Terminology

Table 30.1 Some commonly used terms in congenital heart disease

Term	Definition
ASD	Atrial septal defect. Commonly classified into ostium primum (partial AVSD), ostium secundum, and sinus venosus.
	Ostium primum defects are defects in the inferior septum and comprise the atrial component of AVSD. Secundum defects are absences in the oval fossa region. Sinus venosus defects occur around the superior atrio-caval junction and are associated with pulmonary veins draining anomalously to the superior vena cava.
AVSD	Atrioventricular septal defect, often called AV canal defect or endocardial cushion defect. Defect including primum septal defect and separate atrioventricular orifices (partial), or primum septal defect, ventricular septal defect, and common atrioventricular orifice (complete), or intermediate forms.
Balanced circulation	Relatively equal systemic and pulmonary blood flow.
Blalock-Taussig shunt	Connection of subclavian artery to ipsilateral pulmonary artery. Classical shunt involved transection of subclavian artery and end to side anastomosis to pulmonary artery. Modified Blalock-Taussig shunt uses synthetic interposition graft. Used to increase pulmonary blood flow, albeit using inefficient recirculation of systemic blood.
Concordance	Connection of two structures on the same side morphologically – left atria to left ventricle or right ventricle to pulmonary artery.
Discordance	Connection of morphologically left structure to morphologically right structure – e.g. left ventricle to pulmonary artery.
Double inlet ventricle	Both atrioventricular valves (or greater than 50% of each) connect to one ventricle. Usually left ventricle.
Double outlet ventricle	Both great vessels (or greater than 50% of each) arise from one ventricle. Usually right ventricle.
Fenestration	Surgically-created hole in atrial or ventricular septum or intracardiac baffle. Diverts proportion of blood from right to left heart in situations where normal passage through the lungs is prevented by elevated pulmonary resistance. Cardiac output thereby maintained or increased – at the expense of cyanosis.
Fontan	Surgeon who described the Fontan procedure. Now usually refers to circulatory arrangement whereby systemic veins are connected to the pulmonary arteries – without a right ventricle. The connection may be intracardiac or extracardiac.

Term	Definition
Glenn	Cavo-pulmonary shunt. Connection of the superior vena cava to the pulmonary artery. Bidirectional Glenn refers to connection to joined right and left pulmonary arteries.
Hemitruncus	Right or left pulmonary artery from aorta.
Konno	Enlargement of aortic annulus and left ventricular outflow tract.
Left SVC	Persistence of connection between left subclavian vein and left internal jugular vein with coronary sinus. Coronary sinus usually dilated, and if unroofed or fenestrated associated with intracardiac left to right shunt.
Malposition	Malposition of the atrial or ventricular septum that results in valve overriding the septum.
Mustard	Intra-atrial switch procedure for transposition of the great arteries. Intra-atrial baffles direct pulmonary venous blood to the right ventricle and systemic venous blood to the left ventricle. Results in physiologically appropriate but anatomically incorrect circulation.
Overriding	Valve that is positioned over the ventricular septum.
Rastelli	VSD closure incorporating baffling mitral inflow to (malpositioned) aorta. External conduit or homograft to connect right ventricle to pulmonary artery.
Ross pulmonary autograft	Replacement of the aortic valve with native pulmonary valve. Replacement of the pulmonary valve with cadaveric homograft.
Senning	Similar to Mustard procedure. Intra-atrial baffling to redirect venous blood to the opposite ventricle in transposition of the great arteries.
Single outlet	Single vessel arising from the heart.
Single ventricle	One functional ventricle, although there is usually a second vestigial ventricle.
Straddling	Valve with attachments on both sides of the ventricular septum. Limits anatomical repair.
Transposition great arteries	Ventriculo-arterial discordance. Aorta from right ventricle, pulmonary artery from left ventricle.
Truncus arteriosus	Single arterial vessel arises from the heart. Systemic and pulmonary arteries branch from the single vessel.
Univentricular connection	Both atria connected to one ventricle. Connection is either via two valves or absence of one of the atrioventricular valves and an ASD.

Classification

- Cyanotic.
- Non-cyanotic.

Cyanotic patients often have more comorbid medical problems and experience greater numbers of perioperative complications than non-cyanotics.

- Simple.
- Intermediate.
- Complex.

Table 30.2 Classification of congenital heart lesions

Complex	Moderate	Simple
Conduits	Aorta-LV fistulae	Isolated aortic valve disease
Cyanotic	Anomalous pulmonary veins	Isolated mitral valve disease
Double outlet ventricle	AV canal defects	Isolated ASD
Eisenmenger	Coarctation	Small VSD
Fontan	Ebstein's anomaly	Mild pulmonary stenosis
Mitral atresia	Infundibular RVOTO	Repaired PDA
Single ventricle	Primum ASD	Repaired ASD
Pulmonary atresia	Unclosed PDA	Repaired VSD
Pulmonary vascular disease	Pulmonary regurgitation (moderate/severe)	
Transposition great arteries	Pulmonary stenosis (moderate/severe)	
Tricuspid atresia	Sinus valsalva fistula/aneurysm	
Truncus arteriosus	Sinus venosus ASD	
Other AV or VA connection abnormalities	Sub/supravalvar aortic stenosis	
	Tetralogy of Fallot	
	VSD with other lesion	

Pathophysiology

Table 30.3 Features of congenital heart disease

Primary	Secondary
Shunts	Arrhythmias
Stenotic lesions	Cyanosis
Regurgitant lesions	Infective endocarditis
	Myocardial ischaemia
	Paradoxical emboli
	Polycythaemia
	Pulmonary hypertension
	Ventricular dysfunction

Cyanosis and hyperviscosity
These are associated with:
- Hypoxaemia caused by either right to left shunting or mixing of pulmonary and systemic venous blood in a common chamber. The main adaptive response is secondary erythrocytosis. Blood viscosity increases with haematocrit. Preoperative venesection is no longer practised in the absence of symptomatic hyperviscosity. Haemoglobin concentrations may be greater than 19 preoperatively, and postoperatively drop to approximately 14.
- Brain abscesses.
- Impaired cognitive function.
- Chronic neurologic impairment.
- Aortopulmonary collateral arteries.
- Haematological abnormalities.
- Renal impairment.
- Myocardial scarring.
- Inadequate skin oxygenation and acne or skin infections.

Decreased pulmonary blood flow
Hypoxaemia is minimized by:
- Adequate hydration.
- Maintaining systemic arterial blood pressure.
- Minimizing elevations in pulmonary vascular resistance (avoiding hypercarbia and acidosis).
- Minimizing total oxygen consumption.
- In the presence of a systemic to pulmonary shunt (e.g. modified Blalock-Taussig), pulmonary blood flow is dependent on the size of the shunt and the pressure gradient across the shunt.

Mixing lesions

The peripheral arterial oxygen saturation is dependent on the pulmonary: systemic flow ratio ($Q_P:Q_S$):

$$\frac{Q_P}{Q_S} = \frac{S_aO_2 - S_{SV}O_2}{S_{PV}O_2 - S_{PA}O_2}$$

S_aO_2 = arterial saturation; $S_{SV}O_2$ = systemic venous saturation; $S_{PV}O_2$ = pulmonary venous saturation; $S_{PA}O_2$ = pulmonary artery saturation.

When Q_P is greater than Q_S, S_aO_2 will be higher, but systemic cardiac output will be lower. When Q_S is greater than Q_P, systemic saturations will be lower but cardiac output higher. Thus the systemic saturation can give a useful indication of $Q_P:Q_S$, subject to knowing mixed venous oxygen saturation.

Elevated Q_P (and low Q_S) in a mixing circulation will be suggested by:
- High S_aO_2.
- Systemic hypotension.
- Oliguria.
- Acidosis.
- Increased serum lactate.

If left sufficiently long, increased Q_P can result in characteristic histological changes in the pulmonary vasculature (pulmonary vascular disease).

Ventricular function

- Right ventricle dysfunction is seen more commonly.
- Reduced diastolic compliance is a feature of some right-sided lesions such as tetralogy of Fallot. An extreme is known as restrictive ventricular physiology, when the pulmonary valve opens during diastole as a result of atrial contraction.
- Systemic ventricular impairment may be congenital (systemic right ventricle, hypertrophic cardiomyopathy) or acquired (previous surgery).
- The haemodynamic impact of dynamic ventricular outflow obstruction may be reduced by a modest depression of ventricular function.

Arrhythmias

Patients with diastolic dysfunction or restrictive physiology, as well as those who have lesions that intrinsically limit ventricular filling (atrial switch procedures for transposition of great arteries – Mustard, Senning operations), tolerate loss of sinus rhythm or arrhythmias poorly. Active measures to return sinus rhythm (including early cardioversion) are instituted.

Specific lesions

Tetralogy of Fallot

- Commonest cyanotic lesion in older patients:
  - Ventricular septal defect (VSD).
  - Aortic overriding of the ventricular septum.
  - Variable right ventricular outflow obstruction.
  - Right ventricular hypertrophy.
- The perimembranous outlet VSD allows right to left and bidirectional shunting and consequent cyanosis. The outflow obstruction may be subvalvar (infundibular), valvar, supravalvar (including branch pulmonary artery stenosis), or a combination.
- The aortic annulus and aorta frequently dilate progressively with age.
- A small number of patients have anomalous coronary arteries (e.g. an anomalous LAD coronary artery arising from the right coronary artery).
- Patients who present as adults will usually already have undergone surgery. Unoperated adults largely comprise those with anatomical features unsuitable for repair – usually abnormalities of the pulmonary arteries. Some adult patients will have undergone palliative procedures to improve pulmonary blood flow prior to definitive repair.
- Post-repair sequelae and residua:
  - Rhythm and conduction disorders: predominantly right bundle branch block and ventricular tachycardias.
  - Recurrent right ventricular outflow tract obstruction.
  - Right ventricular outflow tract aneurysm.
  - Recurrent VSD.
  - Pulmonary regurgitation.
  - Impaired right ventricular function.
  - Tricuspid regurgitation.

Atrial septal defect

- Atrial septal defect (ASD) is a common lesion and is often previously undetected in adults. Types include:
  - Ostium secundum.
  - Sinus venosus.
  - Coronary sinus defects.
  - Ostium primum (📖 see also Specific lesions; Atrioventricular septal defect, p. 483).
- Ostium secundum accounts for 70% of ASDs and manifests as an absence of the septum in the region of the oval fossa, usually 1–2 cm in diameter. It is distinct from patent foramen ovale in that the latter comprises a flap-like slit, with no true septal deficiency.
- Superior sinus venosus defects occur around the superior atrio-caval junction. They are associated with partial anomalous pulmonary venous drainage – usually with the right upper pulmonary veins draining directly into the superior vena cava. Rare defects occur near the inferior vena cava junction.

- Pathophysiology involves a left to right shunt. The effect is volume and pressure overload of the right heart, and increased pulmonary blood flow.
- There is a preferential streaming of inferior vena caval blood to a secundum ASD, which places unoperated patients at risk of paradoxical emboli even if the shunt is almost entirely left to right.
- Decline in well-being with age may reflect the onset of hypertension and coronary artery disease, which decrease left ventricular compliance and increase left to right shunting.
- The incidence of arrhythmias, ventricular dysfunction, and pulmonary vascular disease are related to the age at closure. Tachyarrhythmias become increasingly common after the fourth decade.
- If surgical repair is delayed (beyond 40 years), elevation in pulmonary artery pressures may be observed.
- Transcatheter device closure is now routine. It is suitable for secundum defects, less than approximately 30 mm, with a rim around the defect. Long-term comparisons of outcome with surgery are awaited. Endocarditis prophylaxis is not subsequently required.
- Implications of non-operated ASD include paradoxical embolism and elevated work of breathing due to decreased lung compliance. Late atrial arrhythmias may occur, and right heart failure or pulmonary vascular disease occur in approximately 10%.

Transposition of the great arteries

- Transposition of the great arteries (TGA) is defined as atrioventricular concordance and ventriculo-arterial discordance.
- The aorta arises from the anatomical right ventricle and the pulmonary artery arises from the anatomical left ventricle.
- TGA is described as simple in the presence of an intact ventricular septum.
- Complex TGA involves the combination of TGA with VSD and possibly other abnormalities. The pulmonary artery overrides the ventricular septum, and if more than 50% is committed to the left ventricle the abnormality may be described as TGA with VSD, whereas if more than 50% of the pulmonary artery is committed to the right ventricle the correct terminology is double outlet right ventricle.
- Up to 28% demonstrate anomalies of the coronary arteries, which is important for surgical intervention in childhood.
- Adults with this circulation will usually have previously undergone surgery. Very occasionally a degree of subpulmonary stenosis can result in balanced flow, which is compatible with survival to adult life without surgery.
- Simple TGA was originally treated with atrial redirection (atrial switch) operations: the Senning and Mustard procedures. These redirect blood within the atria to the opposite ventricle, resulting in physiologically appropriate circulation pathways.

- The Rastelli operation was originally performed for TGA, VSD, and left ventricular outflow obstruction (subpulmonary stenosis). It involves closing the VSD and simultaneously tunnelling left ventricular blood to the aorta. A valved conduit connects right ventricle to pulmonary artery.
- The arterial switch operation involves transecting the aorta and pulmonary arteries and reconnecting them to the appropriate ventricle.
- Palliative atrial procedures involve redirection of blood at atrial level, while retaining or creating a VSD. This is used in patients who are unsuitable for repair, usually because of pulmonary vascular abnormalities.

Atrial repair

- Late complications include:
  - Arrhythmias.
  - Atrial baffle obstruction and leak.
  - Systemic (right) ventricular dysfunction.
- Systemic or pulmonary venous pathway obstruction occurs in 10–15%.
- Systemic venous obstruction is amenable to balloon dilation with stent insertion if required. Pulmonary venous obstruction is more difficult to treat with dilation. Either type of obstruction may require surgical intervention. Baffle leaks are detected with echocardiography. Closure is indicated if the shunt is severe, and can be achieved either by surgery or with transcatheter devices.

The Rastelli operation

- Closure of the VSD, which incorporates left ventricle to aortic continuity and placement of a right ventricle to pulmonary artery conduit. The conduit may subsequently degenerate with obstruction or regurgitation. There are a variety of conduit substitutes, both synthetic and biological (homograft).
- Many conduits will subsequently require replacing.
- Subaortic stenosis due to the tunnel formed by the VSD patch may necessitate revision.

Arterial switch

- The arterial switch has superseded the atrial switch operation. Normal physiology and anatomical connections are restored, and extensive intra-atrial surgery (and potential for arrhythmia generation) is avoided. The long-term effects are not yet completely defined. The pulmonary root becomes the aortic root, with a 'neo-aortic valve' formed by the original pulmonary valve.
- It requires re-implantation of the coronary ostia and leaves the native pulmonary valve as the systemic neo-aortic valve.
- Neo-aortic regurgitation is possible and aortic root dilation has been reported.
- Supravalvar stenosis of both great arteries can occur.
- Physical obstruction or kinking of the re-implanted coronary arteries is a risk.

Single ventricle

- Univentricular heart describes a number of variant conditions where one dominant and functionally useful ventricular chamber exists. There is usually a second small rudimentary ventricle.
- The characteristic feature of these hearts is that the majority of atrial mass is connected to one ventricle. The connection varies as either atrioventricular connection may be absent (e.g. tricuspid atresia), or more than 75% of the total atrioventricular junction is committed to the dominant ventricle (double inlet ventricle).
- The physiological implication is mixing of systemic and pulmonary venous blood in the dominant ventricle. Pulmonary blood flow and hypoxaemia are dependent on the presence and degree of pulmonary outlet obstruction.

Double inlet ventricle

- Double inlet ventricle implies that both (or more than 75% of the total) atrioventricular valves and junctions are connected to a dominant ventricle.
- The commonest form encountered is double inlet left ventricle with discordant ventriculo-arterial connection (aorta from rudimentary right ventricle, pulmonary artery from left ventricle).
- Systemic blood flow is limited and aortic arch anomalies are common. Unless subpulmonary stenosis is present, pulmonary blood flow will be excessive resulting in pulmonary vascular occlusive disease. Occasionally pulmonary and systemic flows are balanced, and these patients may survive to adult life without surgery.
- 20% of double inlet ventricle hearts comprise double inlet right ventricle. These often involve a single common atrioventricular valve. Chronic volume overload results in abnormal ventricular function, which is also poorer if the dominant ventricle is of right morphology.
- Double inlet left ventricle is associated with a high incidence of congenital and surgical heart block and subaortic stenosis, which may be progressive.
- Treatment depends on the pulmonary blood flow:
  - Cavo-pulmonary connection (see below).
  - Ventricular septation if there is adequate ventricular mass and two atrioventricular valves.
  - Limited pulmonary blood flow can be increased with systemic-pulmonary arterial shunts.
  - Excessive pulmonary blood flow may be restricted with a pulmonary artery band.
  - Increasing systemic blood flow when it is restricted can be achieved by enlarging the VSD or creating an aortopulmonary connection.
- Patients with 'mixing lesions' have systemic and pulmonary venous blood mixing in a common chamber:
  - Some patients have a natural pulmonary blood supply either through pulmonary or collateral arteries.
  - Others have synthetic systemic to pulmonary shunts created surgically.
- Cyanotic single ventricle patients are at high risk for cardiac surgery.

Cavopulmonary connections (Fontan and Glenn circulations)

- The bidirectional Glenn shunt describes connection of the superior vena cava to the pulmonary artery. Inferior vena cava blood usually continues to reach the heart and maintains a right to left shunt with resultant hypoxaemia.
  - The palliative effect diminishes over time, and between 5 and 15 years over 40% require further surgery.
  - Glenn patients can develop venous collaterals, which communicate between the superior vena cava and the inferior vena cava (and provide natural decompression of the high superior vena cava pressures).
  - Glenn procedures are generally unsuitable for adults due to the lower proportion of cardiac output returning via the superior vena cava. This results in inadequate pulmonary blood flow.
- 'Fontan circulation' is a term widely used to generically describe the final result of palliative procedures for patients who will ultimately be limited to a univentricular circulation:
  - These involve diversion of all or part of the systemic venous return to the pulmonary circulation, usually without a subpulmonary ventricle.
  - Flow across the lungs to the left atrium is dependent on the pressure gradient between the systemic veins and the left atrium.

The Fontan operation

- Originally an atriopulmonary anastomosis (APA).
- Superseded by total cavo-pulmonary connection (TCPC).
  - This connects the end of the superior vena cava to the side of the right pulmonary artery, together with a conduit (either intracardiac or extracardiac) connecting the inferior vena cava to the inferior aspect of the right pulmonary artery.
  - Exclusion of the right atrium results in less distension, and diminished turbulence with fewer arrhythmias and less thrombosis.
  - Partial or fenestrated intra-atrial conduits incorporate a fenestration that allows right to left shunting of blood at atrial level. This allows decompression of the systemic venous system and maintains or augments cardiac output, at the expense of increased cyanosis (consequent upon the right to left shunt).
- Continued survival depends on both low pulmonary vascular resistance and left atrial pressure.
- Pulmonary blood flow will diminish in the presence of:
  - Elevated systemic ventricular end-diastolic pressure.
  - Elevations of pulmonary vascular resistance.
  - Atrioventricular valve regurgitation.
  - Loss of sinus rhythm.
- These patients have diminished reserve in terms of ability to increase cardiac output in response to exercise or stress. Cardiac index is decreased both at rest and during exercise. A patient with a completed Fontan circulation often has a peripheral arterial saturation of approximately 95% due to ventilation perfusion mismatching.

- Important factors that influence pulmonary vascular resistance (and hence cardiac output) include pCO_2, pO_2, arterial pH, mean airway pressure, positive end-expiratory pressure, and extrinsic compression (pleural effusions).
- It is important to maintain central venous pressure, utilize positive pressure ventilation with caution, and be aware that reduced contractility and loss of sinus rhythm are poorly tolerated.
- Diastolic function is frequently abnormal. Ventricular relaxation is inco-ordinate, with prolonged isovolumic relaxation, diminished early rapid filling, and dominant atrial systolic filling.
- Late problems include:
  - Arteriovenous fistulae.
  - Arrhythmias.
  - Thrombosis.
  - Peripheral oedema.
  - Protein-losing enteropathy.
  - Pathway obstruction.
- Thrombosis and strokes are particular risks, especially when there are low flow areas within the heart.
- The right atrium is often large and dilated with marked 'spontaneous contrast' – an echocardiographic appearance of 'smoke' and swirling blood that is very low velocity or nearly static.
- An intrinsic thrombotic tendency exists in over 60% of patients, which may be due to protein C deficiency.
- 10–15% will develop a protein-losing enteropathy with hypoproteinaemia by ten years:
  - Clinical features include hepatomegaly, ascites, cirrhosis, peripheral oedema, and pleural and pericardial effusions.
  - It carries a grim prognosis, with 50% of those affected dead at five years.

Atrioventricular septal defect

- Atrioventricular septal defect (AVSD) describes lesions involving a maldevelopment of the atrioventricular septum.
- The embryologic region of the endocardial cushions comprises the inferior portion of the atrial septum, the atrioventricular valves, and the superior and posterior portion of the ventricular septum.
- A complete atrioventricular septal or atrioventricular canal defect comprises a common atrioventricular orifice together with a non-restrictive VSD. Usually, although not invariably, a primum ASD is present.
- A partial atrioventricular septal defect almost always incorporates a primum ASD; there are separate atrioventricular orifices and no VSD. Intermediate forms comprise the spectrum between complete and partial defects.

- Typical morphological pattern – there are five leaflets:
  - Two right-sided leaflets (right anterosuperior and inferior).
  - One left-sided leaflet (mural with one third as opposed to two thirds annular circumference attachment).
  - Two bridging leaflets (superior and inferior), which join the right and left orifices.
  - The left-sided commissure of the bridging leaflets frequently forms a separation – often referred to as a 'cleft' (different from a true cleft of a single mitral valve leaflet).
  - The absence of the true membranous and muscular atrioventricular septum results in 'unwedging' of the aortic outflow tract from between the mitral and tricuspid valves and a narrowed or obstructed left ventricular outflow tract.
- Intervention in patients presenting in adult life is indicated for significant haemodynamic defects, left atrioventricular valve regurgitation causing symptoms, atrial arrhythmias, decreased ventricular function, or significant subaortic obstruction.
- Residua and sequelae include:
  - Residual septal defects.
  - Progressive atrioventricular valve regurgitation.
  - Heart block.
  - Arrhythmias.
  - Left ventricular outflow obstruction.
- Large defects predispose to heart failure and pulmonary hypertension.
- Trisomy 21 patients with untreated AVSDs may demonstrate reactive pulmonary vasculature and pulmonary hypertensive 'crises' similar to those seen in infants. Management comprises opioid sedation, ventilation to hypocapnia, and pulmonary vasodilators such as nitric oxide, inhaled epoprostenol (prostacyclin), and phosphodiesterase inhibitors.

Sequelae

Table 30.4 Sequelae of surgery for congenital heart disease

Condition		Sequelae
ASD		Residual shunt, septal aneurysm, device fracture
Coarctation of aorta		Systolic hypertension, residual gradient, inaccurate left arm BP (subclavian flap repair), aneurysm formation, dissection
PDA		Residual flow, recanalization, laryngeal nerve injury
TGA	Atrial switch	Arrhythmias, systemic ventricular dysfunction, baffle leak, venous pathway obstruction
	Rastelli	Residual VSD, ventricular dysfunction, LVOT obstruction, conduit failure
	Arterial switch	Supravalvar AS/PS, aortic regurgitation, ventricular dysfunction, coronary artery stenosis
Tetralogy of Fallot		Residual VSD, RV outflow tract obstruction, RV dysfunction, pulmonary regurgitation, RBBB/AV block, ventricular arrhythmias, BT shunt – BP inaccurate
Single ventricle		Preload dependence, ventricular dysfunction, cyanosis (fenestration), protein-losing enteropathy, arrhythmias, diminished functional reserve

ASD = atrial septal defect; PDA = patent ductus arteriosus; TGA = transposition of the great arteries; VSD = ventricular septal defect; LVOT = left ventricular outflow tract; AS = aortic stenosis; PS = pulmonary stenosis; BT = Blalock-Taussig; RBBB = right bundle branch block; AV = atrioventricular; RV = right ventricle.

Management

- If a prosthetic (Blalock-Taussig) shunt is present, blood leaving the heart may travel in one of two parallel circulations: either to the systemic circulation via the aorta or to the pulmonary circulation via the shunt. The systemic and pulmonary vascular resistances and the resistance of the shunt determine the flow through each vascular bed. In general the usual goal is to have a 'balanced' circulation (i.e. Q_P: Q_S = 1:1). Depending on the mixed venous oxygen saturations, a balanced circulation is frequently associated with a systemic oxygen saturation of approximately 75% to 85%. Cyanotic patients should have serial haematocrit measurements.
- If pulmonary blood flow is inadequate or appears to be falling, pulmonary vasodilators can be considered. These include control of arterial pCO_2, nitric oxide, epoprostenol (prostacyclin), and phosphodiesterase inhibitors.
- Intravenous induction may be slow when the circulation time is prolonged. Right to left shunts theoretically prolong alveolar to arterial equilibration of volatile anaesthetic gases, but this infrequently appears clinically important in adults.
- Agents that cause vasodilation will increase right to left shunting and reduce S_aO_2, but again in clinical practice this is frequently offset by reductions in total oxygen consumption and consequent elevation of mixed venous oxygen saturation.
- Narcotic-based anaesthesia is the choice of many in the presence of significant ventricular dysfunction.

Monitoring

- Trans-oesophageal echocardiography is useful for following ventricular performance, valvular function, and blood flow velocity.
- End-tidal CO_2 will underestimate $paCO_2$ in the presence of right to left shunting or common mixing.
- Interruption of the IVC or thrombosis following previous instrumentation may preclude femoral vein cannulation.
- In the presence of a subclavian to right pulmonary artery (Blalock-Taussig) shunt, the contralateral arm should be used for arterial pressure monitoring. Meticulous care must be taken to avoid venous air entrainment in patients with shunt lesions as systemic embolization can occur, even when shunting is considered to be predominantly left to right.
- Pulmonary artery catheters do not have a significant role. Anatomical considerations dictate that placement can be technically difficult or even not possible (atrial baffle procedures: Mustard and Senning operations). Thermodilution cardiac output measurements will be inaccurate in patients with right to left shunting.
- Peripheral arterial oxygen saturation will give useful indications of trends in Q_P:Q_S.
- Cavo-pulmonary shunts (Glenn and Fontan) are at risk of venous thrombosis. A single-lumen CVP line is preferable and is removed as early as possible.

Ventilation

- In the Fontan circulation, control of arterial blood gases (particularly $PaCO_2$) is an important influence on pulmonary blood flow. Low airway pressures and early weaning from ventilation are beneficial to transpulmonary flow, although the duration of the inspiratory phase during positive pressure ventilation is usually more important than the absolute level of peak inspiratory pressure. Shortening the inspiratory time (with consequent increase in peak inspiratory pressure) may be an appropriate strategy to maximize the expiratory phase and thus the time available for transpulmonary flow.
- The ventilatory response to $PaCO_2$ is normal in hypoxic patients, hence adequate analgesia and sedation are appropriate. This is important in the presence of labile PA pressures.

Endocarditis

- 20% of adults with infective endocarditis have congenital heart disease. Infective endocarditis requires a susceptible substrate and a source of bacteraemia. Lesions associated with major risk involve high blood flow velocities at sites of significant pressure gradients. Maximum deposition of organisms occurs at either the low pressure 'sink' beyond an orifice or at the site of jet impact.
- Congenital lesions associated with the highest risk include bicuspid aortic valve, restrictive ventricular septal defect, tetralogy of Fallot, and high pressure atrioventricular valve regurgitation.
- Postoperative lesions at particular risk are palliative shunt and prosthetic valves. Low risk lesions include repaired septal defects and patent ducts.
- Antibiotic prophylaxis is recommended in the presence of prosthetic valves, previous endocarditis, systemic to pulmonary shunts, and most cardiac structural abnormalities.

Further reading

1. Baum VC, Stayer SA, Andropolous DB, Russell IA. Approach to the teenaged and adult patient. In: *Anesthesia for Congenital Heart Disease*. Andropoulos DB, Stayer SA, Russel IA, eds. Malden MA, Blackwell Futura 2005, 210–222.
2. Drinkwater DC. The surgical management of congenital heart disease in the adult. *Progress in Paediatric Cardiology* 2003; 17: 81–89.
3. Perloff JK, Warnes CA. Challenges posed by adults with repaired congenital heart disease. *Circulation* 2001; 103: 2637–2643.
4. Srinathan SK, Bonser RS, Sethia B, et al. Changing practice of cardiac surgery in adult patients with congenital heart disease. *Heart* 2005; 91: 207–212.
5. Therrien J, Webb G. Clinical update on adults with congenital heart disease. *Lancet* 2003; 362: 1305–1313.
6. Webb GW, Williams RG. 32nd Bethesda Conference: Care of the Adult with Congenital Heart Disease. *JACC* 2001; 37: 1161–1165.

Hypertrophic cardiomyopathy

Dr M Barnard and Dr B Martin

Pathology *494*
Therapeutic options *496*
Haemodynamic goals *497*
Anaesthetic plan and adverse haemodynamics *498*
TOE essentials *500*
Practice points *502*
Further reading *503*

Pathology

Genetics

- Clinical prevalence estimated at 1 in 500.
- Mendelian autosomal dominant trait.
- Ten gene defects – encoding for sarcomere proteins.
- Three mutant genes account for 50%: beta-myosin heavy chain, myosin-binding protein C, and cardiac troponin-T.
- Over 200 mutations identified.
- Phenotypic expression is very variable – due to influence of environment or other modifier genes.

Morphology

- Characterized by muscular hypertrophy and myocyte disarray.
- Diagnosis established by left ventricular hypertrophy and wall thickening, in absence of another cardiac or systemic cause.
- Hypertrophy usually asymmetric, with predilection for anterior ventricular septum.
- Ventricular chamber non-dilated, hyperdynamic, often with systolic obliteration.
- LV outflow tract obstruction does not occur in all cases – hence the term hypertrophic cardiomyopathy (HCM), now preferred to hypertrophic obstructive cardiomyopathy (HOCM).
- Delayed late onset appearance in older adults is possible (for example with myosin-binding protein C gene).
- Myocardial ischaemia attributed to increase in myocardial mass and non-atherosclerotic thickening of intra-mural coronary arteries.

Pathophysiology

- Outflow obstruction.
- Turbulent flow in left ventricle outflow tract causes systolic anterior motion (SAM) of mitral valve, worsening or precipitating obstruction.
- Obstruction is characteristically dynamic.
- SAM results in mitral regurgitation, usually an eccentric posterior jet.
- There are other hypotheses for the origin of SAM – e.g. abnormal alignment of the papillary muscles.
- Diastolic dysfunction.
- LV hypertrophy causes reduction in compliance and delayed relaxation (diastolic dysfunction).

Assessment of severity

Symptoms

- Outflow tract obstruction – resting gradient >30 mmHg is an independent predictor of disease progression.
- Patients grouped by resting and exercise gradients:
  - Resting gradient >30 mmHg.
  - Resting gradient <30, provocable gradient >30.
  - Resting gradient <20, not provocable >30.

Investigations
- Echo – distribution of hypertrophy, left ventricular outflow tract obstruction, resting gradient, SAM, mitral regurgitation.
- Exercise test – systemic oxygen consumption, increase with exercise.
- Provoked gradient – increase in gradient with dobutamine, isoprenaline, or exercise.

Clinical presentation
- Frequently asymptomatic.
- Shortness of breath.
- Chest pain – particularly after meals, and characteristically after alcohol.
- Syncope and pre-syncope.
- Arrhythmias – heart block, atrial fibrillation.
- Heart failure.
- Sudden death.

Therapeutic options

Medical treatment

The aim is to improve diastolic filling and avoid or reduce myocardial ischaemia. Drug categories include beta-blockers, calcium antagonists (verapamil), and antiarrhythmics (disopyramide). Common to all three groups is negative inotropic effect, which decreases ventricular ejection acceleration, reducing outflow obstruction and pressure gradient. Other antiarrhythmics or anticoagulation may be used for atrial fibrillation.

EPS interventions

The role of dual chamber pacing has yet to be fully evaluated. It will probably be employed in selected subgroups such as advanced age or those unsuitable for surgical intervention. Electrophysiologically inducible ventricular tachycardia or syncopal episodes requires consideration of an implantable cardiac defibrillator.

Alcohol septal ablation

An alternative to surgery in those warranting invasive intervention. A controlled myocardial infarction is produced by injecting small volumes (up to 5 ml) absolute alcohol into septal perforator branches of coronary arteries. Arteries are selected by assessing branch perfusion with contrast echocardiography. Complications include extended infarction, coronary dissection, and heart block.

Surgical myectomy

Indicated in patients refractory to medical treatment, with peak resting gradients >50 mmHg, and unstable symptoms. It involves resection of a small amount of septal myocardium accessed through the aortic valve. Complications include transient and permanent heart block, residual gradient, and (rarely) septal defects.

Haemodynamic goals

Reduced preload and vasodilation are established therapies for other forms of heart failure. In HCM they will increase outflow obstruction. Goals include:

- **Maintain preload** or even slight hypervolaemia – to avoid increasing outflow gradient.
- **Maintain or increase vascular resistance** – to minimize outflow gradient.
- **Sinus rhythm** – atrial contribution important in stiff, non-compliant LV.
- **Avoid increases in contractility** – gradient is dynamic and increased contractility increases the outflow gradient.

Anaesthetic plan and adverse haemodynamics

- Obtain cardiology consultation preoperatively. Check pacemakers and disarm implantable defibrillators. Place arterial line and large intravenous drip prior to induction. Slow intravenous induction predominantly with opioids is common. If blood pressure falls this is often due to vasodilation or increased obstruction. First-line treatment is with (pure alpha) vasoconstrictors or beta-blockers. Norepinephrine infusion is required from induction in approximately 50% of cases. Avoid inotropes, chronotropes, and vasodilators – dobutamine and isoprenaline are used preoperatively to assess dynamic gradients. Keep the patient well filled, the afterload high, and heart rate normal or low.
- Post-bypass a potential complication is temporary or permanent heart block. These patients can leave theatre in sinus rhythm and develop (slow) heart block within the next 24 hours. The non-compliant state of the ventricle compounded by aortic cross-clamping means that this can be poorly tolerated and in extreme cases lead to cardiac arrest. HCM protocols should include two atrial and two ventricular pacing wires for every patient, and *importantly the function and threshold of these should be confirmed prior to chest closure*. The pacing wires should remain *in situ* for at least 48 hours.
- Inotrope support is rarely required – a cause should be sought if they are. If inotropes are genuinely required then phosphodiesterase inhibitors (milrinone, enoximone) are least likely to worsen outflow obstruction and diastolic function.

TOE essentials

Intraoperative TOE is critical to determining surgical strategy (Figures 31.1–31.3). The three key pieces of pre-myectomy information are maximal width of ventricular septum (normal = 11 mm), distance from aortic valve to point of mitral valve contact with septum, and how far distally (into ventricle) turbulent flow originates. Mitral SAM should be recorded and mitral regurgitation quantified. Adequacy of myectomy is assessed by morphology and width of the septum, residual SAM, and residual gradient (ideally none).

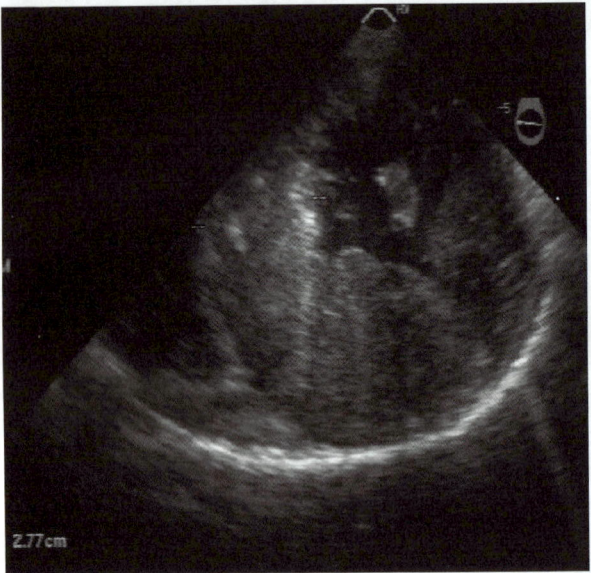

Figure 31.1 Hypertrophic cardiomyopathy – short axis view of the left ventricle. The ventricle is grossly hypertrophied with a thickness greater than 28 mm.

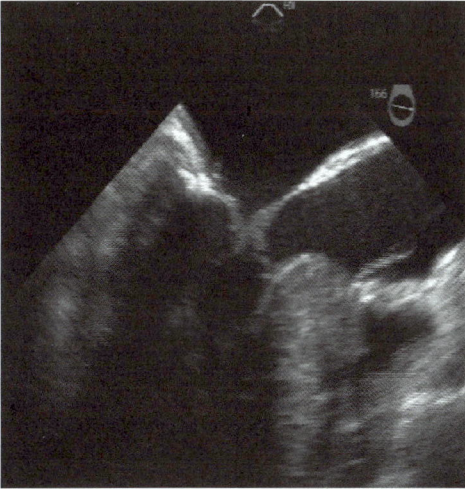

Figure 31.2 Systolic anterior motion (SAM) of the mitral valve with septal contact of the anterior leaflet.

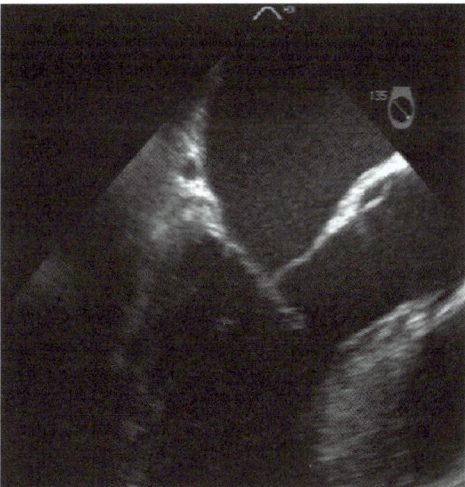

Figure 31.3 Systolic anterior motion of mitral valve in the left ventricular outflow tract.

Practice points

- There may not be any left ventricular outflow tract gradient at rest.
- Inotropes, chronotropes, and vasodilators worsen outflow tract obstruction.
- Vasoconstrictors (phenylephrine) are useful to treat hypotension during anaesthetic induction.
- Sinus rhythm is important. Heart block is poorly tolerated. Facilities for postoperative pacing are essential and should be checked during and after surgery.

Further reading

1. Maron BJ. Hypertrophic cardiomyopathy – a systematic review. *JAMA* 2002; 287: 1308–1320.
2. Maron BJ, McKenna WJ, Danielson GK, et al. ACC/ESC clinical expert consensus document on hypertrophic cardiomyopathy: A report of the American College of Cardiology Task Force on Clinical Expert Consensus Documents and the European Society of Cardiology Committee for Practice Guidelines. *European Heart Journal* 2003; 24: 1965–1991.
3. Spirito P, Seidman CE, McKenna WJ, et al. Medical progress: The management of hypertrophic cardiomyopathy. *New England Journal of Medicine* 1997; 30: 775–785.

Anaesthesia for heart failure and transplantation

Dr S George and Dr A Gaunt

Heart failure *506*
Anaesthesia for patients with severe heart failure *510*
Transplantation *514*
Anaesthetic management of heart transplantation *520*
Rejection and immunology *524*
The previously transplanted patient *526*
Further reading *527*

Heart failure

(📖 see also Chapter 4.) This describes impaired myocardial performance and can be caused by a number of factors, including:

- Valvular disease often leading to volume overload.
- Coronary artery disease leading to ischaemia and myocardial infarction. This leads to necrosis and fibrosis but also areas of limited blood supply that 'hibernate', which have the potential to recover (after weeks) following revascularization.
- Dilated cardiomyopathy is a primary disorder of cardiac muscle; 30% have underlying genetic autosomal dominant predisposition. Aberrant expression of sarcomeric proteins leads to weakness of the myocyte cytoskeleton.
- Hypertrophic cardiomyopathy and restrictive cardiomyopathies. These give rise to diastolic failure where the heart is unable to fill adequately and heart failure can ensue despite 'adequate' systolic function.

Pathophysiology of heart failure (📖 see also Chapter 4)

- Initial adaptive neuroendocrine processes contribute to remodelling of cardiac structure, resulting in ventricular enlargement and loss of normal elliptical shape. Sphericalization of the ventricle results in higher end-systolic wall stress and loss of normal force-length and force-velocity relationships. Changes eventually become self-propagating. **Neuroendocrine activation** results from disruption of the normal baroreflex system. Activation of renin-angiotensin and sympathetic nervous systems results in increased preload and afterload. Levels of norepinephrine, renin-angiotensin, aldosterone, atrial natriuretic factor, and vasopressin are increased. Cytokines and endothelin levels are also increased in advanced heart failure.
- As the heart decompensates there is increasing **volume overload** with fluid retention.
- **Subendocardial ischaemia** can result from high LVEDP, ventricular hypertrophy, increased wall tension, and low coronary perfusion even in the absence of coronary artery disease.
- **Arrhythmias** are common in heart failure due to subendocardial ischaemia, ventricular hypertrophy, ventricular dilation, high sympathetic drive, and diuretics.
- Ventricular thrombus can occur due to blood stasis and systemic propagation of thrombus can occur.
- Progressive enlargement of the ventricle with **sphericalization** leads to dilation of the mitral valve annulus and reduced coaptation of the mitral valve leaflets, leading to **mitral regurgitation** that further compromises cardiac output. This also leads to left atrial enlargement, which can predispose to intracardiac thrombosis and atrial fibrillation.
- **Regional wall motion abnormalities** of the myocardial segments where the papillary muscles are attached contribute to tethering of the mitral valve apparatus.

Medical management of heart failure

- Initial therapy is aimed at identifying the cause and appropriately managing these, e.g. valvular, ischaemic, hypertrophic, and restrictive disease.
- Diuresis to treat volume retention, ß-blockade to reduce sympathetic overdrive, and ACE inhibitors and nitrates to allow vasodilation.
- ACE inhibitors reduce production of angiotensin II and result in fewer hospital admissions and prolonged survival in heart failure. Studies suggest a relative reduction in risk of death of 15–40%.
- Beta-blockers protect the heart from elevated levels of epinephrine and norepinephrine. Reduction in relative risk of death is in the order of 35%.
- Angiotensin receptor blockers have an additive effect on reverse remodelling when used in combination with ACE inhibitors.
- Aldosterone antagonists are recommended in patients who remain in NYHA class III–IV despite ACE inhibitor and beta-blockade.
- Digoxin may improve symptoms, but has no proven role in preventing death from heart failure.
- Nitrates, calcium antagonists, and nicorandil can be used to treat angina symptoms in those patients with heart failure.
- Implantable cardiac defibrillators (ICDs) reduce the risk of death due to arrhythmias by 23%.
- Cardiac resynchronization therapy (CRT) using a biventricular pacemaker in those patients with heart failure and a wide QRS complex can significantly reduce the risk of death or hospital admission for cardiac reasons (19–37%), improve pump function, reduce symptoms, and increase exercise tolerance. Devices combining biventricular pacemakers and an ICD are available.
- Anticoagulation should be considered due to the risk of blood stasis and subsequent thrombosis/thromboembolism.

Surgical management of heart failure

At present orthotopic heart transplantation offers the best long-term survival for severe heart failure, albeit with severely limited availability. Other surgical options are available and can offer some benefit.

Coronary artery surgery

Myocardium that is hibernating may be recruited by revascularization but can be difficult to differentiate from infarcted myocardium. Specific tests are used to identify hibernating myocardium and the likelihood of success of revascularization, including dobutamine stress echocardiography, thallium, and other nuclear medicine studies and MRI. Enough myocardial function needs to be present to cope with the operative process as hibernating myocardium usually needs weeks to recover function.

Mitral valve surgery (📖 see also Chapter 27)

- Mitral valve repair is preferred to replacement on functional and prognostic grounds.
- Mitral valve leaflets are often structurally normal; therefore surgery is aimed at decreasing the annulus size. The mitral valve annulus has dynamic function during closure and a flexible mitral annuloplasty ring preserves this whilst allowing reduction in the annulus size and a subsequent improvement in coaptation and reduction in regurgitation.
- In ischaemic cardiomyopathy scarred papillary muscle apparatus may necessitate a more extensive repair with re-implantation of the papillary muscles and re-fashioning of chordae.
- In mild ischaemic regurgitation, revascularization may be sufficient. Operative mortality of revascularization in the presence of ischaemic mitral regurgitation is approximately 2%, but five-year survival may be as low as 50%.
- Operative mortality of mitral valve repair in dilated cardiomyopathy varies from 0 to 5%, with one-year survival 82–90% and five-year survival approximately 70%. NYHA class, ejection fraction, cardiac output, and end-diastolic volumes may improve significantly.

Ventricular repair

- In the early stages of heart failure, ventricular dilation allows improvement of stroke volume, but in advancing disease ventricular dilation is deleterious, so attempts have been made to reduce ventricular size.
- Partial left ventriculectomy (PLV, Batista procedure) has an operative mortality of 3.2–50%. 32% are dead within two years and 40% by three years. It is no longer offered as a procedure by many centres.
- Left ventricular aneurysmectomy in ischaemic cardiomyopathy (Dor procedure) is more successful. The Cleveland Clinic reported a series of 129 Dor procedures; 87% had CABG also and 50% MV repair. Operative mortality was 1.6% and two-year survival varied from 82.5% for those with akinetic ventricular areas to 98% for those with dyskinetic ventricular muscle. Significant improvements in ejection fraction occurred.
- The ACORN device is a mesh graft that is positioned around the heart and sutured into place to restrict further dilation. Wall stress and myocyte stretch are reduced, but no clear benefit in terms of survival has yet been demonstrated.

Long-term assist devices and artificial hearts (📖 see also Chapter 21)

- Ventricular assist devices are generally used as 'bridges to recovery or transplantation' but the development of smaller and more portable devices has led to the concept of so-called 'destination therapy' as definitive treatment.
- The 2001 REMATCH study showed a 48% reduction in deaths due to end-stage heart failure over a period of 1–8 years using a left ventricular assist device.

Anaesthesia for patients with severe heart failure

Preoperative evaluation

- Standard cardiac anaesthetic evaluation including medical and surgical history, blood tests, cross-match, CXR, ECG, echocardiography and angiography results, airway scoring, reflux, fasting status, dental history, and medication history.
- The presence of pacemakers/defibrillators should be noted. Beta-blockers should not be stopped because of fasting due to the risk of rebound phenomena. Alpha-blockers, ACE inhibitors, and calcium antagonists should be discontinued on the day of surgery due to interactions with anaesthesia-induced vasodilation.
- Sedative premedication is not recommended as patients can have profound responses to sedatives in low cardiac output states.
- Preoperative optimization should be considered. This may include the use of inotropes and phosphodiesterase inhibitors to improve cardiac output with subsequent improvement in renal function and other organ systems. Pulmonary artery catheterization with pressures and cardiac output may even justify volume replacement in the face of overzealous diuresis. Intra-aortic balloon pump (IABP) counter-pulsation can be associated with improved cardiac output and stability.

Pre-induction

Pre-induction monitoring involves monitoring of invasive blood pressure (arterial line) and central pressures and consideration of pulmonary artery catheterization. In those who present *in extremis*, there may be an improvement in haemodynamic condition following induction due to off-loading and reduced sympathetic overdrive.

Induction

- Pre-oxygenation and balanced anaesthesia employing opiates, hypnotics, and muscle relaxation in low doses is used to maintain stability. Fentanyl 3–4 µg/kg, etomidate 0.2 mg/kg, and pancuronium 0.1 mg/kg is a satisfactory approach. Other combinations can be equally satisfactory. Blood pressure should be maintained with vasoconstriction (metaraminol, phenylephrine) or inotropes (epinephrine), which should be drawn and ready to inject. It must be borne in mind that arm-brain circulation times may be very slow in patients with low cardiac outputs.
- Excessive fluid therapy should be avoided as these patients are generally on the falling part of their Starling curve.
- Use of trans-oesophageal echocardiography (TOE) in these patients is highly recommended and allows real-time estimation of left and right ventricular function, assessment of valvular abnormalities, a guide to the success of repairs, and a guide to volume status.

Maintenance

- TIVA and volatile techniques are suitable for maintenance of heart failure patients.
- Volatile agents (isoflurane, sevoflurane) may be of benefit through anaesthetic preconditioning.
- Intraoperative blood loss may be significant depending on the procedure and large falls in preload due to haemorrhage are very poorly tolerated prior to cardiopulmonary bypass. The routine use of antifibrinolytics is recommended.
- Electrolyte levels, especially potassium, must be carefully maintained intraoperatively as arrhythmias are poorly tolerated in this group.
- Anaemia is poorly tolerated as cardiac output cannot be increased to maintain tissue oxygen delivery.
- Procedures may be prolonged, therefore care with patient positioning and pressure area padding are required.

Postoperative

- Adequacy of cardiac output should be continuously assessed with a variety of measures including pulmonary artery catheter-derived cardiac output and S_VO_2, urine output, blood lactate levels, and acid-base status.
- Appropriate treatment should be instituted early and may include increasing inotropic support, phosphodiesterase inhibitors (enoximone, milrinone), inhaled nitric oxide, renal replacement, intra-aortic balloon counter-pulsation, and even ventricular assist devices.
- Recovery can be straightforward and these patients benefit from early weaning and extubation where possible.

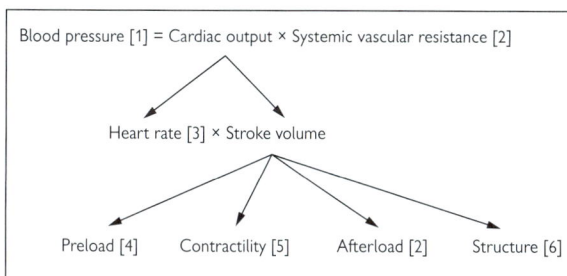

Figure 32.1 Factors that contribute to blood pressure.

	LAP/PCWP	CVP	PAP	SvO$_2$	CO	TOE	Treatment options
1 Spurious reading • Incorrectly positioned or zeroed transducers • Peripheral-central gradient	→	→	→	→	→	Normal	Correct transducer / Measure central pressures (Femoral, direct aorta)
2 Peripheral resistance (afterload) • Vasodilation	→	→	→	→	→↑	↓LVEDA, ↑FAC% Structural disruption e.g. Intimal flap	α1-agonists, vasopressin Surgical repair – dissection
Sepsis, CPB • Pulmonary hypertension	→	↑→	↑↑	→	→	RV RA overload, TR	iNO, PDI, Levosimendan, RVAD
3 Rate and rhythm (Assess ECG)							DC cardioversion to SR Chronotropic agents: isoprenaline, epinephrine
4 Volume status • Hypovolaemia	↓	↓	↓	↓	↓	↓LVEDA, ↑FAC%	Cyrstalloid, colloid, blood
• Hypervolaemia	↑	↑	↑	↓	↓	Bulging atrial septa ↑Chamber sizes	Diuresis, vasodilators, blood removal
5 Contractility decreased • Systolic failure	↑	→	↑	↓	↓	RWMA, ↓FAC%	Inotropes, calcium, IABP, VAD If sig. ischaemia consider angiogram/plasty/revase.
IHD, DCM ↓Myocardial preservation • Diastolic failure	↑	↑	↑	↓		HOCM, LVH	Volume, PDI, β-blockade
• Hypercontractile	↑	↑	↑	↓	↓	Systolic anterior motion of MV (SAM)	Volume, vasocontrictors, PDI β-blockade
6 Structural • Valve disruption, inefficient • Tamponade	↓	↑	↑	↓		Residual Regurg/Stenosis Echo-free space	Surgical correction Restemotomy, drainage
RV-LV interaction RV failure, PHT, ↑	↓	↑	↑→	↓	↓	RA & RV, TR and leftward septal shift	iNO, PDI, Levosimendan, RVAD

Figure 32.2 A structured assessment of hypotension/low cardiac output state and its treatment.

RV: right ventricle; LVH: left ventricular hypertrophy; RA: right atrium; LVEDA: left ventricular end-diastolic area; iNO: inhaled nitric oxide; CPB; cardiopulmonary bypass; DC: direct current; FAC: fractional area change; RWMA: regional wall motion abnormality; HOCM: hypertrophic obstructive cardiomyopathy; SAM: systolic anterior motion (of the mitral valve); IABP: intra-aortic balloon pump; LVAD: left ventricular assist device; PDI: phosphodiesterase inhibitor, e.g. milrinone; PHT: pulmonary hypertension; RVAD: right ventricular assist device; MR: mitral regurgitation; TR: tricuspid regurgitation; LVOT: left ventricular outflow tract; PEEP: positive end-expiratory pressure.

Transplantation

Overview
- Approximately 3400 heart transplants were performed worldwide in 2005 – 900 in Europe.
- Most UK centres carry out between 10 and 19 heart transplants per year with very few performing more than 75.
- Most recipients are in the 50–59 years age group, although the over 60 years rate of transplantation is increasing.
- Five-year survival continues to improve.
- 50% survival at 9.6 years post-transplant.

Indications for heart transplantation
- End-stage heart disease with life expectancy of 12–18 months.
- NYHA grade III or IV heart failure.
- Refractory to medical or surgical therapy.

Contraindications
- Chronic current systemic infection, including endocarditis.
- Chronic extracardiac infection.
- Continued abuse of alcohol or other drugs.
- Irreversible secondary organ failure unless considering for combined transplant.
- Psychiatric history likely to result in non-compliance and/or persistent non-compliance with medical therapy.
- Severe peripheral or cerebrovascular disease.
- Malignancy.
- Other life-threatening medical condition likely to cause death within five years.

Relative contraindications
- HIV (subject to discussion with Medical Director at UK Transplant).
- Hepatitis B/C.
- Acute pulmonary embolus (within three months).
- Obesity BMI >30.
- COPD with FEV1 <50% predicted.
- Pulmonary vascular resistance greater than 4 Wood units.
- Transpulmonary gradient greater than 12 mmHg.
- Chronic renal impairment with GFR <50 ml/min, unless candidate for combined renal transplant.
- Diabetes with target organ damage.
- Hypercholesterolaemia or other lipid diseases refractory to diet or drug therapy.
- Severe osteoporosis (bone mineral density >2 SDs less than predicted for age).
- Amyloidosis.
- Continued smoking.
- Giant cell myocarditis.

Table 32.1 Risk factors for one- and five-year mortality (📖 see also ishlt.org for more information)

Risk factors for one-year mortality	Risk factors for five-year mortality
Congenital heart disease	Repeat transplant
Temporary circulatory support	Ventilator
Ventilator	Dialysis
Dialysis	Diabetes
Hospitalized at time of transplant	Hospitalization at time of transplant
Donor history of cancer	Infection requiring IV antibiotics within two weeks of transplant
Female recipient and male donor	
Donor CVA	HLA DR mismatch
Female recipient and female donor	Pre-transplant CAD
Pulsatile chronic VAD	Previous transfusions
Repeat transplant*	Female recipient
Pre-transplant CAD	IV inotropes
PRA >10%*	Recipient age <30 or >55**
HLA DR mismatch*	Donor age >32**
IABP usage*	Recipient weight <70 kg or >90 kg**
HLA B mismatch*	Recipient BMI <23 or >27
Infection requiring IV antibiotics within two weeks of transplant*	Donor: recipient weight ratio <1**
	Transplant centre volume <22**
Prior transfusion*	Ischaemia time >3 hours**
IV inotropes	Pre-transplant serum creatinine >1.4 mg/dl**
Recipient age >55**	Pre-transplant bilirubin >0.9 mg/dl**
Recipient weight <70 kg**	
Donor age >35**	
Donor:recipient weight ratio <1**	
Transplant centre volume <20**	
PA diastolic >22**	
Ischaemia time >3 hours**	
Pre-transplant bilirubin >0.9 mg/dl**	
Pre-transplant serum creatinine >1.4 mg/dl**	

* Not significant in the 2000–2003 cohort.

** Relative risk increases above 1 at the values quoted.

Table 32.2 Factors not significant for one- and five-year mortality

Factors not significant for one-year mortality	Factors not significant for five-year mortality
Recipient factors: Pneumothorax, sternotomy, thoracotomy, ventricular remodelling, pregnancy, pulmonary embolism, prior malignancy, pulmonary vascular resistance, PCW, PA systolic.	*Recipient factors:* VAD, gender, pulmonary vascular resistance, PA systolic, PA diastolic, thoracotomy, sternotomy, pregnancy, history of malignancy, pneumothorax, pulmonary embolism, symptomatic cerebrovascular disease/ cerebrovascular event.
Donor factors: Clinical infection, history of diabetes, height, history of hypertension.	*Donor factors:* Gender, history of diabetes, history of cancer, clinical infection, cause of death, history of hypertension.
Transplant factors: ABO identical/compatible.	*Transplant factors:* Donor/recipient BMI ratio, ABO identical/ compatible.

Table 32.3 Recipient characteristics for thoracic organ transplantation

	Heart transplant	Heart-lung transplant
Mean age group	60–64 years	35–49 years
Male	73%	41%
Female	26%	58%
Common diagnoses	Cardiomyopathy 40%	Congenital heart disease 32%
	Coronary artery disease 29%	Primary pulmonary hypertension 25%
	Congenital heart disease 6%	Cystic fibrosis 15.5%
	Re-transplant 2.6%	Acquired heart disease 4.3%
	Valvular heart disease 1.9%	COPD 4%

Box 32.1 Routine tests prior to transplantation

- Height/weight.
- NIBP.
- Bacteriology.
- 24-hour urine for creatinine clearance.
- Chest radiograph.
- ECG and 24-hour Holter.
- Echocardiogram.
- Full blood count, urea, and electrolytes, liver function, thyroid function, viral screen, clotting profile, issue typing, blood group.
- HIV test.
- Left and right heart catheter.
- Lung function.
- VQ scan
- Arterial blood gas
- Exercise test.

The donor

- Following improvements in road safety and critical care, there has been a significant drop in the number of organs donated for transplantation. Donors have a mean age of 31, are typically male, and common pathologies include subarachnoid haemorrhage/stroke and head trauma. The number of heart transplants declined from 4460 in 1994 to 3355 in 2008.
- Active malignant disease outside the CNS is a contraindication to donation.
- Following an initial diagnosis of brain death, relatives are approached to ascertain the donor's wishes regarding transplantation. The donor co-ordinator is then contacted, and they will liaise with the family regarding the necessary tests prior to donation. Donors are screened for infections including HIV and hepatitis. UK Transplant then offers the organs to a transplant centre. The decision to transplant rests with the transplanting surgeon. The organs are assessed to determine their suitability for transplantation. Hearts undergo TOE +/- haemodynamic assessment.
- The donor is taken to theatre and the transplant team (consisting of transplant harvest surgeon, anaesthetist, scrub nurse, and perfusionist) proceed to harvest the organs. Although the patient is dead, it may be necessary to administer muscle relaxants to prevent spinal reflex movement and vasodilators to control hypertension. Brain death can be a source of significant intraoperative instability and cardiovascular support may need to be instituted to maintain organ perfusion.
- Efforts to increase the donor pool include active donor management, which aims to make borderline organs transplantable, as well as promotion of the organ donor register.
- The co-ordinator at the transplant centre is responsible for the organization of the transplant. Timing can be critical and it is a significant undertaking to have everyone ready at the appropriate time.

Surgical essentials (heart transplant)

- Chest is opened and the heart is exposed, dissected, and cannulated (bicaval) prior to arrival of donor heart.
- Additional time in theatre may be required prior to the arrival of the donor heart in patients requiring a redo sternotomy. This can be difficult if the donor's hospital is nearby.
- Before commencing cardiopulmonary bypass, the donor heart is inspected to confirm that it is suitable. Errors in harvest rarely happen, but sometimes it may be necessary abandon the transplant if the donor heart is damaged in transport.
- Anastomoses required are pulmonary artery, aorta, right atrium, and left atrium. The bicaval technique anastomoses the SVC and IVC (rather than at the right atrial level).
- De-airing is critical and at least three cycles are recommended. TOE can be a useful guide to removal of intracardiac air.
- A left atrial line or a pulmonary artery catheter gives useful information about left and right heart function.
- Atrial and ventricular pacing wires are required even if the heart is in sinus rhythm.
- The aim is for less than three hours donor organ ischaemic time.
- The heart is reperfused for 20 minutes per 60 minutes ischaemia. A reperfusion period longer than 60 minutes is probably not necessary.
- If right heart failure occurs post-transplantation, LA pressure, PCWP, and TOE are useful guides to avoid over-filling.

Anaesthetic management of heart transplantation

Assessment
- Standard anaesthetic assessment including anaesthetic/medical/surgical history, medication, allergies, dental assessment, airway status, and reflux. Specifically note recent renal function, and any evidence of deterioration or cardiac events after the last clinic assessment.
- History of cardiac pathology.
- Fasting status (due to the nature of transplantation, patients may arrive un-starved).
- Previous echo and angio results. Patients with a high PVR or TPG (transpulmonary gradient = mean PA pressure – LA pressure (or PAOP)) may require right heart support.
- Avoid sedative pre-medication; there is usually insufficient time for it to be effective and responses can be unpredictable. Profound sedation can occur in those with heart failure. Initial immunosuppression is prescribed by transplant physicians, and is given orally.

Pre-induction preparation
- Induction agents – propofol, thiopental, or etomidate.
- Opiates – fentanyl, alfentanil, or sufentanil (not licensed in UK).
- Paralysis – pancuronium, vecuronium, atracurium, rocuronium.
- Suxamethonium may be required for rapid sequence induction.
- Resuscitation drugs – metaraminol or phenylephrine, calcium chloride, atropine, epinephrine 1/100,000.
- Heparin 300 IU/kg.
- Immunosuppression and antibiotic prophylaxis guided by local protocols.
- Lidocaine 1%.
- Maintenance drugs e.g. propofol, remifentanil.
- GTN infusion.
- Inotropes guided by policy (see below).
- TOE machine with probe.
- Nitric oxide if high PVR (especially with documented reversibility), high TPG, heart size discrepancy.
- Request 6 unit cross-match and platelets to be available.

Induction

Methods of induction may vary somewhat from unit to unit:
- Induction in theatre recommended for unstable patients.
- Judicious sedation (e.g. midazolam) can be used if the patient is very anxious.
- Lines under local anaesthetic – 20 G radial arterial line, 14 G peripheral IV cannula.
- Central venous access prior to induction is not essential, but is policy in some centres. Those who are very unstable may already have central lines and inotropic support running.
- Pre-oxygenation.
- Modified rapid sequence induction if full stomach.
- Slow IV induction, remembering that arm-brain circulation times can be prolonged in heart failure.
- Judicious fluid management with vasoconstriction and inotropes will help to maintain arterial blood pressure; those on preoperative diuretics may have low circulating volumes.
- Intubation with single lumen endotracheal tube.
- Temperature probe, eye protection, and urinary catheter.
- Central venous lines if not already sited. Use of the left internal jugular vein preserves the right for subsequent myocardial biopsies. Four- or five-lumen central line.
- Insertion of TOE probe.
- Half of the methylprednisolone dose administered at induction.
- Nasogastric tube inserted (may need to delay until TOE probe is removed) to allow postop immunosuppression and nutrition.

Induction factors in patients with ventricular assist devices

- Siting a radial arterial line can be difficult, especially with the axial flow pumps as there is no pulse pressure. It is usually feasible to reduce the flow through the device temporarily to allow the heart to eject so that a pulse can be felt; all but the most badly damaged hearts will eject somewhat. If this is not possible, then an ultrasound-guided approach can be used for either the brachial artery or the femoral artery. Remember that one femoral artery and vein may be required for cardiopulmonary bypass in those having repeat sternotomy.
- Central access may take longer as the internal jugular veins may have been cannulated previously.
- In the event of a haemodynamically significant arrhythmia, most modern devices are defibrillator safe.
- The mean arterial pressure (less the central venous pressure) rather than the normal systolic/diastolic pressure is used as a guide to perfusion pressure.
- The cardiac output is determined by the VAD flow.
- Drive lines and insertion sites may be infected or colonized and its manipulation can lead to a significant microbial and toxic load.

Management prior to cardiopulmonary bypass

- Inhalational and intravenous techniques are all suitable for maintenance prior to bypass.
- A balanced approach using opiates, muscle relaxation, and either intravenous or inhaled anaesthetics is suitable. ACE inhibitors, alpha-blockers, and calcium antagonists all exacerbate anaesthesia-induced vasodilation.
- Excessive fluid therapy prior to CPB should be avoided as the patient will receive bypass prime and is often already fluid-overloaded.
- Adequacy of arterial blood pressure is best judged by urine output and indices of tissue oxygenation. An evolving metabolic acidosis or lactic acidosis indicate poor peripheral perfusion.
- Baseline thromboelastography can be done prior to heparinization. A chronic inflammatory reaction in VAD patients can lead to a prothrombotic state, whereas chronic liver congestion can cause a clotting factor deficiency.
- Heparin 300 IU/kg is given prior to cannulation.
- In those patients anticoagulated with warfarin, it is not necessary to reverse the anticoagulation with FFP prior to CPB.

Management during cardiopulmonary bypass

- Anaesthesia is maintained by intravenous techniques. Propofol and remifentanil infusions are suitable.
- Mean arterial pressure is maintained using pressor agents (e.g. metaraminol) or volatile agents (e.g. isoflurane).
- Regular ACT and ABG every 30 minutes.
- Haemoglobin maintained above lower limit as per unit protocol (8.0 g/dl).
- Assess the need for vasoconstriction while on cardiopulmonary bypass, especially as protective donor cardioplegia is added to the circulation and ventricular assist devices are being mobilized. Consider infusion of norepinephrine or vasopressin.

Weaning from cardiopulmonary bypass

- The potassium level should be 3.5–4. Newly transplanted hearts are very sensitive to extracellular potassium levels and rapid administration can lead to VF, so a lower limit is tolerated compared with other types of cardiac surgery.
- The denervated heart rate is usually around 100. If the rate is lower then AAI or DDD pacing should be used. Higher heart rates limit ventricular filling time and ventricular wall stresses.
- Inotropic support should be running at low levels to facilitate weaning.
- The echo probe should be positioned in either four-chamber view, to give an overview of left and right heart function, or in transgastric short axis, as a guide to LV filling and function.
- The pump flow is reduced slowly and venous return clamped early, to come off bypass with minimal ventricular filling. TOE, left atrial pressure/PCWP, and CVP are then used as a guide to filling 'up the Starling curve'.

Haemodynamic compromise following weaning

- A structured assessment of haemodynamic compromise will enable appropriate therapy (Figure 32.1).
- A low-dose epinephrine infusion is commonly started. At-risk patients (high PVR/transpulmonary gradient or heart size mismatch) should have phosphodiesterase inhibitors (enoximone/milrinone) and inhaled nitric oxide to hand. The newer calcium channel agonist levosimendan has shown promise, although is not licensed in the UK.
- Significant vasodilation may require norepinephrine or vasopressin.
- Intra-aortic balloon counter-pulsation or the use of ventricular assist devices may need to be considered if inotrope requirement progressively increases.

Common pitfalls following heart transplantation

- Right heart failure is relatively common following transplantation. Signs include hypotension, rising CVP (particularly with a falling PAOP), low urine output, and indices of poor tissue perfusion (acidosis, lacate).
- Right heart failure has been associated with administration of blood products, particularly platelets.
- Reperfusion injury can manifest as global heart failure; the typical echo appearance is that the tissues affected become brightly echogenic. Short-term VAD support may be required.
- Hyperacute rejection can occur in cases of ABO compatibility, but is rare.
- Bleeding is common and excessive losses must be addressed surgically whilst coagulation defects are addressed.

Intensive care following heart transplantation

- A short period of stability prior to weaning and extubation is appropriate. Reperfusion injury and myocardial oedema peak at four hours postop and it may be judicious to delay weaning until after this.
- Inotropic support should not be weaned prematurely despite good haemodynamics, as once ventricular failure occurs, it is a self-propagating phenomenon. Good haemodynamics on support is preferable to compromised haemodynamics without the need for support.
- Ventricular failure can occur rapidly.
- Administration of nitric oxide precludes weaning of ventilatory support until either right heart failure subsides or other medication is used to offload the right ventricle (sildenafil).
- Oliguria is an early sign of right heart dysfunction as well as impending renal failure.
- Patients on immunosuppression are susceptible to infections and sepsis; prophylactic antibiotics are usually continued long-term.
- The addition of immunosuppression (e.g. ciclosporin (cyclosporine)) with antibiotics predisposes to renal dysfunction, which may be exacerbated by low cardiac output and withdrawal of diuretics. Oliguria should be addressed early and renal replacement used if required.
- Routine echocardiography is recommended at 24 hours and myocardial biopsies are performed at one week to assess rejection.

Rejection and immunology

Acute rejection
- Rare in the first week, but can occur at any time.
- Episodes tend to become less common in the years following transplantation, but are the main cause of death within the first year.
- Symptoms include fever, malaise, and poor exercise tolerance. Signs include cardiac failure and arrhythmias.
- Diagnosed by endomyocardial biopsy with characteristic findings of lymphocyte proliferation and myocyte necrosis. Histological features are graded as a guide to treatment. Mild acute rejection in the absence of symptoms may require only surveillance.
- Treatment is aimed at reducing the expansion of the cytotoxic T-cell pool. Pulsed steroids (methylprednisolone) and optimization of immunosuppressive therapy are used in the first instance.
- OKT3 (a monoclonal antibody directed against cytotoxic T-cells) may be given. In severe cases, plasmaphoresis is considered.

Chronic rejection
- Refers to the long-term changes that occur in the transplanted heart.
- Features include coronary artery disease and myocardial fibrosis.
- Accelerated coronary heart disease occurs in 30% of patients at five years and 45% at eight years. Ischaemia is often silent in the denervated heart. Coronary artery bypass grafting may be undertaken.
- Myocardial fibrosis causes a restrictive filling pattern on TOE (small or absent A wave on transmitral flow). This means that although ejection fraction is well maintained, increased filling pressures are poorly tolerated, and can precipitate right heart failure. Signs include congestive cardiac failure, tricuspid murmurs, and liver congestion.
- Treatment of chronic rejection is by prevention and expeditious treatment of episodes of acute rejection. Simvastatin may have a role in the prevention of chronic rejection due to its lipid-lowering properties and suppression of T-cell function.

Intercurrent pathologies post-transplantation
- 70% develop hypertension at one year post-transplantation that may be difficult to control.
- 25–30% develop renal dysfunction within one to five years. Most manifest as elevated creatinine; some may require dialysis or renal transplantation.
- 50–60% have hyperlipidaemia within one year, increasing to 85% at five years.
- 25% develop diabetes/abnormal glucose tolerance within one year.
- Malignancy rates are high in post-transplant patients, especially skin and lymphatic. 3% at one year rising to 16% at five years and 26% at eight years.

Immunosupressant medications

Table 32.4 Immunosuppressant medications

Medication	Mode of action	Side effects
Ciclosporin (Cyclosporine) A	Calcineurin inhibitor, inhibits cytotoxic T-cell response	Renal impairment, hypertrichosis, headaches, tremor, hepatic dysfunction
Tacrolimus	Calcineurin inhibitor, inhibits cytotoxic T-cell response	GI disturbance and ulceration, hepatic dysfunction, hypertension, tachycardia, angina
Mycophenolate mofetil	IMPDH inhibitor; reduces lymphocyte counts and clonal expansion in lymphocytes	GI disturbance, influenza-like syndrome, elevated creatinine
Corticosteroids	Reduces synthesis of interleukins and interferon	GI disturbance and ulceration, pancreatitis, osteoporosis, hirsutism, weight gain, myopathy
Azathioprine	Purine analogue that blocks DNA synthesis	Interstitial nephritis, marrow suppression, hepatic impairment
Sirolimus	Prevents T-cell expansion, but not a calcineurin inhibitor; acts synergistically with cyclosporin	Oedema, abdominal pain, thrombocytopenia
Daclizumuab	Il-2 receptor antibody, monoclonal. Prevents T-cell expansion	
Muromonab-CD3 (OKT3®)	Anti-CD3 antibody that binds to cytotoxic T-cells and blocks antigen recognition	Risk of excessive immunosuppression, anti-OKT3 antibodies neutralize the effect
RATG	Polyclonal antibodies that bind to circulating lymphocytes	Fever, rigors, anaphylaxis, serum sickness, immune complex glomerulonephritis
Simvastatin	Suppresses T-cell function	GI disturbance

The previously transplanted patient

- 2% of heart transplants worldwide are re-transplantations.
- Outcome is worse than first time transplantation. 50% survive at seven years compared to 9.6 years for first-time transplantation.
- >80% survive more than one year if re-transplanted after five years compared to less than 50% survival if re-transplanted within one year.
- Operative implications are the same as those for a redo-sternotomy.

Further reading

1. Hunt S. ACC/AHA guideline update for the diagnosis and management of chronic heart failure in the adult. *Journal of the American College of Cardiology* 2005; 46: e1–e82.
2. Lee D, Austin P, Rouleau J, et al. Predicting mortality among patients hospitalized for heart failure. *JAMA* 2003; 290: 2581–2587.
3. Massad M. Current trends in heart transplantation. *Cardiology* 2004; 101: 79–92.
4. Mehra M, Kobashigawa J, Starling R et al. Listing criteria for heart transplantation: International Society for Heart and Lung Transplantation guidelines for the care of cardiac transplant candidates. *The Journal of Heart and Lung Transplantation* 2006; 25: 1024–1042.

Urgent cardiac procedures

Dr K Grebenik

Cardiac tamponade *530*
Chest trauma *534*
Blunt trauma *536*
Aortic transection *538*
Pulmonary embolism *540*
Cardiac tumours *542*
Practice points *543*
Further reading *544*

Cardiac tamponade

Pathology
- Acute tamponade – early post-cardiac surgery, penetrating or blunt trauma, aortic dissection, or iatrogenic injuries.
- Chronic tamponade – late post-cardiac surgery, infection, malignant disease, uraemia, or post-radiotherapy.

Pathophysiology
Pericardial pressure is normally subatmospheric and becomes more negative during inspiration. Accumulation of fluid within the pericardium raises intrapericardial pressure. Initially the cardiac output can be maintained by increasing heart rate and atrial and ventricular filling pressures. As further fluid accumulates within the pericardium, pericardial pressure increases above the ventricular filling pressure causing a reduction in stroke volume and cardiac output. The pressure–volume curve for the pericardium is dependent on the rate of accumulation of fluid – large volumes (up to one litre) can be accommodated if fluid accumulation is slow so that the pericardium stretches. In contrast, volumes of 150 ml may produce tamponade acutely.

Cardiac chamber compression causes pulsus paradoxus – a decrease in systolic blood pressure of more than 10 mmHg during inspiration (exaggeration of the normal inspiratory decrease in arterial pressure). The x descent of the CVP is accentuated, but the y descent is flattened or absent, as cardiac filling is severely restricted during diastole. Pulsus paradoxus may be absent in tachycardia or profound hypotension. Ascites may be seen in association with chronic tamponade.

Clinical presentation
Acute post-surgery tamponade
- Occurs postoperatively when chest drains block in the presence of excessive bleeding.
- Can occur in presence of localized clot compressing the atria despite an open pericardium and without other widespread compression.
- Fall in cardiac output initially responds to volume loading and inotropic support – but eventually becomes refractory to therapy.
- Classical clinical signs (Beck's triad) – hypotension, neck vein distension, and muffled heart sounds. Of these, only hypotension may be detectable.
- Electrical alternans may be seen on the ECG.
- Diagnosis is primarily clinical. Any patient who requires increasing amounts of inotropic support and rising filling pressures without a dramatic change in regional wall motion should be assumed to have tamponade. Trans-oesophageal echo (TOE) is helpful in distinguishing tamponade from ventricular failure.
- Always consider tamponade. If you remember it, you will never forget it.

Acute tamponade after injury

If the neck veins are distended in association with low blood pressure after chest trauma, the differential diagnosis is:

- Tamponade.
- Tension pneumothorax.
- Myocardial contusion.
- Myocardial infarction.
- Air embolism.

Chronic tamponade

- Signs of low cardiac output and high venous pressure.
- Classical clinical signs (Beck's triad) – hypotension, neck vein distension, and muffled heart sounds.
- Pericardiocentesis of even small volumes of pericardial fluid may dramatically improve the patient's condition.

Treatment for chronic pericardial disease with effusion is initially medical. Pericardiocentesis is performed under echo control. Occasionally open pericardotomy with insertion of a drain is necessary, or for chronic effusions, creation of a pleuro-pericardial window. This may be done thoracoscopically.

Haemodynamic goals in acute tamponade

Maintain blood pressure with fluid loading, intropes, and vasoconstrictors ('**full**, **fast**, **and squeezed tight**') until surgical release.

Anaesthetic plan

- Acute post-surgical tamponade requires early re-sternotomy.
- Induction of anaesthesia and re-intubation should take place in the operating theatre with surgeons scrubbed, as haemodynamic collapse is likely.
- Induction with low doses of induction agent and relaxant may be the least likely to exacerbate hypotension. Ketamine may be useful.
- Small doses of metaraminol (0.5 mg) or phenylephrine may be needed to maintain perfusion pressure.
- Once the chest is opened, there is likely to be rebound hypertension. At this point, anaesthesia can be deepened and inotropic support decreased.
- Lifting the heart to deal with surgical bleeding may cause major disturbance.
- Coagulation should be normalized with the help of thromboelastography.
- Antibiotic cover is needed since reopening of the sternotomy is associated with a considerably increased risk of wound infection.

Surgical essentials

Rarely, it may be necessary to immediately reopen after cardiac surgery to distinguish between tamponade and primary cardiac failure, although this should not occur in the era of TOE. When thoracotomy is undertaken emergently for trauma-related tamponade, evacuation of pericardial haematoma should be followed by careful inspection of the heart for bleeding. This can often be controlled by digital pressure to allow time for resuscitation prior to definitive treatment.

TOE essentials

There will always be a certain amount of clot present around the heart following cardiac surgery; echo signs of tamponade may be subtle but include:

- Fluid or clot collection around the heart.
- Early diastolic collapse of the right ventricular free wall.
- Late diastolic collapse of the right atrium.
- Small chamber sizes with moderate or vigorous ventricular contraction.
- Reciprocal changes with respiration between right and left ventricular chamber size.

TOE should be interpreted in relation to the patient's clinical condition – whilst TOE alone may be misleading, the combination of clinical appearance of low cardiac output with TOE evidence of fluid accumulation around the heart is pathognomic of tamponade.

Chest trauma

Chest trauma may be due to blunt (chest wall remains intact) or penetrating (chest wall integrity is breached) injury – the ratio of the two will vary. In the USA levels of gun use make penetrating trauma considerably more common than in the UK.

As always, priority must be given to maintenance of the airway, breathing, and circulation, and stabilization of the cervical spine. Good multidisciplinary care will help to secure the best possible outcome for these patients; it may be difficult to prioritize investigation and immediate treatment, especially if there is associated head, abdominal, or pelvic injury. A high index of suspicion for chest injury occurring in blunt trauma, coupled with an aggressive diagnostic and therapeutic approach, remains the basis of management.

Any patient with severe chest trauma and hypotension disproportionate to estimated loss of blood or with an inadequate response to fluid administration should be suspected of having a cardiac cause of shock. The diagnosis of tamponade in the presence of hypovolaemia is difficult. Haemodynamic instability may supervene rapidly and require urgent intervention prior to definitive diagnosis. However, emergency thoracotomy for attempted resuscitation of patients who present with absent vital signs is futile; such heroics should be limited to patients who have sustained penetrating chest injuries but who retain signs of life. Closed chest cardiopulmonary resuscitation is ineffective in these circumstances. Cardiopulmonary bypass is rarely needed in the initial management of penetrating cardiac injuries and thoracotomy should not be delayed to wait for availability of CPB.

Immediately life-threatening chest injuries include:
- Massive haemothorax.
- Tension pneumothorax.
- Cardiac tamponade.
- Aortic transection.
- Tracheo-bronchial disruption.
- Lung contusion.
- Flail chest.
- Cardiac contusion or laceration.
- Coronary or valvular injuries.

A complete primary survey should be performed to avoid missing injuries.

Investigations

- CXR – severe chest trauma can be present even in the absence of rib or other thoracic bony fractures. However, abnormalities of the mediastinum on the plain film, including widening of the mediastinum, tracheal displacement, or deviation of a nasogastric tube to the right at the T4 level and depression of the left main-stem bronchus below 40 degrees from the horizontal, are signs associated with a high sensitivity but low specificity for aortic rupture. In other words, if the mediastinum is 'funny looking' then further investigation is needed.
- CT scan is considerably more sensitive than CXR in detecting injuries after blunt chest trauma. CT scanning provides detailed information

about the size, location, and extent of aortic injury, as well as involvement of the mediastinal structures and pericardial and pleural spaces. With intravenous contrast, the aorta and its branch vessels can be imaged, and aortic true and false lumens readily distinguished. The cardinal signs of aortic injury are calibre change of the aorta, intraluminal abnormality, and abnormal outer contour (perivascular haematoma).

- Transthoracic echo (TTE) has low diagnostic yield in severe blunt chest trauma.
- TOE gives better image quality than TTE. TOE is accurate in diagnosis of aortic injuries, although tracheal shadowing may limit visualization of the proximal and distal aortic arch; it can distinguish cardiac tamponade from myocardial dysfunction secondary to contusion. TOE is inexpensive, relatively non-invasive (assuming that the patient has already been intubated), does not interfere with other diagnostic or therapeutic procedures, and can be carried out without transferring the patient from the emergency room.
- Aortography may be needed to assess aortic continuity if TOE is unavailable. In addition to being invasive, time-consuming, and requiring nephrotoxic contrast material, angiography only shows the flow lumen. It gives little information about the aortic wall, and no information about the mediastinum or pleural and pericardial spaces. Additionally, it requires transport to an angiography suite, and specialist personnel who may not be continuously on site.
- Magnetic resonance imaging (MRI) offers many of the advantages of CT scanning and produces superb image quality without the need for ionizing radiation or nephrotoxic contrast media. However, MRI suites are often distant from emergency departments, frequently require lengthy examination times, are restrictive in terms of accompanying metallic equipment, and may not be continuously available nights and weekends.

Blunt trauma

Myocardial contusion

Myocardial contusion is common and presents as a spectrum of injuries of varying severity. The right ventricle is most commonly involved because of its anterior position. Sinus tachycardia, dysrhythmias, bundle branch block, or non-specific ST segment abnormalities may be seen – occurring within the first 24 hours after the injury. Treatment is supportive; associated injuries must be dealt with and the haemodynamics supported. Myocardial contusion carries a favourable prognosis, although occasionally infarction may occur. An elevated troponin level is a sensitive indicator of myocardial damage.

Structural cardiac injuries

Structural cardiac injuries (i.e. chamber rupture or perforation) carry a high mortality rate and patients rarely survive long enough to reach hospital. Chamber rupture is present at autopsy in 36–65% of deaths from blunt cardiac trauma, whereas in clinical series it is present in 0.3–0.9% of cases and is an uncommon clinical finding.

Haemothorax

Haemothorax is present in 25–50% of cases with blunt chest trauma. Initial treatment is with intercostal drain. Bleeding is usually from torn low pressure pulmonary vessels and frequently subsides spontaneously. Thoracotomy is indicated for massive initial blood loss or for continuing losses >200 ml/hour after the first four hours. Large central pulmonary vessels or systemic thoracic veins or arteries are the usual cause of such life-threatening bleeding.

Aortic transection

Clinical presentation and assessment

Rupture or laceration of the thoracic aorta is one of the most dramatic and dangerous consequences of chest trauma. The majority of ruptures occur at the aortic isthmus just distal to the origin of the left subclavian artery, where the aorta is relatively fixed. Patients with ascending aortic rupture rarely survive to reach hospital. When transection is complete, death from haemorrhage is virtually instantaneous. Survival to arrival in hospital implies a contained rupture. Approximately 10–15 per cent of individuals with traumatic rupture survive temporarily; if the lesion is promptly diagnosed appropriate surgical treatment may be life-saving. Diagnosis may be difficult and at times the rupture may remain clinically silent for variable periods.

Clinical history is an important pointer. Traumatic aortic transection is caused by massive deceleration forces, e.g. high-speed motor vehicle crashes. The use of an airbag or seat belt does not eliminate risk. The injury can also occur at low severity impacts, particularly in side impacts.

Patients with blunt aortic injury tend to fall into three major categories, as outlined in Table 33.1.

Table 33.1 Presentation and management of aortic injury

Presentation	Injury type	Management
Dead	Aortic transection with free rupture	
Haemodynamically unstable	Aortic haemorrhage or bleeding from other injuries	Control haemorrhage, prioritize emergency surgical management
Haemodynamically stable	Contained aortic injury	Blood pressure control, decide treatment priority and urgency

Haemodynamic goals

Early arterial cannulation with careful intravascular pressure monitoring is vital. Fluid resuscitation should be limited to that required to keep systolic blood pressure around 80–90 mm Hg (permissive hypotension), i.e. minimum blood pressure required to maintain vital organ function. Hypertension may cause rupture. If necessary, treatment with ß-blockade (e.g. esmolol or labetalol infusion) and vasodilators (glyceryl trinitrate or nitroprusside) should be started to lower blood pressure whilst essential investigations are performed and arrangements made for transfer to theatre.

Anaesthetic plan

- Preoperative considerations include the effects of other injuries, the correction of hypovolaemia, and institution of appropriate monitoring.
- Avoidance of hypertension is crucial.

- Intravenous access should be sufficient to allow rapid transfusion in case of catastrophic intraoperative haemorrhage.
- Intraoperative management is similar to that for elective aortic surgery.
- Postoperative hypertension should be treated vigorously to reduce strain on suture lines.

Surgical essentials

There is controversy over the timing of treatment for aortic transection when it occurs in association with other life-threatening injuries. It may be necessary to delay definitive aortic surgery in order to deal with more urgent problems. Early operative repair is needed in case of:

- Large volume haemorrhage from chest drains.
- Rapidly expanding mediastinal haematoma.
- Penetrating injury of the aorta.

Open surgical repair is hazardous, with mortality rates reaching over 20%. Techniques for repair of aortic transection are similar to those described for thoracic aortic surgery. Repair of transection using simple aortic cross-clamping alone is feasible in the majority of patients without increased mortality or spinal cord injury.

Emergency stent repair to control haemorrhage in patients with an acute thoracic aortic rupture is an attractive, rational, and less invasive treatment option, especially if associated lesions or comorbidity may interfere with the surgical outcome. Compared to open procedures, reports suggest that mortality and paraplegia may be reduced significantly after endovascular treatment of traumatic thoracic aortic disruption – but skill and experience in these techniques may not be available at all times and in all centres. The technology associated with this procedure is evolving.

TOE essentials

- TOE has 93% sensitivity, 98% specificity, and 98% accuracy in detection of aortic rupture.
- The aorta is usually surrounded by haematoma and a false aneurysm may be seen.
- Intimal disruption may resemble atheroma – but this is uncommon in patients under the age of 50.
- The presence of apparently severe localized atheroma in a young person is suggestive of aortic rupture.

Pulmonary embolism

Pathophysiology

Pulmonary embolism (PE) causes acute right ventricular overload and pulmonary hypertension from a combination of mechanical obstruction and release of vasoconstrictor mediators, such as serotonin and thromboxane A2. The effects depend on the degree of pulmonary vascular obstruction and the prior state of the heart and lungs.

When more than 75% of the pulmonary vascular tree is obstructed, mean pulmonary artery pressure approaches the maximum that can be generated by a normal right ventricle (45–50 mmHg); this leads to right ventricular (RV) dilation, increased right atrial pressure, and a decreased cardiac index, associated with low left atrial pressure. Hypoxaemia results from ventilation/perfusion mismatch.

Clinical presentation and diagnosis

Commonly presenting symptoms include chest pain, breathlessness, and anxiety. Massive PE causes syncope, hypoxaemia, hypotension, and cardiac arrest.

Ventilation/perfusion scanning is the cornerstone of PE diagnosis, but for those patients with suspected massive PE who are too sick to move, echo may confirm or refute the diagnosis. TOE can visualize a clot in the main pulmonary arteries, has sensitivity of 80% to 90%, and specificity of nearly 100% for the detection of massive pulmonary embolism, but is dependent on the expertise of the echocardiographer. CT angiography is very useful.

Acute massive pulmonary embolism is associated with a high mortality rate. Prompt diagnosis and treatment are mandatory for a successful outcome. Although thrombolysis is effective, it is associated with a high rate of bleeding complications.

The indications for surgery are:
- Life-threatening circulatory instability, when thrombolysis is contraindicated or has been unsuccessful.
- Occasionally as a resuscitative manoeuvre in patients with intractable or recurrent cardiac arrest where embolism is deemed to be the cause.

Early aggressive surgical treatment of pulmonary embolus is recommended by some authorities, and may be associated with improved long-term survival.

Anaesthetic plan

- Patients presenting for surgical embolectomy are likely to be *in extremis*. Induction of anaesthesia should take place in theatre with surgical staff scrubbed and ready. Further haemodynamic compromise should be anticipated following induction.
- High inspired oxygen concentrations are needed to reduce hypoxaemia. PEEP should be avoided, since it will add to right ventricular afterload.
- Noradrenaline infusion is used to support the arterial pressure and improve right ventricular perfusion.

- Severe coagulopathy may be anticipated in those in whom thrombolytic therapy has already been tried. This requires support with antifibrinolytics, clotting factors, and platelets.
- In some centres percutaneous supportive bypass may be set up to assist the circulation before definitive surgery.

Surgical essentials

Open pulmonary embolectomy is performed on bypass. The main and branch pulmonary arteries are opened and disobliterated as far as possible. A patent foramen ovale or atrial septal defect should be closed at the time of surgery to prevent passage of any further emboli into the left heart. Prevention of further emboli is important and insertion of a vena caval filter may be considered.

TOE essentials

- It may be possible to visualize large central emboli and to differentiate fresh from old thrombus.
- High RV afterload will be manifest as RV dilation and hypokinesis, frequently with functional tricuspid regurgitation.
- Paradoxical motion of the interventricular septum may be seen due to a shift by a dilated right ventricle.
- The left heart is usually empty and vigorous.

Cardiac tumours

The commonest cardiac tumours are secondaries from lung, oesophagus, breast, or lymphoma, but these rarely require surgical intervention. Myxoma is the commonest benign tumour of the heart.

Pathology

Myxomas are usually solitary; 75% arise in the left atrium, 20% in the right atrium. Macroscopically they are soft, rounded, or polypoid tumours, often gelatinous or semi-translucent.

Clinical presentation

- Cardiac failure due to valve obstruction or regurgitation.
- Systemic or pulmonary emboli.

Patients who have recently suffered embolic events may present for urgent surgery to reduce the risk of further embolization.

Preoperative investigation

Diagnosis is achieved by echo. Cardiac catheterization is contraindicated because of the risk of tumour fragmentation.

Anaesthetic plan

Standard anaesthetic management applies. In right atrial myxoma it may be wise to avoid passing the Seldinger wire from a CVP into the right atrium since it could potentially cause tumour fragmentation.

Practice points

Cardiac tamponade

- Always consider tamponade in the differential diagnosis of low cardiac output state following surgery.
- Do not delay when tamponade is suspected – the patient will not improve until the tamponade is released.

Aortic transection

- Emergency room thoracotomy in dead patients is dramatic but pointless.
- Hypotension in polytrauma may be multifactorial. Look for other injuries besides the obvious.
- Permissive hypotension will minimize the risk of aortic rupture and may improve outcome.
- Early TOE and/or CT scan will help to delineate cardiac and aortic injury.
- When dealing with patients for urgent cardiac procedures, close cooperation is needed between surgeon and anaesthetist.

Further reading

1. Bell RE, Reidy JF. Endovascular treatment of thoracic aortic disease. *Heart* 2003; 89: 823–824.
2. Holt R, Martin T, Hess P, Beaver T, Klodell C. Jehovah's witnesses requiring complex urgent cardiothoracic surgery. *The Annals of Thoracic Surgery* 2004; 78: 695–697.
3. Sybrandy KC, Cramer MJM, Burgersdijk C. Diagnosing cardiac contusion: Old wisdom and new insights. *Heart* 2003; 89: 485–489.
4. Orford VP, Atkinson NR, Thomson K, et al. Blunt traumatic aortic transection: The endovascular experience. *Annals of Thoracic Surgery* 2003; 75: 106–112.

Anaesthesia for electrophysiology procedures

Dr E Ashley

Permanent and temporary pacemakers *546*
Anaesthesia for pacemaker and ICD insertion *550*
Indwelling pacemakers, ICDs, and anaesthesia *552*
Anaesthesia for DC cardioversion *554*
Anaesthesia for electrophysiology and catheter
   ablation procedures *556*
Further reading *561*

Permanent and temporary pacemakers

Patients now present for cardiac and non-cardiac surgery with sophisticated pacing devices. Temporary pacing is frequently employed after cardiac surgery to maximize cardiac output. The cardiac catheter laboratory and catheter-mediated arrhythmia surgery present unique problems for the cardiac anaesthetist.

Epicardial pacing

Patients who have undergone valve surgery or complex cardiac surgical procedures are at risk of developing complete heart block or bradycardia in the postoperative period and may require pacing. Most anaesthetists treat sinus bradycardia after coronary artery surgery with epicardial pacing, whereas others prefer chronotropic drugs.

Temporary epicardial wires are placed on the heart prior to separation from bypass. Atrial wires are attached to the right atrial appendage and ventricular wires to the epicardial surface of the right ventricle. Conventionally atrial wires emerge through the chest wall on the right and ventricular on the left. An active and an indifferent connection are required to pace a chamber and these are connected to the temporary pacing box. It is possible to pace with only one pacing wire. A skin indifferent is created by attaching a pacing wire to the patient's skin and connecting this to the second terminal of the pacing lead connector. The single wire is the active lead, and the skin indifferent completes the circuit. The perceived advantage is that it decreases the risk of bleeding on removal. However, the uninitiated may be unsure of how to connect up the wires and do not understand that a skin indifferent has to be placed to complete the electrical circuit. This can cause confusion and delay pacing in an emergency.

One or two chambers may be paced in asynchronous (fixed-rate) or demand modes. Atrial wires do not work in chronic atrial fibrillation, but in general dual chamber sequential pacing is preferable to reproduce a paced sinus rhythm and maintain atrial contribution to ventricular filling. Asynchronous pacing can be hazardous if it competes with a patient's intrinsic rhythm. Demand pacing senses the heart's intrinsic activity, and inhibits pacing if a predetermined voltage is detected.

Pacing modes of temporary devices have the same nomenclature and coding as implanted devices. The first letter indicates the chamber **paced**, the second the chamber **sensed**, and the third the **response** to sensing (Table 34.1).

Table 34.1 Temporary pacing modes

Pacing mode	I	II	III
Asynchronous atrial	A	0	0
Demand atrial	A	A	I
Asynchronous ventricular	V	0	0
Demand ventricular	V	V	I
Asynchronous dual pacing	D	0	0
Sequential with ventricular sensing	D	V	I
Sequential with dual sensing	D	D	D

A = atrium; V = ventricular, I = inhibit; D = dual; 0 = neither (sense nor inhibit)

Complications

Pacing failure

This may be due to inadequate voltage output, lead failure, pacing box failure, detachment of wires, or electrical shorting of epicardial wires. Pacing thresholds increase if fibrosis, oedema, or haematoma occur around temporary wires, which may necessitate replacement by a permanent system in pacing-dependent patients. ECG interference due to diathermy in theatre can inhibit demand pacing. **Pacing thresholds should be checked daily** and epicardial wires generally become unreliable after seven days.

If pacing fails, a solution should be sought by checking all components of the pacing system, checking the position of the epicardial wires if the chest is still open, increasing the output voltage, and considering switching to an asynchronous mode if diathermy use persists. If this is unsuccessful, give chronotropic drugs (atropine or isoprenaline), commence external pacing, or prepare for transvenous pacing. Asynchronous pacing is often necessary when the chest is open due to frequent interference, not only from diathermy but also direct handling of the heart. If this situation arises, it is essential to frequently review the underlying rhythm to avoid pacing competing or interfering with the native rhythm. Once the chest is closed, demand pacing should be reinstated.

Arrhythmias

These can be due to competition with a patient's own rhythm. This can arise as above when asynchronous pacing is employed and there is inadequate sensing of the native rhythm. R on T phenomena, i.e. pacing on top of a T wave, can lead to ventricular fibrillation.

Removal of epicardial wires

This infrequently causes bleeding or tamponade, particularly in anti-coagulated patients, Wires should be removed in a cardiac centre early in the day, with maximal staff availability, in case of complication or requirement for emergent re-sternotomy.

External pacing

This can be useful in emergencies and is a function available on most modern defibrillators. ECG recording, sensing, and pacing occur via adhesive defibrillator pads applied to the chest wall. The pulse generator causes painful shocks and is not well tolerated in awake patients. The efficacy of this technique is highly variable.

Transvenous pacing

This is achieved by passing a temporary pacing wire into the right atrium, right ventricle, or coronary sinus via a central vein, often under X-ray control. A ventricular wire is optimally positioned at the lateral wall of the right-ventricular apex. If the wire points towards the left shoulder it may be positioned in the coronary sinus. An atrial wire takes on the form of a 'J' in the right atrium. The patient is asked to cough or take large breaths to check that pacing is maintained and confirm wire stability. Asynchronous or demand pacing modes can be achieved with this system and sensing and pacing chambers depend on wire position.

Complications of transvenous pacing
- Complications of central venous line insertion.
- Complications of epicardial pacing systems, i.e. box lead and connector failure (as above).
- Atrial and ventricular ectopics and arrhythmias.
- Perforation leading to tamponade.
- Endocarditis.
- Pericarditis.
- Diaphragmatic pacing.

Balloon-directed pacing catheter

Balloon-directed pacing catheters are available that incorporate a pacing electrode at the catheter tip. This enables emergency pacing of the right ventricular outflow tract. Flotation-pacing catheters can be quickly inserted into the right ventricle via a venous sheath without X-ray guidance in an emergency situation. If the patient is critically unstable, simply insert a right internal jugular pacing sheath and push the flotation catheter with balloon inflated through it until pacing can be achieved at any output voltage. Repositioning for stability and to minimize voltage threshold can then occur when haemodynamic stability returns.

Permanent pacemakers

Evidence-based indications for insertion of permanent pacemakers are graded from class I to class III by the American College of Cardiology. Class I indications are:
- Acquired third degree heart block associated with bradycardias or arrhythmias.
- Symptomatic acquired second degree heart block.
- Chronic bifascicular and trifascicular block.
- Post-myocardial infarction infranodal atrioventricular block.
- Sinus node dysfunction with symptomatic bradycardia.
- Sustained ventricular tachycardia in which the efficacy of pacing has been documented.

- Hypertensive carotid sinus syndrome.
- Patients with HOCM or dilated cardiomyopathy who have sinus node dysfunction or atrioventricular block.
- After cardiac transplantation, if symptomatic bradyarrhythmias persist.

Pacemakers are usually situated subcutaneously or sub-pectoral below the left clavicle. Leads pass current to the myocardium as well as relay information back to the pacing box. Modern pacemakers contain a microprocessor that can be programmed via the manufacturer's interrogation system. A wand is placed over the pacemaker and functions such as pacing mode, pacing rate, voltage output, sensing, rate-responsiveness, and anti-tachycardia functions can be changed. Pacing modes are similar to those generated by epicardial wires (Table 34.1). In addition there are letters IV and V for permanent devices; IV indicates programmability and rate modulation, and the defibrillation function is indicated by V (Table 34.2).

Anaesthesia for pacemaker and ICD insertion

Table 34.2 The NASPE/BPEG generic (NBG) pacemaker code

Letter position	I	II	III	IV	V
Category	Chamber paced	Chamber sensed	Response to sensing	Programmability and rate modulation	Anti-tachyarrhythmia functions
Letters	0 = none	0 = none	0 = none	0 = none	0 = none
	A = atrium	A = atrium	T = triggered	P = simple programmable	P = pacing
	V = ventricle	V = ventricle	I = inhibited	M = multi-programmable	S = shock
	D = dual (A + V)	D = dual (A + V)	D = dual	C = communicating	D = dual (P + S)
				R = rate modulation	

Example: VVIR = Rate responsive ventricular demand pacing.

Indications for implantable cardiac defibrillator (ICD) insertion

Primary
- Previous myocardial infarction (MI) and left ventricular ejection fraction (LVEF) <30–35%, and either non-sustained ventricular tachycardia (VT) on Holter monitoring with inducible VT on electrophysiology study (EPS) or QRS >120 ms.
- Conditions associated with high risk of sudden death, e.g. long QT syndrome, hypertrophic cardiomyopathy, Brugada syndrome, arrhythmogenic right ventricular cardiomyopathy, and congenital heart disease.

Secondary
- Post-VT or ventricular fibrillation (VF) cardiac arrest.
- Spontaneous VT causing syncope or haemodynamic compromise.
- Sustained VT without syncope or arrest with an ejection fraction less than 35%.

Patients and preoperative assessment

Look out for:
- Patients can be sick with poor ejection fractions and are at risk of ventricular arrhythmias.
- Post-myocardial infarction.
- Hypertrophic cardiomyopathy.
- Left ventricular failure.

- Occasionally young, fit, and asymptomatic with normal ventricular function.
- Preoperative assessment should include an assessment of ejection fraction and the patient's ability to lie flat. Electrolytes should be checked including potassium.

Intraoperative

Some cardiologists sedate their own patients for ICD insertion. However, the enlightened ones enlist anaesthetic support. NICE guidelines suggest that ICDs are inserted under sedation with local anaesthesia. The box is usually placed sub-pectoral on the left side. The leads are inserted via the left cephalic vein and positioned in the right ventricle or the coronary sinus; the latter enables pacing of the left side of the heart. Testing the device at the end of the procedure demands deeper sedation so that external defibrillation can be employed if necessary. Revisions or replacements of a pacemaker box with ICD can be more difficult and uncomfortable and often require general anaesthesia.

General comments concerning the problems of anaesthesia in the catheter lab apply (📖 see also Anaesthesia for electrophysiology and catheter ablation procedures, p. 556).

- Monitoring should be appropriate for the cardiovascular status of the patient. If concerned, insert and monitor an arterial line when awake. External defibrillator pads attached to a defibrillator and ECG monitoring are essential. Careful anaesthesia or sedation using midazolam or a target-controlled infusion (TCI) of propofol are appropriate (aim for 2–3 µg/ml target plasma concentration for sedation).
- The airway may be maintained with a laryngeal mask and spontaneous respiration, but paralysis and intubation are appropriate in compromised or larger patients. Access to the airway is limited during the procedure due to the proximity of the surgical field.
- Depth of anaesthesia can be conveniently titrated with TCI propofol to facilitate device testing.
- If the device fails to defibrillate during testing, external paddles must be used. The patient may be hypotensive after a period of induced VF and require vasoconstrictors.
- Antibiotic prophylaxis should be considered. Infection is a disaster in implantable devices.

Indwelling pacemakers, ICDs, and anaesthesia

300,000 patients have a permanent pacemaker in the UK, with approximately 300 new implants per million population per year. ICD implants are increasing. These devices pose unique problems for anaesthesia and surgery.

Patients and preoperative assessment

- Patients will hopefully produce a 'European Pacemaker Patient Identification Card'. This should contain patient data, date of original implantation, primary and secondary symptoms, ECG characteristics, and aetiology of the rhythm. It should contain useful details of the pacemaker centre, cardiologist, and GP, details of the device, pacing mode, leads, and date of implantation.
- The other extreme is that the patient will not inform anybody that they have a pacemaker and you will discover it on examination of the chest, from the ECG or on the chest X-ray!
- The pacemaker should be checked prior to anaesthesia. If there is no information available about the device, cardiac technicians can identify the device manufacturer from the device's default magnet rate (Table 34.3). They can then interrogate the pacemaker and reprogram it with the appropriate apparatus. Anti-tachycardia and defibrillator functions should be deactivated in ICDs, as well as rate-responsiveness. It is usually unnecessary to reprogram to a fixed-rate mode and indeed this may be dangerous if pacing competes with native rhythm.
- Investigations include:
  - 12-lead ECG: evidence of pacing, evidence of capture (pacing spike followed by an electrical complex), underlying rhythm.
  - Chest X-ray: position of the pacing box, integrity and position of the leads, lead fracture. Also cardiac size and evidence of cardiac failure.
  - Electrolytes: correct before surgery as abnormalities might interfere with capture.

Intraoperative management

- Monitoring: standard, according to the complexity of the surgery, but consider an arterial line to confirm beat-to-beat capture. Central venous lines must be inserted carefully to avoid dislodging newly implanted pacing wires. The ECG should be in 'pacing-mode' if available so that pacing spikes are not interpreted as complexes, giving erroneous heart rates, or even reporting a heart rate when the pacemaker is failing to capture and the patient is asystolic.
- Induction: careful; suxamethonium can cause fasciculations, which will be falsely sensed as ECG activity.
- Diathermy: bipolar only if possible. A unipolar diathermy plate should be positioned as far from the pacing box as possible. The direction of the current pacing from the diathermy to the earth plate should be perpendicular to the pacing leads to avoid induction currents. Unipolar diathermy should be restricted to short bursts. This is the

most useful strategy if diathermy interference is occurring despite these precautions.

- Magnets **can** be used on newer programmable pacemakers and ICDs. The effect of magnet placement for common pacemakers is listed in Table 34.3. A circular magnet should be available in theatre and this is taped over the pacing box on the patient's chest. Default fixed-rate modes will be induced.
- Contingency measures in the event of pacing failure include isoprenaline infusions, external pacing via the defibrillator pads, transvenous temporary pacing, and epicardial wires after cardiac surgery.

Postoperative management

Get the device checked and reprogrammed. Functions such as rate responsiveness and defibrillation modes should be reactivated.

Table 34.3 Default settings in response to magnet placement

Pacemaker type	Magnet rate	Magnet mode
CPI/Guidant	100 bpm	DOO or VOO
ELA	96 bpm	DOO or VOO
Medtronic	85 bpm	DOO or VOO
St. Jude Medical	90 bpm	DOO or VOO
ICD		All tachy-therapies disabled

Placement of a magnet will turn off rate-responsiveness in all devices

Anaesthesia for DC cardioversion

Patients present with acute or chronic atrial fibrillation or flutter for DC cardioversion. Atrial fibrillation can be inducible, paroxysmal, persistent, or permanent and each type carries a different prognosis for successful cardioversion, or electrophysiological ablation. Atrial flutter has an atrial rate of 280–320 bpm with a variable AV node conduction block, determining the ventricular rate. 2:1 block with a ventricular rate of 150 bpm is common.

Preoperative

- Check potassium (K^+ ≥4.5 mmol/l). If it is low the procedure is less likely to be successful.
- Check anticoagulation. If the patient has been in AF for more than 48 hours, anticoagulation for four weeks is necessary prior to cardioversion or left atrial thrombus should be excluded by TOE. An INR of ≥2.5 is desirable.
- Digoxin toxicity is a relative contraindication as it reduces successful cardioversion.
- Note the cause of the AF (recent MI, ischaemic heart disease, valvular heart disease, congenital heart disease, thyroid disease).
- Asses the extent to which the cardiac output is compromised by the arrhythmia.

Intraoperative

- Remote site considerations, e.g. coronary care unit, catheter lab.
- Take and check all equipment and an assistant!
- If a TOE is required it is usual to intubate the patient.
- If not, a spontaneously breathing, mask anaesthetic is appropriate unless there is an aspiration risk.
- Induction with full non-invasive monitoring using a small dose of propofol or etomidate. A short-acting muscle relaxant such as mivacurium or a small dose of atracurium can be used if intubation is required.
- Defibrillation is more likely to be successful if the pads are placed in a front to back position (anterior/posterior chest). Some cardiologists prefer to press hard with paddles to reduce chest impedance (especially in obese patients or those with emphysematous lung disease), whereas others used adhesive pads. With monophasic defibrillators commence at 200 Joules in AF increasing to 360 Joules on the third shock. In flutter commence at 50 Joules. These values can be significantly reduced if a biphasic defibrillator is used.
- Remove oxygen during defibrillation.
- Analgesia is unnecessary although the nurses like to rub 1% hydrocortisone cream into the patient's chest after the procedure!

Postoperative

- Recovery facilities may be inadequate in the catheter laboratory and it may be necessary to recover the patient yourself or transfer to the main recovery facility.
- Atrial stunning (impaired atrial contractility) can occur after successful cardioversion. The suggested mechanisms include tachycardia-induced atrial myopathy and chronic atrial hibernation.
- Atrial stunning does not occur after unsuccessful attempts at cardioversion.
- The patient can be discharged according to day-care criteria.

Internal cardioversion

External cardioversion may be unsuccessful in obese patients or patients with emphysematous lung disease or asthma. Some cardiologists may attempt internal cardioversion between a right heart catheter (positioned under X-ray screening via the femoral vein) and a back plate. A small synchronized shock of 10–20 Joules is delivered to the heart via the catheter. This technique may also be used in patients with implanted devices that could be damaged by high-energy shocks. Anaesthetic considerations are similar to those for external cardioversion. Anaesthesia or sedation should be deepened before the shock is delivered.

Anaesthesia for electrophysiology and catheter ablation procedures

(📖 see also Chapter 13.)

Patients and preoperative assessment

Many EP procedures can be carried out under local anaesthesia and sedation, but some are lengthy and require the patient to lie still and cooperate for several hours. Consequently some patients and/or cardiologists request general anaesthesia. Patients who may require general anaesthesia include:
- Children and adolescents.
- Anxious adults.
- Adults with congenital heart disease and complex cardiac anatomy.
- Patients requiring left atrial ablation via a trans-septal puncture.

Associated risk factors to be aware of on preoperative assessment include:
- Cardiovascular disease.
- Ischaemic heart disease.
- Valvular disease (particularly mitral causing left atrial enlargement).
- Hypertension.
- Hypercholesterolaemia.
- Thyroid disease.
- Obesity.
- Diabetes.
- Excessive alcohol consumption.
- Impaired LV function.
- Cardiomyopathy.
- Congenital heart disease.
- Previous cardiac surgery.
- Antihypertensive and antiarrhythmic medication.
- Anticoagulation.

The patient may be anticoagulated. It is important to establish how long the patient has been in an atrial arrhythmia and how long he or she has been effectively anticoagulated, to assess the need for exclusion of left atrial thrombus by TOE. Longer than 48 hours without anticoagulation mandates TOE or deferment for four weeks with warfarin.

Catheter laboratory

The environment
- Hazardous.
- Isolated.
- Noisy, crowded, distractions.
- Staff can be unfamiliar with general anaesthesia.
- Non-tipping cardiac catheter tables (tipping tables are available).

Procedures and requirements
- Protracted (1–6 hours).
- Non-stimulating.

- Require absolute immobility.
- Potential for arrhythmias.
- Maintenance of temperature.
- Positioning.
- Fluid overload.
- Volatile vs. total intravenous.
- Monitoring of neuromuscular block (movement can dislodge catheters).
- Oesophageal temperature measurement (local temperature rises might be associated with oesophageal injury).
- Nasogastric tube or oesophageal temperature probe to assist operator in defining oesophageal relationship.

Anaesthesia for catheter ablation surgery

There are usually no anaesthetic rooms in catheter laboratories and so anaesthesia induction has to take place in the lab. The procedures require extensive ECG monitoring and the application of adhesive defibrillator pads. These depend on the ablation system in use. The front and back monitoring is applied by cardiology technicians prior to induction. The pads must have good contact to avoid electrical burns. Standard anaesthetic monitoring should be commenced, including non-invasive blood pressure recording and pulse oximetry. Some catheter laboratory tables do not tip. If the table tips, the radiographer who is familiar with the table controls must be immediately available during induction, otherwise anaesthesia should be induced on a trolley.

Induction is tailored to the cardiovascular status of the patient. Intravenous induction with a judicious dose of propofol and a non-depolarizing neuromuscular blocker is standard. Intubation is usual for prolonged procedures and when TOE is required. Positioning and protection of pressure areas requires careful attention, and securing arms in position to allow lateral X-rays, but avoiding brachial plexus injury, is important. Maintenance is controversial as volatile agents have been implicated in the suppression of arrhythmias. A total intravenous anaesthesia (TIVA) technique with propofol may therefore be desirable, although the difference between volatile techniques and TIVA is probably not clinically relevant. General anaesthesia can interfere with inducibility of AV node re-entrant tachycardias, which makes it very difficult to diagnose this condition under anaesthesia. There are some effects of general anaesthesia on pulmonary vein isolation confirmation when treating atrial fibrillation, and little if any effect when treating atrial flutter.

The procedures are non-stimulating with little postoperative pain, and analgesia requirements are minimal. Left-sided procedures such as AF ablation in the left atrium involve a trans-atrial septal puncture. This increases the risk of cardiac perforation and tamponade. The patient is anticoagulated with heparin and the ACT maintained at >250–300 seconds during ablation to decrease the risk of thromboembolic complications related to the large-bore catheters.

Vasoconstrictors are frequently necessary during the procedure to maintain blood pressure. The cardiologist will usually infiltrate with local anaesthetic at percutaneous catheter insertion sites. It is important to monitor neuromuscular block during the procedure to avoid coughing during catheter ablation. Although ablation systems compensate for respiratory variation, minimal tidal volumes are desirable whilst ablating in the left atrium to reduce posterior left atrial motion and catheter movement.

A radio-opaque nasogastric tube indicates the position of the oesophagus and monitoring oesophageal temperature at the distal end of the nasogastric tube alerts the cardiologist to excessive local oesophageal heating during left atrial ablation. This is most likely when ablating the posterior left atrium. There have been reports of oesophageal perforation and late oesophageal-atrial fistula. There have also been reports of peri-oesophageal nerve damage, resulting in acute pyloric spasm, abdominal pain, and delayed gastric emptying.

The ablation catheters are cooled with a saline infusion and significant volumes of saline can be infused into the patient. The anaesthetist must be aware of volumes used and reduce IV infusion rates accordingly. A urinary catheter may be required. Heat conservation is an issue during prolonged procedures and a heat moisture exchanger and forced-air-warming blanket are useful.

Reversal of anaesthesia and extubation requires concentration; the table is narrow and patients can roll. Sitting the patient up or extubating them in the left lateral position is limited by the need for groin compression to prevent haematoma formation. Coughing increases venous pressure and is thought to increase the likelihood of groin haematoma. The laboratory staff are less familiar with anaesthetized patients and therefore require direction during lifting and transfer to prevent injury to limbs and loss of lines, etc. They also tend to focus on groin bleeding rather than the airway!

Recovery

- Monitoring: O_2, SaO_2, BP, and ECG.
- Postoperative echo to exclude pericardial effusions and tamponade.
- Pain control with simple analgesia.

Complications

Anaesthesia related

- Hypotension.
- Suppression of arrhythmia.
- Coughing and dislodgement of the ablation catheter.
- Movement of ablation catheter associated with IPPV.
- Problems on emergence and extubation.
- Unable to sit up after extubation because of control of groin haematoma.

Ablation related

- Complications of arterial and venous puncture, bleeding, haematoma.
- Cardiac perforation and tamponade, especially in cases involving trans-septal puncture.
- Left to right atrial shunting after trans-septal puncture.
- Mitral valve damage.
- Oesophageal perforation.
- Pyloric spasm and delayed gastric emptying.
- Left recurrent laryngeal nerve palsy following AF ablation.
- Arrhythmias, atrial and ventricular.
- Bundle branch block.
- Embolic complications due to clot.
- Air embolus (air entrainment via catheters).
- Brachial plexus injury due to positioning.

Postoperative

- Late tamponade.
- Arrhythmias.
- Atrial stunning and spontaneous echo contrast in the LA. This resolves within three weeks of the procedure.
- Left ventricular failure.
- Pulmonary vein stenosis due to circumferential ablation in the LA around the pulmonary vein ostia.

Surgical treatment of arrhythmias

Atrial fibrillation can be treated surgically when medical therapy has failed, or the patient is haemodynamically compromised or at risk of embolic events. It can occur as an isolated procedure or at the time of mitral valve repair or replacement or coronary artery surgery.

The Cox-Maze procedure

This involves the surgical creation of functional left-atrial myocardium for AV conduction while the interposed surgical scar tissue interrupts routes of electrical re-entry that are the substrate for atrial fibrillation. Multiple full-thickness atrial incisions are created around the sinus node and then re-sutured. This procedure has to be carried out on bypass, with bicaval cannulation. It is 90% successful in restoring sinus rhythm. Complications include:

- Atrial flutter.
- Attenuated heart rate responsiveness.
- PPM dependence.
- Fluid retention due to reduced secretion of atrial natriuretic peptide, increased antidiuretic hormone, and aldosterone.

The modified Maze procedure

Linear transmural scars can now be produced from the epicardial atrial surface using cryoablation, radiofrequency, or microwave energy. This is quicker and less technically demanding than formal surgical Maze. It can also be performed off-pump. Oesophageal injury has been reported after surgical left atrial radiofrequency ablation. Elimination of fibrillation occurs in only 60–75% of patients. It is more successful in paroxysmal fibrillation. The advantage of this technique is that using bioimpedance measurements it is possible to be certain that a transmural lesion has been created.

Anaesthetic considerations

Anaesthetic management is similar to any cardiac surgery case. If a 'modified Maze' procedure is carried out with the heart beating the patient must be anticoagulated with heparin to reduce the risk of embolic complications (ACT >300 seconds).

Further reading

1. American Society of Anesthesiologists Task Force on Perioperative Management of Patients with Cardiac Rhythm Management Devices. Practice advisory for the perioperative management of patients with cardiac rhythm management devices: Pacemakers and implantable cardioverter defibrillators. *Anaesthesiology* 2005; 103: 186–198.

2. Blomström-Lundqvist C, Scheinman M, Aliot E, et al. ACC/AHA/ESC guidelines for the management of patients with supraventricular arrhythmia. Executive summary: A report of the American College of Cardiology/American Heart Association Task Force on Practice Guidelines and the European Society of Cardiology Committee for Practice Guidelines. *Journal of the American College of Cardiology* 42: 1493–1531.

3. Buxton A, Calkins H, Callans D, et al. ACC/AHA/HRS 2006 Key data elements and definitions for electrophysiological studies and procedures. A report of the American College of Cardiology/American Heart Association Task Force on Clinical Data Standards. *Journal of the American College of Cardiology* 2006; 48: 2360–2396.

Cardiac disease in pregnancy

Dr F Walker

Background 564
High-risk lesions 565
The current spectrum of maternal heart disease 566
Hierarchy of antenatal care (ANC) 568
Practice points 570
Further reading 571

Background

The UK Confidential Enquiry into Maternal and Child Health (CEMACH) report identifies heart disease as the second most common cause of maternal death – more common than thromboembolism. It also charts the decline of rheumatic heart disease (RHD) over the past 40 years (most recently 0 deaths compared with 250 deaths between 1952 and 1960). There are five main cardiac causes of maternal death:

- Dilated cardiomyopathy – idiopathic; a result of previous peripartum cardiomyopathy or myocarditis.
- Aortic dissection – secondary to connective tissue diseases (Marfan or Ehlers-Danlos syndrome) or congenital heart lesions (coarctation of the aorta).
- Pulmonary hypertension – primary or secondary (Eisenmenger syndrome).
- Myocardial infarction (coronary atheroma 40%, spasm/normal coronaries 30%, thromboembolism 20%, coronary artery dissection 20%).
- Other causes – includes complex congenital heart disorders, endocarditis, and severe valvar lesions.

High-risk lesions

- Pulmonary hypertension/pulmonary vascular disease – mortality remains 30–50%.
- Severe aortic or mitral stenosis (pre-pregnancy MVA <1.0 cm^2, AVA <1.0 cm^2, or peak gradient >50 mmHg) – mortality is 2–10%.
- Marfan syndrome/Ehlers-Danlos syndrome with aortic root dilation (>40 mm) – mortality 1–20%.
- Mechanical heart valves – maternal mortality ~2–10%.
- Poor left ventricular function and ejection fraction <30% – mortality ~1–20%.
- Highly complex congenital heart disorders (Table 35.1) – mortality 1–5%.

Women with any of the above cardiac lesions should be advised against pregnancy until they are reviewed by a physician/cardiologist with expertise in maternal medicine. Of course, risk must be considered in the context of a 1:10,000 maternal mortality for a healthy woman.

The current spectrum of maternal heart disease

Congenital heart disease

Congenital heart disease (CHD) in pregnancy (0.8%) is more common than acquired heart disease (0.1%). In the UK, by 2010 there will be approximately 166,000 adults with CHD, of whom 15,000 will have complex lesions. The majority with simple or moderately complex CHD do well in pregnancy with good maternal and foetal outcome. Those with complex lesions need careful pre-conceptual assessment.

Inherited cardiac disorders

There is now improved prognosis and survival for familial cardiomyopathies (hypertrophic/dilated/arrhythmogenic right ventricular dysplasia) due to improved diagnosis, genetic screening, and risk stratification for sudden cardiac death (SCD). The majority do well in pregnancy, with outcome related to ventricular function and the severity of outflow tract obstruction.

Marfan syndrome – those with cardiac involvement, in particular aortic root dilatation (>50 mm), are operated on electively to prevent aortic dissection. Fifty per cent of all aortic dissections in females under 40 years old occur in pregnancy, which is therefore relatively contraindicated if the maximal aorta root diameter is >40 mm.

Rheumatic heart disease

Valvar aortic or mitral obstruction is an important cause of maternal morbidity (pulmonary oedema, stroke, and arrhythmia). Those with mild valvar obstruction usually tolerate pregnancy well (valve area >1.5 cm^2). Moderate mitral stenosis (mitral valve area >1.1–1.5 cm^2) requires optimal medical management (beta-blockade and anticoagulation) to avoid complications. Those with severe valve obstruction (valve area <1.0 cm^2) presenting in pregnancy will often require percutaneous balloon dilation if pregnancy is to proceed without maternal decompensation (best performed in second trimester). Regurgitant lesions tend to be better tolerated.

Mechanical heart valves

There is no ideal anticoagulant for mechanical valves in pregnancy. Warfarin is associated with less thromboembolic risk for the mother but causes embryopathy and foetal loss, while heparin has a higher maternal thrombotic risk, albeit with less foetal wastage. The balance of risks needs to be discussed and choice of anticoagulant considered on an individual patient basis.

Acquired heart disease

Atherosclerosis is becoming more prevalent in women of childbearing age. Those with a past history of myocardial infarction but well-preserved LV systolic function usually do well, as do those with stable controlled exertional angina. The majority will require coronary arteriography, risk stratification, and definitive treatment prior to conception.

Hierarchy of antenatal care (ANC)

A hierarchical model of ANC for women with heart disease (Table 35.1) can be derived by modifying the current recommendations of the European Society of Cardiology (ESC) and others for the care of adults with CHD, in conjunction with the Toronto risk predictor score (Box 35.1).

Table 35.1 Hierarchy of ANC for women with heart disease

Level I Exclusive care in specialist unit with multidisciplinary team	Repairs with conduits, Fontans, Marfan, Ebstein, pulmonary atresia, Eisenmenger syndrome, repaired TGA (arterial switch or atrial switch), CCTGA, PHT, cyanotic CHD, native CoA, AS, TOF with PR (moderate), VSD/AR, mechanical valves, HCM, DCM, Toronto score ≥1
Level II Shared care between specialist cardiologist and local obstetric team	CoA repaired, AVSD, AS, PS/PR (mild), TOF with minimal residua, VSD/AR, Toronto score 0
Level III Shared care between general adult cardiology unit and local obstetric team	Repaired PDA, mild PS, small VSD, repaired ASD, Toronto score 0

Box 35.1 Toronto risk markers for a maternal cardiac event

- Prior episode of heart failure, TIA, CVA, or arrhythmia.
- NYHA ≥ II or cyanosis.
- Left heart obstruction (MVA <2 cm^2, AVA <1.5 cm^2, peak LVOTO >30 mmHg on echo).
- Reduced LV function (EF <40%).

0 risk markers: risk of a cardiac event is 5%

1 risk marker: risk of cardiac event is 27%

>1 risk marker: risk of cardiac event is 75%

These recommendations ensure that the majority of women with moderate or highly complex disease are reviewed at least once in a specialist centre. This review will define a lesion-specific labour and delivery management plan, and detail the requirement for haemodynamic monitoring and anaesthetic considerations (Figure 35.1).

Obstetric Cardiac Case
Name: *LS*
D.O.B.:
G2P1
EDD: *30/07/2004*
Diagnosis: *Transposition of the great vessels.* *Mustard repair 1975.* *LV–PA conduit for LVOTO 1984.* *Replacement conduit 1993.* *DDDR pacemaker for tachy–brady syndrome 1998.* 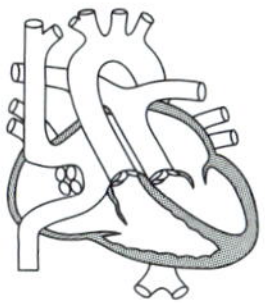
Pre-pregnancy status:
Medications:
Clinical examination findings:
Current status @ x/40:
Past obstetric history:
Recent investigations: *TTE/ETT/MRI/Angio.*
Haemodynamic issues:
Delivery plan:
Labour and delivery: • *Elective CS planned for 38/40 with epidural anaesthesia (previous CS).* • *Endocarditis prophylaxis to be given at induction.*
Drugs to be available on labour ward:
Haemodynamic monitoring and intrapartum care:
Postpartum care and monitoring:
Discharge plan and follow-up:
Plan provided by: Dr Fiona Walker, Consultant Cardiologist (Fiona.walker@uclh.org) after discussion and consensus from

Figure 35.1 Template for high-risk cardiac obstetric report.

Practice points

- All women with a history of cardiac disease should be referred for specialist pre-conceptual assessment and counselling.
- Those with high-risk lesions should be advised against pregnancy until they have had specialist assessment.
- Antenatal care should be stratified by lesion complexity and predicted risk.
- Pregnancy physiology may have a profound impact on cardiac disease and the anaesthetist must equip himself or herself with sufficient understanding of the dynamic pathophysiology, recruiting specialist help if needed.

Further reading

1. Drenthen W, Pieper W, Roos-Hesselink J, et al. Outcome of pregnancy in women with congenital heart disease. *Journal of the American College of Cardiology* 2007; 49: 2303–2311.
2. Yentis SM, Steer PJ, Plaat F. Eisenmenger's syndrome in pregnancy: Maternal and fetal mortality in the 1990s. *British Journal of Obstetrics and Gynaecology* 1998; 105 (8): 921-922.
3. Chan WS, Anand S, Ginsberg JS. Anticoagulation of pregnant women with mechanical heart valves: A systematic review of the literature. *Archives of Internal Medicine* 2000; 160 (2): 191–196.
4. Elkayam U, Tummala PP, Rao K, et al. Maternal and fetal outcomes of subsequent pregnancies in women with peripartum cardiomyopathy. *New England Journal of Medicine* 2001; 344 (21): 1567–1571.
5. Siu SC, Sermer M, Colman JM, et al. Prospective multicenter study of pregnancy outcomes in women with heart disease. *Circulation* 2001; 104: 515–521.
6. Thorne S. Heart disease in pregnancy. *Heart* 2004; 90: 450–456.

Further reading

Index

ablation 192
  atrial fibrillation
    ablation 192, *193*
  alcohol septal
    ablation 496
  catheter ablation
    procedures 556–9
abnormal gases 318
acid-base management 280
acidosis 319
actin 20
action potentials *16*
acute coronary
    syndromes 53, 171
  treatment 54
acute lung injury (ALI) 145
acute phase reaction 112
acute renal failure 126
  acute tubular
    necrosis 127
  cardiac surgery 127, 131
  definition 126
  diuretics 133
  dopamine agonists 132
  future strategies 133
  glycaemic control 131
  grading system *126*
  intravascular volume
    expansion 130
  key points 135
  maintenance of renal
    blood flow and
    renal perfusion
    pressure 130
  N-acetylcysteine
    (NAC) 133
  natriuretic peptides 133
  nephrotoxic agents
    127, 131
  non-pharmacological
    strategies 130
  pathophysiology 127
  perioperative renal
    protection 134
  pharmacological
    strategies 131, *132*
  postoperative
    complications 131
  prevention 130
  risk factors 127, *128*
  vascular surgery 127
  vasodilator agents 133
Acute lung injury ALI 145
acute respiratory
    distress syndrome
    (ARDS) 145
adrenaline 41, 46, 312

adrenergic agents
  mixed agonists 46
  selective agonists 46
  α-adrenergic antagonists 49
  β-adrenergic antagonists 43
alcohol septal
    ablation 496
amiodarone 38
amlodipine 44
anaesthetic considerations
  anomalous
    pulmonary venous
    connections 447
  aortic dissection
    Type A 392
  aortic transection 538
  aortic valve surgery 360,
    364, 457
  arterial switch
    operation 443
  assessment 334
  atrial septal defect 437
  atrioventricular septal
    defect (AVSD)
    closure 453
  cardiac tamponade 531
  cardiac
    transplantation 465
  cardiac tumours 542
  coarctation repair 462
  haemodynamic goals 338
  heart failure 510
  heart transplantation 520
  hypertrophic
    cardiomyopathy 498
  hypoplastic left heart
    syndrome 448
  interrupted aortic arch
    repair 455
  MIDCAB 341
  mitral valve surgery
    402, 406
  off-pump surgery 340, 351
  on-pump surgery 340
    see also
      cardiopulmonary
      bypass
  pacemaker and ICD
    insertion 550, 552
  paediatric cardiac
    anaesthesia 428
  paediatric cardiac surgical
    procedures 463
  paediatric cardiac
    transplantation 465
  patent ductus arteriosus
    closure 438–9

  percutaneous coronary
    intervention 177
  placement of ventricular
    assist devices 302
  preoperative
    investigations 337
  redo surgery 341
  risk factors 334
  routine CABG
    surgery 340
  tetralogy of Fallot
    correction 441
  trans-oesophageal
    essentials 344
  tricuspid valve
    interventions 414, 416
  truncus arteriosus
    correction 445
  ventricular septal defect
    (VSD) closure 452
analgesia 328
angina 55, *56*
  stable angina 171
angiography 172
  long-term
    complications 175
  peri-procedural
    complications 173
  post-procedural
    complications 175
angiotensin 31
anomalous
    pulmonary venous
    connections 446, *446–7*
antenatal care *see* cardiac
    disease in pregnancy
anticoagulation 106
  off-pump CABG 351
antifibrinoloytics 97
antioxidants 121
antiplatelet therapy
    172, 176
antithrombotic drugs 94
aortic arch surgery 382
aortic dissection 390
  assessment 390
  causes 390
  classification *391*
  pathology 390
  pathophysiology 390
  Type A 391
  Type B 394
aortic regurgitation
  aortic stenosis and 412
  clinical presentation 362
  haemodynamics 363–4
  investigations 362

aortic regurgitation (*cont.*)
mitral regurgitation
and 412
pathology 362
pathophysiology 362
practice points 374
requirement for
intervention 363
severity assessment 363
surgical essentials 367
trans-oesophageal
echocardiography 370
aortic stenosis
aortic and left ventricle
pressures and
gradients 359
aortic regurgitation
and 412
clinical presentation 359
haemodynamics 360
mitral regurgitation
and 412
mitral stenosis and 412
paediatric congenital heart
disease 456
pathology 358
pathophysiology 358
practice points 374
severity assessment 358
surgical essentials
and therapeutic
options 366
trans-oesophageal
echocardiography
370, *371*
aortic transection 538,
538, 543
aortic valve 8–9
aortic valve surgery
360, 364
haemodynamic
monitoring 360, 363–4
postoperative
morbidity 361
preoperative
investigations 359
surgical essentials
and therapeutic
options 366
trans-oesophageal
echocardiography 370,
371–2
aprotinin 97, 121
arrhythmias
congenital heart
disease 477
heart failure 506
pacemakers 547
surgical treatment 559
see also electrophysio-
logical procedures;
perioperative
arrhythmias
arterial cannulation 228

arterial pressure
monitoring 228
arterial pressure waveform
abnormal 229
normal 229, *229*
systolic pressure
variation 230, *230*
arterial switch
operation 443, 480
arterial trunks 9
arterial valves 9
arteries see coronary
arteries
artificial hearts 509
aspirin 94
atelectasis 142
atherogenesis 52
atherosclerosis 170, 332
atrial chambers 4
atrial contraction 22
atrial fibrillation 61
ablation 192, *193*
causes and risk
factors 326
chemical
cardioversion 327
electrical
cardioversion 327
incidence and
significance 326
management 61, 326
postoperative care 326
prevention 61, 326
rate control 62
rhythm control 62
substrates 61
atrial flutter 61, 192
atrial septal defect 436,
436, 478
atrial septum 5
atrial switch
operation 480
atrioventricular nodal
re-entrant tachycardia
(AVNRT) 192
atrioventricular re-entrant
tachycardia (AVRT) 192
atrioventricular septal
defect (AVSD) 453,
453, 483
atrioventricular valves 8
atropine 38, 314
autonomic system 30

bacteria *155*
balloon atrial
septostomy 181
balloon counter-pulsation
see intra-aortic balloon
counter-pulsation
balloon dilation of
arteries 462
balloon-directed pacing
catheter 548

balloon valvuloplasty
182, 366
baroreceptor reflexes 30
beta-agonists 40
Blalock Taussig shunt 460,
460
bleeding 96
antifibrinolytics 97
blood conservation 96
cell salvage 99
choice of CPB
equipment 99
coagulopathy after
cardiac surgery in
children 432
desmopressin 98
investigation of cause
102, *103*
non-surgical 103
PEEP (positive
end-expiratory
pressure) 99
postoperative
care 324
recombinant factor
VIIa (rFVIIa:
'Novoseven') 98
red cell transfusion 104
Surgical Blood Ordering
Schedule (SBOS) 100
surgical
re-exploration 104
topical sealants 99
treatment options 103
blood pressure 30,
424, *511*
blood transfusion see
transfusion
blunt trauma 536
bradycardia 314
brain injury see central
nervous system injury
bypass surgery see CABG;
cardiopulmonary
bypass

CABG (coronary artery
bypass grafting)
anaesthesia 300
see also anaesthetic
considerations
intraoperative
arrhythmias 60
neuroprotection 81, 83
off-pump see off-pump
coronary artery bypass
surgery
risk indices 210
calcium 42
calcium channel
blockers 44
calcium overload 200
cAMP-independent
agents 42

Cardiac Anaesthesia Risk
        Evaluation 212
cardiac catheterization 219,
        219–20
    paediatric 462
cardiac cycle 22, *23*
cardiac disease in
        pregnancy 564
    acquired heart
        disease 566
    congenital heart
        disease 566
    hierarchy of antenatal
        care 568, *568*
    high-risk lesions 565
    inherited cardiac
        disorders 566
    mechanical heart
        valves 566
    practice points 570
    rheumatic heart
        disease 566
    template for high-risk
        cardiac obstetric
        report 569
    Toronto risk markers *568*
cardiac muscle 20, *21*
cardiac output 26
    afterload 27
    blood pressure 30
    contractility 28, *28*
    heart rate 29
    lithium dilution cardiac
        output 236
    monitoring 236
    oesophageal Doppler
        cardiac output 236
    preload 26
    pulse contour
        analysis 237
    stroke volume 26
    SVR (systemic vascular
        resistance) 29
    thermodilution cardiac
        output 236
cardiac physiology 14
    blood flow 32
    cardiac cycle 22
    cardiac muscle 20, *21*
    electrophysiology 16
    output *see* cardiac
        output
cardiac surgery
    conduct of surgery 198
    emergency surgery
        see urgent cardiac
        procedures
    minimally invasive cardiac
        surgery (MICS) 204
    myocardial preservation
        see myocardial
        preservation
    new techniques 206

off-pump coronary
        artery bypass
        (OPCAB) surgery 83,
        120, 203
    reoperative surgery 205
    risk assessment 196
cardiac tamponade 199,
        530, 543
cardiac transplantation *see*
        transplantation surgery
cardiac tumours 542
cardiac valves 88
cardioplegia 201
cardiopulmonary bypass
    anaesthesia checklist 263
    anaesthetic support 340
    arterial cannula-
        aortic dissection
        detection 267
    blood pressure
        control 266
    carotid/subclavian
        occlusion 267
    children 430
    choice of equipment 99
    circuits 262
    circulatory control 265
    complications 267
    drugs 269
    fluid management 269
    haemodilution 268
    heart transplantation 522
    initial checklist 264
    left ventricular
        distension 266
    maintenance
        checklist 264
    massive air embolism 267
    neuroprotection 82, *83*
    oxygen failure 268
    perfusionist's
        checklist 263
    pharmacokinetics 269
    priming solution 262
    pump-oxygenator
        failure 268
    renal protection 134
    reservoirs and bonded
        circuits 99
    reversed cannulation 267
    temperature 270
    venous return
        obstruction 267
    volatile anaesthetic
        agents 269
cardiovascular drugs
    control of contractility 40
    control of heart rate and
        rhythm 38
    control of preload and
        afterload 46
cardioversion
    chemical 327

    electrical 327
catheter ablation
        procedures 556–9
cavopulmonary
        connections 482
cell salvage 99
    off-pump CABG 352
central nervous system
        injury 74
    cardiopulmonary bypass
        management 82, *83*
    clinical spectrum 76
    diagnosis 86, *87*
    diffuse-microfocal
        injury 79
    aetiology 78, *79*
    focal injury 79
    global injury 79
    incidence 78, *78*
    inflammatory
        response 118
    management 87
    neurological
        monitoring 84, *84*
    off-pump coronary artery
        bypass (OPCAB)
        surgery 83, 354
    pathophysiology 79
    pharmacological
        neuroprotection 84
    prognosis 88
    risk factors 80, *81*
    routine clinical
        monitoring 82
    watershed injury 79
central venous pressure
        monitoring 230, 234
cerebral metabolism
        276, *277*
cerebral perfusion
        techniques 282
cerebral reperfusion
        injury 276
chest trauma 534
chest x-ray 168
clopidogrel 94
clotting tests 102, *103*
coagulation-
        fibrinolysis 115
coagulation-fibrinolytic
        system activation 112
coagulation pathways 92
    alternatives to
        heparin 93
    deep hypothermic
        circulatory arrest 281
    heparin management 92
    heparin-induced
        thrombocytopaenia
        (HIT) syndrome 93
    heparin resistance 93
    protamine
        management 92

coagulopathy in
children 432
coarctation of the
aorta 184
paediatric congenital heart
disease 458
cognitive dysfunction 76
off-pump CABG 354
commissurotomy 366
comorbidities 208
complement inhibitors 122
complement system 114
complex shunts 433
computed tomography
(CT) 218
conduction pathway 18
congenital heart disease
(CHD) 180, 470
arrhythmias 477
assessment 471
atrial septal defect 436,
436–7, 478
atrioventricular septal
defect (AVSD) 453,
453, 483
balloon atrial
septostomy 181
balloon valvuloplasty 182
cavopulmonary
connections 482
classification 474
coarctation 184
cyanosis and
hyperviscosity 476
decreased pulmonary
blood flow 476
double inlet
ventricle 481
endocarditis 490
see also infective
endocarditis
fistulae 186
Fontan circulation
461, 482
Glenn shunt
460, 461, 482
management 488
mixing lesions 477
monitoring 488
pregnancy 566
primary and secondary
features 476
septal defects 183
sequelae 486, 486
single ventricle 481
terminology 472, 472
tetralogy of Fallot 440,
440, 478
transposition of the great
arteries (TGA) 181,
442, 442, 443, 479
valves 185
ventilation 489
ventricular function 477

see also paediatric
congenital heart
disease
congestive heart failure
(CHF) 64–5
continuous coronary
perfusion 201
continuous wave
Doppler(CWD)
246, 247
contractility 28, 28
cardiovascular drugs 40
contraction 21
coronary arteries 10, 10
circumflex 11
left anterior
descending 10
left main stem 10
right coronary
artery 11
variations in anatomy 11
coronary artery bypass
grafting see CABG
coronary artery disease
acute coronary
syndromes 171
angina 55, 56, 171
atherosclerosis 170, 332
clinical presentation 336
preoperative
investigations 337
stable angina 171
see also ischaemic heart
disease
coronary artery
surgery 508
coronary circulation 32
coronary intervention see
percutaneous coronary
intervention
coronary thrombosis 52
coronary vascular
resistance (CVR) 32
autoregulation 33
endothelial control 33
metabolic control 32
myogenic control 33
neurogenic control 33
coronary veins 11
corticosteroids 121
Cox-Maze procedure
559–60
cytokines 114

DC cardioversion 554
deep hypothermic
circulatory arrest
(DHCA) 274, 278
acid-base
management 280
anaesthetic
considerations 278
cardiopulmonary bypass in
children 430

cerebral metabolism
276, 277
cerebral perfusion
techniques 282
cerebral protection
281, 382
cerebral reperfusion
injury 276
coagulation 281
cooling and
rewarming 280
general effects 278
glucose homeostasis 281
hyperoxia 280
indications 274
monitoring 279, 279
outcome 284
spinal cord
protection 283
thoracic aortic
surgery 382
delirium
central nervous system
injury 76
postoperative 329
desmopressin 98
diastole 22–3
diltiazem 44
diuretics 133
dobutamine 40, 313
dopamine 40, 46, 313
Doppler imaging CP17.S2.3
Doppler principle 243, 243
Drew-Anderson
technique 120
drugs
agents for
bradycardia 314
agents for tachycardia 314
analgesia 328
antithrombotics 94
cardiopulmonary
bypass 269
control of contractility 40
control of heart rate and
rhythm 38
control of preload and
afterload 46
corticosteroids 121
immunosuppressant
medications 525
inotropes 312
paediatric cardiac
anaesthesia 428
perioperative
medications 209
postoperative care 312
sedation 328
vasodilators 47, 133, 313
vasopressors 312

echocardiography
aortic regurgitation 363
diagnoses 68

preoperative
assessment 218, 337
trans-oesophageal see
trans-oesophageal
echocardiography
ejection 22
elastase 116
electrical cardioversion 327
electrical conduction 16
electrocardiography
atrial ECG leads 224
colour coding
systems *224*
diagnosing myocardial
ischaemia 224
filter modes 224, *225*
lead location *224*
lead selection 217, 224
non-standard limb
leads 216
perioperative
monitoring 224
preoperative
assessment 214,
214, 337
signal gain 225
standard limb leads 215
subendocardial
versus transmural
ischaemia 226
electophysiological
procedures 190, *191*
ablation 192
catheter ablation
procedures 556–9
Cox-Maze
procedure 559–60
DC cardioversion 554
diagnoses 191
hypertrophic
cardiomyopathy 496
indications 190
pacemakers see
pacemakers
patient preparation 190
supraventricular
arrhythmias 191
surgical treatment of
arrhythmias 559
ventricular
tachycardia 191
embolization
procedures 463
emergency surgery
see urgent cardiac
procedures
end diastolic volume
(EDV) 22
endocarditis see infective
endocarditis
endotoxin 113
end systolic volume
(ESV) 23

enoximone 313
epicardial pacing 546
epidural analgesia 330
Epinephrine (adrenaline)
46, 312
esmolol 43
etomidate 428
EuroSCORE 210, *211*, 334
exercise testing 217
extracorporeal circuit
112, 120

fast action potentials 16, *16*
fentanyl 428
filling pressures 232
first heart sound 22
foetal circulation 422
Fontan circulation 461, 482
fungi 155

Glenn shunt 460, *461*, 482
glucose homeostasis 281
glyceryl trinitrate (GTN) 47
glycoprotein IIb/IIIa
receptor
antagonists 94

haematology
coagulation see
coagulation pathways
postoperative
anticoagulation 106
preoperative
antithrombotic
drugs 94
see also bleeding; transfusion
haemodynamics
anaesthesia for coronary
artery disease 338
aortic regurgitation 363–4
aortic dissection
Type A 392
aortic stenosis 360
aortic transection 538
arterial pressure
monitoring 228
causes of adverse
haemodynamics 342
central venous pressure
monitoring 230, 234
filling pressures 232
heart transplantation 523
hypertrophic
cardiomyopathy
497–8
left ventricular end-
diastolic pressure
(LVEDP) 232, 234, *234*
mitral valve
surgery 401–2, 405–6
off-pump CABG 351
pulmonary artery
catheterization 231

pulmonary stenosis 418
technical
considerations 228
transmural pressures
232, *233*
tricuspid
regurgitation 414
tricuspid stenosis 416
ventricular
compliance 232, *233*
haemothorax 536
heart failure 64, 506
acute 67
anaesthetic
management 510
arrhythmias 506
blood pressure *511*
causes 65
chronic 65
clinical features 66–7
coronary artery
surgery 508
differential diagnosis 67
echocardiographic
diagnosis 68
hypotension/low cardiac
output state *512*
long-term assist
devices and artificial
hearts 509
medical management 507
mitral regurgitation 506
mitral valve surgery 508
neuroendocrine
activation 506
pathophysiology 65, 67
signs 66
surgical management 507
symptoms 66
symptom severity *64*
treatment 66, 68
ventricular repair 508
volume overload 506
heart rate 29
cardiovascular drugs 38
heart sounds 22–3
heart transplants see
transplantation surgery
heparin
alternatives 93
anti-inflammatory
effects 112
clotting tests 102, *103*
management 92
resistance 93
heparin-coated circuits 120
heparin-induced
thrombocytopaenia
syndrome (HIT) 93
hibernation 333
hydralazine 48
hypercarbia 319
hyperoxia 280

hypertrophic
cardiomyopathy
alcohol septal
ablation 496
anaesthetic plan 498
assessment of
severity 494
clinical presentation 495
electrophysiological
interventions 496
genetics 494
haemodynamic
goals 497–8
medical treatment 496
morphology 494
pathophysiology 494
practice points 502
surgical myectomy 496
trans-oesophageal
echocardiography 500,
500–1
hypoplastic left heart
syndrome 448, 448–9
hypotension 322
hypothermia 238
see also deep hypothermic
circulatory arrest
hypoxaemia 318

immunosuppressant
medications 525
implantable cardiac
defibrillators
(ICDs) 550, 552
infection
antibiotic prophylaxis 152
early postoperative
period 151
impaired local immune
response 151
operative procedures 153
postoperative
procedure 153
preoperative preparation
and screening 152
risk factors 150, 150
sternal wound
infections 160
wound contamination 150
infective endocarditis
aetiology 154
clinical features 155
congenital heart
disease 490
definition 154
Duke diagnostic
criteria 155
enterococcal disease 157
epidemiology 154
investigations 155
microbial causes 155
mortality rates 156
pathogenesis 154

prevention 158
sites 154
staphylococcal 157
streptococcal 157
surgical treatment
157, 158
symptoms and signs 156
treatment 157
inflammatory response 110
acute phase reaction 112
air-blood mixing 112
antioxidants 121
aprotinin 121
blood transfusion 113
cardiac effects 118
cellular response 114
central nervous system
injury 118
coagulation-fibrinolytic
system activation 112
complement
inhibitors 122
complement system 114
corticosteroids 121
cytokines 114
design of the
extracorporeal
circuit 120
diagnosis 110
Drew-Anderson
technique 120
elastase and
myeloperoxidase 116
endotoxin 113
genetic predisposition 113
heparin and
protamine 112
ischaemia-reperfusion
injury 112
kallikrein-kininogen-kinin
system 115
nitric oxide (NO) 115
off-pump coronary
bypass 120
pulmonary effects 118
reactive oxygen species
(ROS) 116
renal effects 118
surgical trauma 112
inotropes 312
intermittent cross-clamp
fibrillation 201
interrupted aortic arch
454, 454
interventional cardiac
catheterization
(ICC) 462
interventional cardiology
see percutaneous
coronary intervention
intra-aortic balloon counter-
pulsation 288
complications 295

contraindications 289
indications 289
management 292
placement 290
timing and common
inflation/deflation
errors 293
weaning and removal 295
intracoronary shunts 350
intraoperative
arrhythmias 60
ischaemic heart disease
acute coronary
syndromes 53
treatment 54
atherogenesis 52
current therapies
slowing of disease
progression and
perioperative
medication 54
treatment of angina
55, 56
diagnosis 57
ECG monitoring 224, 226
hibernation 333
infarction 333
interventions 55, 56
myocardial function 333
pathology 52
perioperative ischaemia
see perioperative
ischaemia
plaque rupture
and coronary
thrombosis 52
preconditioning 333
risk factors 54
stunning 333
ischaemic-reperfusion
injury 112, 200
isoprenaline (isoprotenerol)
38, 41, 314
isovolumetric
relaxation 23
isovolumetric ventricular
contraction 22

kallikrein-kininogen-kinin
system 115
ketamine 428

labetalol 43, 314
Law of Laplace 27
left atrium 5
left ventricle 6
left ventricular end-diastolic
pressure (LVEDP) 232,
234, 234
left ventricular failure
(LVF) 64–5
leucocyte depletion 120
levosimendan 43

lithium dilution cardiac output 236
lysine analogues 98

magnetic resonance imaging (MRI) 218
mechanical heart valves 566
mechanical ventilation 141
metaraminol 46, 312
microorganisms 155
midazolam 428
MIDCAB (minimally invasive direct coronary artery bypass) 341
minimally invasive cardiac surgery (MICS) 204
mitral regurgitation 400
 aortic regurgitation and 412
 aortic stenosis and 412
 clinical presentation 401
 haemodynamics 401–2
 heart failure 506
 pathology 400
 pathophysiology 400
 practice points 409
 preoperative investigations 401
 severity assessment 400
 trans-oesophageal echocardiography 403
mitral stenosis
 aortic stenosis and 412
 clinical findings 405
 clinical presentation 404
 haemodynamics 405–6
 pathology 404
 pathophysiology 404
 practice points 409
 preoperative investigations 405
 presenting features 405
 trans-oesophageal echocardiography 406
mitral valve 8–9
mitral valve surgery 398
 anaesthesia 402, 406
 haemodynamic monitoring 401–2, 405–6
 heart failure 508
 mixed mitral valve disease 408–9
 practice points 409
 preoperative investigations 401, 405
 surgical technique 402, 406
 therapeutic options 402, 406
 trans-oesophageal echocardiography 403, 406

mixed mitral valve disease 408–9
monitoring
 cardiac output see cardiac output
 deep hypothermic circulatory arrest 279, 279
 ECG see electrocardiography
 haemodynamic see haemodynamic monitoring
 neurologic 239
 paediatric heart disease 429
 temperature see temperature monitoring
 trans-oesophageal echocardiography 250, 250
MRI (magnetic resonance imaging) 218
myeloperoxidase 116
myocardial contusion 536
myocardial ischaemia 224
myocardial oxygen supply-demand balance 34
myocardial
 preservation 200
 calcium overload 200
 cardioplegia 201
 continuous coronary perfusion 201
 intermittent cross-clamp fibrillation 201
 ischaemic reperfusion injury 200
 oxidative stress 200
 practical considerations 202
 techniques of delivery 201
myosin 20

N-acetylcysteine (NAC) 133
natriuretic peptides 133
neonatal physiology 424
nephrotoxic agents 127, 131
neurological monitoring 84, 84, 239
neuroprotection see central nervous system injury
nifedipine 44
nitric oxide (NO) 115
nitroglycerin (GTN) 313
nitroprusside 48, 314
Norepinephrine (noradrenaline) 41, 47, 312

Norwood Stage 1 operation 449, 449
nuclear cardiology 218

oesophageal Doppler cardiac output 236
off-pump coronary artery bypass (OPCAB) surgery 120, 203, 355
 anaesthesia 340, 351
 anticoagulation 351
 blower-misters 350
 cell salvage 352
 contraindications 348
 emergence and extubation 352
 graft patency 355
 haemodynamic stability 351
 history and evolution 348
 intracoronary shunts 350
 neurological injury 83, 354
 outcome 354
 patient selection 348
 positioning the heart and grafting 350
 postoperative care 353
 stabilizers 350
 temperature maintenance 352
oliguria 320
opioids
 adjuncts 330
 epidural analgesia 330
 intrathecal 330
 intravenous 330
oxidative stress 200
oxygen supply-demand balance 34

pacemakers
 anaesthesia for pacemaker and ICD insertion 550, 552
 arrhythmias 547
 balloon-directed pacing catheter 548
 complications 547
 default settings in response to magnet placement 553
 epicardial pacing 546
 external pacing 548
 pacing failure 547
 permanent pacemakers 548, 550
 removal of epicardial wires 547
 temporary 546, 547
 transvenous pacing 548

paediatric cardiac surgical
procedures
anaesthetic
considerations 463
cardiac
catheterization 462
embolization
procedures 463
Fontan circulation 461
interventional
procedures 462
occlusion procedures 462
risks 463
transplantation 464
paediatric congenital heart
disease
anomalous pulmonary
venous connections
446, 446–7
aortic stenosis 456
atrial septal defect
436, 436–7, 447
atrioventricular septal
defect (AVSD)
453, 453
Blalock Taussig shunt
460, 460
cardiopulmonary
bypass 430
classification 433
coagulopathy after cardiac
surgery 432
coarctation of the
aorta 458
complex shunts 433
drugs used in
anaesthesia 428
equipment and
monitoring 429
foetal circulation 422
Glenn shunt 460, 461
hypoplastic left heart
syndrome 448, 448–9
interrupted aortic
arch 454, 454
left to right shunts 433–4
neonatal physiology 424
patent ductus arteriosus
(PDA) 438, 438
premedication for cardiac
surgery 427
preoperative
assessment and
premedication 426
right to left shunts
433, 435
tetralogy of Fallot
(TOF) 440, 440
transposition of the great
arteries (TGA) 181,
442, 442, 443
truncus arteriosus
444, 444

ventricular septal defect
(VSD) 452, 452
pain control 328
neonatal physiology 425
pancuronium 428
paravalvar prosthetic
leaks 186
Parsonnet score 210
patent ductus arteriosus
(PDA) 438, 438
patent foramen ovale
(PFO) 183
percutaneous balloon
valvoplasty 366
percutaneous coronary
intervention 172
anaesthetic support 177
antiplatelet therapy
172, 176
development 166
long-term
complications 175
non-cardiac surgery
and 176
peri-procedural
complications 173
post-procedural
complications 175
stents 166, 167
stent thrombosis
167, 168
perioperative
arrhythmias 60
intraoperative
arrhythmias 60
postoperative
arrhythmias 61
perioperative ischaemia 56
causes 57
prevention 58
risk factors 56
treatment 58
perioperative
medications 209
phenoxybenzamine 49
phentolamine 49
phenylephrine 46, 312
phosphodiesterase
inhibitors 41
phrenic nerve paralysis 143
plaque rupture 52
pneumonia 143
pneumothorax 146
positron emission
tomography (PET) 218
postoperative
arrhythmias 61
postoperative care 308
abnormal gases 318
agents for
bradycardia 314
agents for tachycardia 314
analgesia 328

atrial fibrillation 326
see also atrial fibrillation
bleeding 324
patient handover 308
delirium 329
hypotension 322
inotropes 312
investigations 309
mechanical
ventilation 316
off-pump CABG 353
oliguria 320
sedation 328
transfer to ICU 308
vasodilators 313
vasopressors 312
pregnancy see cardiac
disease in pregnancy
preoperative assessment
aortic dissection
Type A 392
aortic valve surgery 359
cardiac
catheterization 219,
219–20
cardiac evaluation 208
comorbidities 208
computed tomography
(CT) 218
echocardiography 218
electrocardiogram
(ECG) 214, 214
exercise testing 217
magnetic resonance
imaging (MRI) 218
mitral regurgitation 401
mitral stenosis 405
non-invasive testing 214
nuclear cardiology 218
paediatric congenital heart
disease 426
perioperative
medications 209
positron emission
tomography (PET) 218
risk indices see risk indices
thoracic aneurysms 380
pressure-volume loop 24
propofol 428
protamine 92
anti-inflammatory
effects 112
pulmonary artery
catheterization 231
pulmonary embolism
145, 540
pulmonary function tests
(PFTs) 140
pulmonary oedema 144
pulmonary
regurgitation 418
pulmonary stenosis 418
pulmonary valve 8–9

pulsatile flow 120
pulse contour analysis 237
pulsed-wave Doppler 245, 245–6

radionuclide studies
  nuclear cardiology 218
  positron emission tomography(PET) 218
Rastelli operation 480
reactive oxygen species (ROS) 116
recombinant factor VIIa (rFVIIa:'Novoseven') 98
red cell transfusion 104
redo surgery 205
re-entrant arrhythmias 192
regional anaesthesia 343
regional wall motion abnormality (RWMA) 57, 58
renal failure see acute renal failure
renin-angiotensin system 31
reoperative surgery 205
respiratory
  complications 138
  ARDS/ALI 145
  atelectasis 142
  barotraumas 146
  intraoperative management of mechanical ventilation 141
  phrenic nerve paralysis 143
  pneumonia 143
  pneumothorax 146
  postoperative respiratory function 142
  preoperative assessment 140
  pulmonary embolism 145
  pulmonary oedema 144
  tracheostomy 146
rheumatic heart disease 566
right atrium 54
right ventricle 6
right ventricular failure (RVF) 64–5
right ventricular outflow tract (RVOT) 192
risk indices 210
  Cardiac Anaesthesia Risk Evaluation 212
  EuroSCORE 210, 211, 334
  Parsonnet 210
  STS (Society of Thoracic Surgeons) 210

sedation 328
septal defects 183

see also congenital heart disease; paediatric congenital heart disease
septum
  atrial 5
  ventricular 6
sevoflurane 428
shunts 350
  Blalock Taussig shunt 460, 460
  Glenn shunt 460, 461, 482
  left to right 433–4
  right to left 435
  slow action potentials 16–17,17
sodium nitroprusside 314
spinal cord injury see central nervous system injury
stable angina 171
Staphylococcus aureus see infection; infective endocarditis
Starling's Law 26, 27–8
STEMI (S-T elevation MI) 53
stents 166, 167
  paediatric cardiac surgical procedures 462
  thoracic aorta 388
stent thrombosis 167, 168
sternal wound infections 160
stroke 76, 77
  diagnosis 87
  incidence 78
  risk factors 81
stroke volume 26
STS (Society of Thoracic Surgeons) 210
stunning 333
subendocardial ischaemia 226
supraventricular arrhythmias 191
Surgical Blood Ordering Schedule (SBOS) 100
SVR (systemic vascular resistance) 29
systole 22
systolic pressure variation 230, 230
systolic ventricular wall stress 27

tachycardia
  pharmacological manipulation 314
  see also electrophysiological procedures; perioperative arrhythmias

temperature
  monitoring 238
  cardiopulmonary bypass 270
  neonatal physiology 425
  off-pump CABG 352
tetralogy of Fallot (TOF) 440, 440, 478
TGA (transposition of the great arteries) 181, 442, 442, 443
thermodilution cardiac output 236
thiopentone 428
thoracic aneurysms 380
  ascending aorta aneurysms 382
  clinical presentation 380
  descending thoracic aneurysms 386
  pathology 380
  preoperative investigations 380
thoracic aortic stents 388
thoracic aortic surgery 378
  anaesthetic plan 382, 386
  aortic dissection see aortic dissection
  ascending aorta 382
  complications 388
  deep hypothermic circulatory arrest (DHCA) 382
  descending thoracic aneurysms 386
  indications for surgery 382, 386
  practice points 395
  surgical techniques 383, 387
  trans-oesophageal echocardiography 384, 388, 393
thromboelastography (TEG) 102
thrombosis 52
tissue Doppler imaging (TDI) 247
topical sealants 99
transcutaneous aortic valve implantation (TAVI) 367
transfusion 96
  blood conservation 97
  cell salvage 99
  choice of surgery 99
  inflammatory response 113
  predonation 99
  Surgical Blood Ordering Schedule (SBOS) 100
transmural ischaemia 226
transmural pressures 232, 233

trans-oesophageal
  echocardiography (TOE)
  2D imaging 244
  3D imaging 247
  anaesthesia for coronary
    artery disease 344
  aortic dissection
    Type A 393, 394
  aortic transection 539
  aortic valve surgery 370,
    371–2
  cardiac tamponade 532
  cardiopulmonary
    bypass 370
  complications 256
  continuous wave Doppler
    (CWD) 246, 247
  Doppler imaging 245
  Doppler principle
    243, 243
  examination
    sequence 252, 253
  hypertrophic
    cardiomyopathy
    500, 500–1
  imaging modes 244, 244
  imaging planes 252,
    252, 258
  mitral regurgitation 403
  mitral stenosis 406
  M-mode 244, 244
  monitoring applications
    250, 250
  pulsed-wave Doppler
    PWD) 245, 245–6
  thoracic aortic
    surgery 384, 388
  tissue Doppler imaging
    (TDI) 247
  ultrasound physics
    CP17.S1
  uses and indications
    248, 248
transplantation surgery 514
  anaesthetic
    management 520
  common pitfalls
    following heart
    transplantation 523
  contraindications 514
  donors 517
  immunosuppressant
    medications 525

indications 514
intensive care
  following heart
  transplantation 523
intercurrent
  pathologies post-
  transplantation 524
paediatric 464
recipient characteristics
  for thoracic organ
  transplantation 516
rejection 524
re-transplantations 526
risk factors for one-
  and five-year
  mortality 515–16
routine tests prior to
  transplantation 517
surgical procedure 518
transposition of the great
  arteries (TGA) 181, 442,
  442, 443, 479
tricuspid regurgitation 414
tricuspid stenosis 416
tricuspid valve 8
troponin 20
truncus arteriosus
  444, 444
tumours 542
Type A aortic
  dissection 391
Type B aortic
  dissection 394

ultrafiltration 121
ultrasound physics 242
urgent cardiac
  procedures 199
  aortic transection 538,
    538, 543
  blunt trauma 536
  cardiac tamponade 199,
    530, 543
  cardiac tumours 542
  chest trauma 534
  pulmonary embolism
    145, 540

valve disease
  mixed valve lesions 412
  pulmonary
    regurgitation 418
  pulmonary stenosis 418

tricuspid
  regurgitation 414
  tricuspid stenosis 416
  see also aortic
    regurgitation; aortic
    stenosis; mitral
    regurgitation;
    mitral stenosis
valve replacement 366
valves 8
  congenital heart
    disease 185
vasodilators 47, 133, 313
vasopressin 47
vasopressors 46, 312
venous drainage 11
ventilation 141
  extubation criteria 317
  postoperative care 316
ventilator-associated
  pneumonia 144
ventricles 6
ventricular arrhythmias 62
  management 62
ventricular assist
  devices(VADs) 298, 509
  anaesthetic management
    during placement 302
  anaesthetic
    management of heart
    transplantation 521
  complications 304
  extracorporeal/
    paracorporeal 301
  indications 299
  intracorporeal 301
  percutaneous 301
  types and characteristics
    300, 300
ventricular compliance
  232, 233
ventricular repair 508
ventricular septal defect
  (VSD) 452, 452
ventricular septum 6
ventricular
  tachycardia 191–2
verapamil 44
volatile anaesthetic
  agents 269

warfarin 94